Rebalancing

Professor Neal Maskrey

Front cover designed by Hannah Wroe, Neal Maskrey, and Nick Neal and Chris Paine from www.iseeyouonline.co.uk using Microsoft Copilot™

Simply a magnificent achievement. Grounded and readable throughout.

Professor Richard Lehmann.
Former GP, former Visiting Professor of Shared Understanding in Medicine, Birmingham University, and hero to many for his long running weekly BMJ column.

This is a masterpiece. Should be required reading for policy makers who seem to want to ignore decades of research evidence. I'll re-read; probably twice.

Professor Alf Collins.
Formerly NHS England's Clinical Director, Personalised Care Group.

ABOUT THE AUTHOR

Neal Maskrey was a general practitioner on the east coast of Yorkshire for about twenty years, the last eight of which he also worked for North Yorkshire Health Authority helping to develop primary care in the county. He then spent a decade as Medical Director of the National Prescribing Centre, followed by becoming Programme Director of the Medicines and Prescribing Centre at the National Institute for Health and Care Excellence, and Visiting Professor of Evidence-informed Decision Making at Keele University.

Gradually he worked out that understanding how humans make decisions was a very important thing, and that making decisions for populations is very different from making decisions for individuals. Only late in his career was he paid to undertake research, but is still in the top 6% worldwide of healthcare researchers according to ResearchGate. He has been writing this book for ten years and hopes that medicine might be a little better balanced by the time he really, really needs it.

He lives in Birkdale in the Northwest of England with his wife Helen, Muffin the cat, and Billy the ex-cat (in the yard).

PROLOGUE

Joan's Paradox

Joan had lived for twenty years in the small bungalow she and her late husband Herbert had bought when they retired. But when she was in her mid-80's maintaining even that had become difficult. It was an easy decision to move into a small retirement apartment nearer her son, and where there was a built-in community and social life. Her son did her heavy shopping, and she had been delighted to be scooped up and recognised for her own talents by his and his family's friends. It had been decades since she'd stayed up until the early hours at a New Year's Eve party, this time with her new neighbours. She was independent, her pensions easily covered her modest needs, and she could do just what she wanted when she wanted. It was better than ok.

Herbert had been five years older than her. In the late 1940s he was single, bright, well thought of, and hard working as a finance officer who spent his days calculating teacher's pay, pensions and taxes. He wasn't a conventional heart throb, but he was kind and smiled a lot. In the war, Herbert had been called up into the Infantry, fighting in North Africa, Italy, and - rumour had it - he was in the second glider down at Arnhem, the biggest ever airborne troop landing and a military disaster, subsequently known to many as "The Bridge Too Far". After five days of defending the drop zones from German counter attacks and then fighting his way from one foxhole to another in a desperate retreat, it seems he volunteered to go looking in darkness for a Dutch ferry which might have helped get the tattered and by now heavily outnumbered remnants of the First Airbourne Division back across the Lower Rhine to safety. They did not find the ferry, and trying to get back to report that failure he was shot through the thigh with a machine gun bullet. He had spent the rest of the war – about seven months - in a prison camp with 90,000 others in what became East Germany, living on thin cabbage soup and the odd red Cross parcel. He came back weighing about 7 stones (100lb) and with expert status as a cribbage player, because playing games of cribbage was pretty much all he had to keep him occupied.

Joan and Herbert got married in June 1948. It was a glorious, sunny day and the reception, held in a marquee in the grounds of the water works where Joan's father was an engineer, was plagued by wasps. Just before the war started, Herbert had put down a deposit on a newly built, small, detached house in his village where most people worked "down the mine". He lived there with his mother and one of his step-brothers Ralph (always pronounced Rafe), and it was there he returned after he had been discharged from the Army. And so Joan had set about managing the tricky role of becoming Herbert's wife in an already-established household of three other adults, and where her new-mother-in-law had, up to that point, been in charge of all things domestic.

Emotions and feelings were not people's strong suit in a North Midlands pit village at the end of the 1940s. Average life expectancy in the UK for people born around 1920 was 56 for men and 60 for women.[i] Factor in the local demographics, and life expectancy in the Potteries was even lower. Two World Wars, the constant threat of injury and death in the mines and the other local heavy industries, and the threat from infectious diseases such as polio, diphtheria and tuberculosis, and there wasn't much of a price placed on feelings. Life was truly tough, you were grateful for what you had, and you were expected to get on with it as cheerfully as you could.

Joan rapidly learned not to ask Herbert about the war. The briefest of mentions and he would have nightmares every night for weeks. And then Herbert and Joan had a son. Babies can put marriages under enormous strain, or they can make them. And in this case, it cemented Joan and Herbert as a proper team with drive and a rock-solid common purpose. Money was still tight, and the pace of post-war progress was glacial. But they got there. They bought a tiny black and white television in 1953 to watch the Queen's coronation. Infectious disease was an ever-present

2

threat, and Joan queued in the rain outside the village health clinic to get her four-year-old son vaccinated in the 1956 polio epidemic. In 1959 Herbert's brother-in-law Fred, who'd been best man at their wedding, was killed in a roof fall in the mine. Huge sigh. But they just had to get on with it.

Their son was bright and diligent, just like them. He loved sport, and on 28th October 1961 Herbert took the small boy for a birthday treat to see the return of 40 year old Stanley Mathews to play for his home town team Stoke City. The crowd was 35,974. That was 27,565 up on the attendance at the previous match, and the returning hero was instrumental in a thumping 3-0 victory over Huddersfield that was never to be forgotten. Their son passed the entrance examination to the grammar school and thanks to the 1944 Education Act, Joan and Herbert only had to find the money for the uniform. But even that was not easy.

Joan had returned to work as a school secretary a few years before. It was great to get out of the house and let's face it, away from her mother-in-law. The years rolled by. Much to everyone's surprise, the shy 51 year old Ralph had married the delightfully chatty 38 year old Mavis and they bought a new, small, semi-detached house in the village. And despite the years of frosty relationships, Joan and Herbert nursed his mother at home throughout her final illness. By then their son had gone to university to study medicine with a taxpayer-funded student grant. For the first time in their marriage, after nearly 30 years, it was just the two of them.

And then Herbert had a heart attack aged just 62. He needed a defibrillator three times in hospital and was lucky to come out alive. He retired on grounds of ill health, and was glad to do so. Herbert's stable local office had become unstable, bigger, and was now in the next town. He didn't enjoy the work now because he no longer personally knew the teachers he was trying to help. He'd rather have avoided the heart attack, but he was glad to have the opportunity to retire. Joan's school had merged to form a huge educational consortium; she was a small cog in a big wheel and spent her days trying to help people who thought they knew better than her, except they didn't. She hated it. At the first opportunity she took her own occupational pension a few years early and left the world of work.

And most importantly, they moved into the bungalow nearer to their son and had the chance to see lots of first one, then two and finally three granddaughters. Joan had never stopped cooking and sewing, and now she had a new generation to teach and inspire.

And then one sunny but terrible June morning, Herbert suddenly died. He was walking home from the local shop. Joan knew something had happened. It was the first day of the first Test cricket match of the summer, and in those days it was always live on the BBC. Herbert would not have missed a ball being bowled in the entire five day match. There had been an hour of play before she heard why her husband hadn't come home, and why he never would again. A shocked passer-by had called an ambulance and Herbert was pronounced dead on arrival at the local hospital. Joan and her son sobbed for 10 minutes in the biggest hug they'd had in years. And then they just got on with it.

Joan had had her own first heart attack aged 68 and the second a few years later. Increasing angina in her 70s led to a quadruple heart bypass, and after that she developed heart failure which had eventually responded well to a cocktail of medicines. She bounced back every time, continuing to live independently, helping with the grandchildren and enjoying gardening, sewing, cooking, knitting much as she had done throughout her adult life. Mavis and other relatives visited; Ralph had died suddenly of a stroke; whilst they didn't think about it in these terms, they were all victims of the cardiovascular epidemic which peaked in the UK in 1979. Joan went away each summer with a friend on a coach trip – usually to Scotland. But they were both getting older. Every year Joan wondered if this was to be their last time enjoying the scenery, the company, and a little whiskey.

She didn't bounce when she fell in the street when shopping and fractured her wrist. Then she got her foot tangled in the electric blanket flex and she didn't bounce again – the fall fractured her hip. Hip fractures in older people are an especially serious matter. In the first year after a hip fracture about a third of older patient die, and of those that survive up a fifth of those who were living independently before the fracture are unable to regain their ability to live independently.[ii] But the orthopaedic surgeons had put a metal rod into her femur, she recovered, convalesced at her son's, and quickly got back to her quiet life in her quiet but determined way.

All this meant she was taking 17 tablets and capsules every day. Some of these she needed to control the symptoms of her heart disease, and some served a dual purpose of also giving her some protection against further heart attacks or strokes. Others were pure prevention – calcium, vitamin D and a drug to strengthen her bones in the hope of preventing another fracture. Joan was benefitting from 40 years of intensive scientific and clinical research and new approaches to manage and prevent heart and bone disease. None of the medicines were a cure, and they didn't benefit everybody who took them, but in proper scientific experiments called randomised controlled trials, on average a population with one of her problems did better if they were on the medicines than if they were not.

Of course, that came at a cost, and not just in terms of the cost of the medicines to the NHS. Controlling rather than curing suited the pharmaceutical companies who had funded the research and development. A medicine someone needed to take long term made them more money than a medicine that a patient takes for a few days and the condition is cured. The cost to Joan was the constant reminder that she wasn't young anymore, and there was the drudge of taking tablets, getting her prescriptions, and going for check-ups. She hated it.

And then for a few weeks she had been feeling occasionally a little faint and dizzy, and she had also noticed palpitations – a fluttering feeling in her chest. No pain; she would have been really worried about pain. But she had struggled the last couple of days to prepare a meal, and certainly couldn't think about going shopping for food. And then one morning she felt unsteady on her feet and had nearly fallen in the shower. Joan desperately wanted to keep her independence, she didn't want to be a burden to anyone, and she didn't want to fall and break another hip, naked, in the shower.

It was soon obvious what the problem was. Joan's pulse was irregular. One of the GPs from her practice came round and an electrocardiograph (ECG) confirmed her suspicion that she had developed atrial fibrillation (AF) – one of the most common forms of abnormal heart rhythm. Nearly a fifth of people over the age of 80 have AF[iii], and whilst some of them have symptoms, many others don't. Joan's GP checked out the rest of her cardiovascular system and was relieved to find that there were no signs of worsening heart failure.

One of the biggest problems with AF is that it significantly increases the risk of a stroke and other blood clot-related complications. There was a clinical guideline for AF produced by the National Institute for Health and Care Excellence (NICE). About a quarter of people who have a stroke due to AF die in the acute episode[iv], AF is responsible for 1 in 6 strokes,[v] and only 40% of people who have an AF-related stroke survive for five years.[vi]

The guideline emphasised the importance of considering anticoagulation for most people with AF – adding a medicine to prevent blood clots forming in the left upper chamber of the heart. Anticoagulation would prevent about two thirds of AF-related strokes, and the NICE guideline and the previous European guideline both now took the view that instead of looking at all patients with AF and deciding who should be anticoagulated, anticoagulation was now to be the norm for almost everyone. According to the guideline, there were very few people with AF in whom anticoagulation should not be considered.

The guideline was new but the message was clear. There was a conversation to be had about the AF, and the need to add another medicine to prevent Joan having a stroke.

That conversation did not get very far. Joan's eyes flashed, her lips narrowed, and entirely uncharacteristically she held up her hand and interrupted the conversation. "Look, I don't want any more tablets" she said. "I take 17 a day already. Preventing something that might or might not happen in the future isn't important to me."

"Strokes in people with AF were preventable" was the clear message in the guideline. Healthcare professionals were failing if anticoagulation was not started, and quickly. Anybody who working in the NHS had seen plenty of people who were severely disabled post-stroke or who had died. A stroke was a really bad thing. If people survived most of them had a very poor quality of life; the health and social care resources required to look after them was considerable. To say nothing of the distress and strain on the patient's family and friends.

The conversation wasn't easy for Joan and her voice faltered as she said "I'm hearing what you say, but I feel weak and wobbly, I can't stand a cook a meal, I couldn't make it to the shops and get food. That's what matters to me now. My husband was on something to thin his blood – the anti-thing you talk about. It was awful. Blood tests and bruising and trying not to eat the wrong foods. He loved a glass of whiskey at night, just the one. But he had to give it up to try and get the blood tests to behave. He really missed that, and it did no good. He had another massive heart attack and died anyway. So, I'd like you to tell me which of my tablets are controlling my symptoms and let's stop the rest. I'm 84. I'll take my chances, thank you". The unconscious nodding of the head and the pursed lips indicated that the was Joan's final word on the matter.

Suddenly this wasn't so straightforward. The science was unequivocal. Up-to-date technical information, including a national clinical guideline told everybody clearly what do. What was the problem? And compliance with such guidelines was measured. Thanks to the 2005 Quality and Outcomes Framework quite a big chunk of a general practice's income depended on complying with national guidelines including anticoagulating most people with AF. If Joan was not anticoagulated, the GP would have to "exception report" her. Otherwise, the practice income could potentially suffer.

In this consultation there was one person with technical knowledge about diseases and their treatment, and one with huge experience of living with diseases and their treatment. The technical knowledge was based upon three centuries of medicine becoming predicated upon science and the scientific method. Those approaches are about proof and certainty; this sounds intuitively a good thing, and in many ways it is. That Joan was still alive might well have been down to clever and dedicated scientists in universities and pharmaceutical companies developing a vastly expanded range of medicines for many conditions including ischaemic heart disease. Joan was alive more than fifteen years after her initial heart attack, and in large part taking her medicines conscientiously had increased the probability of that good outcome.

Once they had been developed, those medicines were tested using the scientific method called a randomised controlled trial (RCT). A group of people taking the new medicine had been scientifically proven to live longer or better than a group of people who were not given the new medicine. Again, undoubtedly a very good thing, and since the first modern RCT performed in the UK just after the Second World War that approach, which was a cornerstone of what was now called evidence-based medicine, had come to dominate medical decision making including the recommendations made in the more than 300 national clinical guidelines from NICE.

Except that Joan wasn't "a group". She was an individual. Joan's paradox encapsulated some of the current challenges in medicine. Making decisions for individuals is very different from making decisions for populations. For populations, we have the

8

science and the evidence. We know the application of that science to a group of patients improves the probability of a good outcome – or at least in the case of AF one important and easily measured outcome. That has to be a very good thing. But not everyone who takes an anticoagulant will benefit. Of course, more people will live linger or better in the group that are anticoagulated, but we cannot predict in advance whether Joan as an individual will benefit.

If she takes an anticoagulant and does not have a stroke it is likely that both Joan and the health care professionals looking after Joan will attribute the absence of the stroke to her treatment. But the reality is that the probability of Joan having an AF-related stroke in the next year is about 5%. That means if there are 100 people like Joan, 95 of those 100 will not have a stroke. It is obviously a devastating event for most of the five people who do have a stroke.

Anticoagulation reduces the number of strokes by about 60%, which sounds and is impressive. But what that means is the number of people with a stroke in the next year would go down from around five in a hundred to two in a hundred. But most people with AF do not have a stroke, even without treatment. And it is not possible to identify the three people who benefit in advance. It is all based on probability, not certainty. The three people who do not have a stroke because of treatment are indistinguishable from the 95 who were never going to have a stroke even without treatment. We simply don't know in advance whether Joan would be one of the 95 who are fine without treatment, one of the three who benefit if all 100 are anticoagulated, or one of the two who still have a stroke despite all 100 people being anticoagulated. There is irresolvable uncertainty in such decision making. And of course, anticoagulants are not without risk. There might be several people treated with an anticoagulant who get no benefit but experience a side effect from the treatment, some of those being serious and possibly fatal.

Making decisions for a population is often relatively straightforward with well-established frameworks being in place and organisations established to make such assessments. There is often good quality, scientific evidence from randomised controlled trials describing the benefits. The safety data may not be as good as the RCT data on effectiveness but there is usually enough for an assessment to be made with reasonable certainty. And in the last thirty years a new science of health economics has developed approaches when enable judgements to be made about the affordability of new medicines and technologies by health systems. Those three elements map across to the ethical constructs in medicine of beneficence (always try and do good), non-malfeasance (first, do no harm), and equity (benefit should be available to all, not a few). At the level of the population the decision can be dichotomous – use or not use in the treatment of a condition.

What is missing from that assessment is the fourth ethical construct - patient autonomy. Making decisions for a population is fundamentally different from making decisions with and for an individual. Individual decisions are, well, individual. There cannot be a rule in medicine of "never" or "always". People are very different one from another. We cannot know in advance whether preventing the stroke is the priority for that individual or not. For many, it might well be. But for others, like Joan, at least for now there are other more pressing matters – her need for support with activities of daily living, maintaining her independence, and reducing the burden imposed on her by her medicines. To impose a population-based decision of anticoagulation would be unethical. It would contravene patient autonomy and be an assault.

And that's fine, apart from the uncomfortable fact that if we don't try and prevent strokes in people like Joan and the strokes occur, then the costs and the burden of her care after a stroke fall not only on her and her friends and family. They also fall on society, because it's society that will be paying for large parts of her care, and the time spent looking after her when she's had a stroke could be spent looking after someone else.

10

There is unresolvable uncertainty. Nobody can predict what will happen to Joan if she accepts anticoagulation, and nobody can predict what will happen if she does not accept anticoagulation. From a population perspective Joan's decision could even be regarded as selfish. From an individual perspective, it must be respected.

****

I have spent much of my spare time in the last fifteen years thinking about this difference between population decision making and decision making for individuals. There is no doubt that for well-intentioned reasons, in medicine we have ended up with lots of decisions being made of the basis of "the guideline says". And sadly that is pretty much where thinking about individualising patient care begins and ends. Good medicine has come to be associated with "following the rules", and many health care professionals deviating from them in response to individual patients' needs or wants feel very uneasy, perhaps for very good reasons. Laura Marshall-Andrews, a GP in Brighton, recognised the importance of listening to patients and working with them with their approaches alongside conventional treatments sometimes had amazing results. In 2022 she wrote about the development of her thinking, and how difficult it was to create a GP practice based on those new principles and approaches in her book called "What Seems to be the Problem". Her practice won national awards, but shockingly she also faced a "Fitness to Practice" hearing having been referred to the General Medical Council by local health managers on the basis that her prescribing sometimes temporarily and for individual patients deviated from accepted guidelines. If a doctor is found guilty at a Fitness to Practice hearing they are no longer a doctor. Dr Marshall-Andrews was exonerated, but it is of great concern that her devotion to individualised care put her in such a position.

There are good reasons for science and the scientific method dominating medicine, but if medicine only says, "What's the matter?" and does not also say "What matters to you?", it is failing patients. This book is about how we have ended up in this situation, how has the science developed, why have we relied on it so much, and why is it necessary but not sufficient for great care?

Some of the difficulties arise because health care professionals and patients are humans, and it is now clear from the work of cognitive psychologists that humans much prefer certainty to uncertainty. Uncertainty is sometimes talked about a little in relation to health and health care, but often in hushed tones. After all, being uncertain of a diagnosis or uncertain about whether treatment will help or has helped a patient is almost a complete contradiction to modern ways of thinking about health and disease. Science and the scientific method are about dispelling uncertainty, the aim being proof and certainty. Many people will accept that there might be some uncertainty on some occasions – perhaps an atypical presentation of a rare disease will require some time and effort before the differential diagnoses are refined down to a single condition. Or perhaps when two courses of chemotherapy have not produced any measurable therapeutic response, the cancer patient, her relatives, and the health care professionals looking after her will all recognise the uncertainty about prognosis as the third treatment option is being considered.

Uncertainty is therefore largely generally regarded as an occasional problem - something that from time to time may disrupt the smooth certainty of diagnosis or treatment. Health care professionals often do not recognise that a state of certainty is frequently achieved only after the passage of time and multiple scientifically and technologically based investigations. When it comes to treatment, we have evidence-based clinical guidelines that apparently determine with great certainty what the management of a wide range of conditions should be. The certainty of "guideline-recommended treatment" provides cognitive relief from the complexity of selecting the best option from multiple management options, especially with limited time in a health system where demand far outstrips available resources.

Yet we worship a false idol in seeking certainty in medicine. Uncertainty is not an occasional instance in health care. As John Launer has written, uncertainty "doesn't come occasionally, singly, or in isolated categories. It's the ocean in which we swim for most of our working lives." [vii]

And there's more. In medicine the dilemma we now have not only revolves around treatment options. We also have many treatments we can prescribe to prevent disease occurring, and tests we can use to screen for pre-symptomatic disease. The same issue arises there. If we do identify potential disease early, what about the people who have an abnormal test but turn out in the end to have had a false alarm. After further tests, they turn out not to have the disease, despite a positive initial screening test. Some of them may be grateful, but others will made anxious or even traumatised by the screening process. Then there are the people who test negative, but who are subsequently found to have the disease. The result of the screening test was falsely negative. How do they feel? Did the potentially false idol of "prevention" work well for them? And then there are the individuals who say "I'll take my chances" - not everyone wants the "prevention".

Is it always appropriate to prescribe the evidence-based treatment or to screen for or prescribe medicines to prevent future disease? Whether it's treatment or prevention, we're starting to recognise that what is good for the population may not be the right thing for the individual. Understanding how medicine has reached this point and then working out what are the approaches that will turn us little by little more to making decisions for and with individuals instead of following rules is no easy or simple task. It means nothing less than rebalancing medicine.

And still there is more. There are other big forces at work making healthcare headlines now almost every day, and however important better decision making is for individuals and for health systems, the rebalancing needed looks to be broader than shared decision making and cognitive psychology. Firstly, the financial crash of 2008 and the general election of 2009 have resulted in significantly lower increases in the annual budget for the NHS. The NHS as a health system held up very well by all international comparisons until the last 15 years of austerity.

William Kissick's iron triangle of health care describes how the three competing priorities of health care delivery – cost, quality, and access – are interdependent and form a zero-sum game.[viii] In order to improve access and quality costs must rise, unless there are major gains in efficiency. On international comparisons, in 2008 the NHS was already delivering a lot for comparatively modest costs. Kissick's model tells us that if costs are squeezed by fiscal austerity then either access to health care is more difficult for patients, or quality of care deteriorates, or both happen. If demand for access increases, then costs must rise, or quality will deteriorate. If we want to improve access, we must improve capacity. Since health care is inevitably delivered in therapeutic relationships by individual people, capacity depends on having enough people. And those people need to have the optimum blend of skills to best meet the needs of the population they serve. These trade-offs are well documented, but are seldom acknowledged explicitly by governments and health policymakers.

In simple terms, with many years of public sector cost constraints, the NHS and social care has not had the annual increases in funding to provide sufficient quantities of care of adequate quality. This has not been a few difficult years. It has now been a decade and a half, the flexibility in the system is used up, and the health and social care workers who saw us through the dark days of the coronavirus pandemic, often putting themselves at personal risk, have seen real world reductions in their earnings of up to 35%. That changes the culture of professions.

Kissick's triangle applies to primary care and general practitioners. There are now fewer general practitioners than there were ten years ago, and yet millions more appointments are being provided than before the pandemic. Demand for care has massively increased, and if care is not available instantly then rudeness and even aggression have become far more common. Something fundamental has happened in society. Some days 4% of patients registered with a GP will request care. If the GP has a fairly modest 1500 patients, that's 60 people needing care when the accepted safe limit is 25. The deadlines for not one but two political promises of thousands of more GPs have come and gone with a continued decline in GP numbers. Attempts are being made to increase capacity in primary care by encouraging nurses, pharmacists and others to take up newly designed posts working in GP practices. The limited evidence is that whilst many individuals in the new posts can provide a valuable service to patients, there has not been any easing of pressure on the GPs. There have been many bad times in the NHS in my professional lifetime, but I have never seen it as bad as it is now. Doctors are walking away and giving up their practices, and almost anyone who can retire does. It is frankly scary if action is not taken and things do not improve, and quickly.

Given Kissick's triangle, after 15 years of austerity it isn't surprising that there many people in hospital beds who could be in care homes if only there were places in care homes and sufficient, well trained care home staff. That means there are no empty hospital beds for the new people arriving at the hospital with acute illnesses. In turn that means those people who are acutely ill waiting in the Accident and Emergency department or in some holding area perhaps called a Clinical Decision Unit before being transferred to a ward. Patients then move wards, sometimes a number of times, due to endless pressure from newer, and perhaps sicker patients. Someone recently described their hospital stay as being "like Bedlam, in the literal meaning of the word". The amazing thing is that many people still get excellent clinical care when they are very sick with complex conditions when they are moving to wards where new nurses don't know them and the senior doctors looking after them struggle to find which ward their patients have been moved to.

Care is sometimes poorly coordinated, or simply not good enough. It is a miracle it remains as good as it is.

But it cannot be just a matter of "Give the NHS more money" endlessly. Unless the national economy grows at the same pace as the NHS budget, assuming the NHS principles remain intact (and let me say very clearly that I strongly believe they should), in time the NHS budget becomes unaffordable via any funding route.

In any case, it is not just about money. There are now fewer young people to work in the NHS and in social care looking after mostly older people. Increasing life expectancy is a triumph and medicine, predicated as it is upon science, has played its part. But there are now many more people with multiple, long term conditions. Medicine has therefore incrementally become more complex, with proportionally more people needing more long term care. The NHS was created to largely deal with single, acute, and often infectious disease – and not large numbers of people with multiple, long-term conditions.

The NHS has huge numbers of long term, unfilled vacancies. The money matters but it isn't just about the money. The NHS needs more people, but it needs to do things differently too. If we are rebalancing medicine then looking at how things are done and what is done and by who all have to be part of the equation.

We cannot look at healthcare, or at any aspect of society, and not consider the effects of the pandemic. Its mere mention touches raw emotions for many people, but we cannot pretend the pandemic has not had profound effects. In the early months of 2020 people working in the NHS literally put their lives on the line. Many healthcare workers died from coronavirus. Many others went to work, never thinking when they joined the NHS or care system that they would ever have to put their bodies in harm's way. But despite knowing the risks they were running they still went. Some people left their own families and slept at work – with their residents in their Care Home for example - to keep the patients, residents and their own families as safe as they could. In the early days of course, they were begging and borrowing makeshift personal protective equipment (PPE) – little knowing the shady dealings and contracts for PPE that were being exchanged, only for the PPE never to arrive or be of such poor quality that it could not be used.

Of course, many people working in health and social care did get covid and recovered, but some of them got long covid. There are large numbers of people unable to return to work in the NHS and social care – and right across society - because of long covid. That accounts for some of the vacancies. Other people in the NHS and elsewhere have re-evaluated their work – life balance and reduced their hours. And still more carry the scars, many of them psychological, from that period. It all means that hospitals in particular have struggled to return to their pre-pandemic levels of activity. It is almost as if they gave their all and they still remain battered and bruised in so many ways from a dreadful experience.

Such issues have of course not been restricted to medicine and healthcare. The pandemic has impacted right across society. A schoolteacher I know almost certainly caught covid the first time on a Christmas class trip to a pantomime – undertaken when cases were rising rapidly in her locality. She was seriously ill in the acute phase with at times a heart rate of 230 per minute and her oxygen saturation dipped to 83%. Her family spent a good part of the next eight weeks looking after her, she needed months of further recovery from that episode, and struggled to get back to work part time before the end of the school year. Another autumn term of full time teaching, and she got covid a second time. Another miserable Christmas isolating and ill was followed by a second bout of long covid. And then, just as she was able to begin returning part time as part of her recovery, her school made her redundant. Shocked to the core by her callous employers, on the advice of her Union instead she resigned with an agreed three months' pay. To her credit, after a period of supply teaching, she is now back teaching with a permanent contract at a different school.

I tell her story just as one, personal illustration of the sort of horrible physical, emotional, and economic effects the pandemic has had on households and their extended families right across the world. At least in my family, no one has died from covid; we didn't, for example, have to say a goodbye to a loved one from a hospital car park using an iPad and be unable to hug one another at their funeral. Yet many of the people providing care have experienced things they never expected to, and have themselves experienced a life of quiet desperation for far too long. And that is a big factor to consider when rebalancing medicine.

And finally, there is the prospect of Artificial Intelligence (AI) and its impact on health care and across society. Whilst it remains difficult to envisage exactly how AI will change our lives, the one certain thing now is that it will rapidly spread its influence in many ways. From being a pipedream five years ago, there are now large language models (LLMs) that can replicate healthcare decision making and perhaps do so with greater empathy (as assessed by patients) than those patients experienced from a human doctor. The LLMs are not perfect, but then neither are humans. They make mistakes, and sometimes they make things up – a phenomenon referred to as an AI "hallucination" – and even those designing and training the LLMs are unable to yet determine how and why such hallucinations arise. We are not there yet, and I roll my eyes at those who enthuse unreservedly about how AI will save healthcare. When our local A&E department, designed for 30 patients, has 100 patients and senior staff are called down to the department to ensure the patients get cups of tea so they stay hydrated and can be helped to the toilets, I don't think talking to the A&E staff about how AI is going to solve all of their problems would be wise. But we cannot ignore AI, because in truth it has serious potential to make big changes in how healthcare is delivered.

The difficulties described are not unique to the NHS. Capacity of health and care systems to meet demand in many developed countries is stretching those health systems and the people who provide care as never before. What is clear is that rebalancing medicine is no longer just about better consultation skills, or about using shared decision making alongside the best available evidence and clinical expertise. It's now also about the balance between health and social care, the balance between access to care for acute illness and the resources used for prevention, about the limited effectiveness of health care in the face of social determinants of health such as poor education, poverty and the unequal distribution of wealth across our society, about helping people with multimorbidity and polypharmacy better, about overdiagnosis and overtreatment, about reducing the carbon imprint of health care, and especially about supporting a tired and dispirited health care workforce many of whom are struggling or unable to continue within the current system. If we don't take these issues seriously, if leaders don't show some leadership and soon, the future for health and care is frankly terrifying.

There is enormous complexity, and in complex systems, there are no simple solutions. But in the face of complexity, some things are better than others. And there are some great stories along the way.

CHAPTER ONE

Maths. Science. Histories.

When did modern medicine begin? If I ask people, they suggest Alexander Fleming and penicillin (1928), or René Laennec and the stethoscope (1816), or the discovery of X-rays by William Röntgen (1895) . But for me, medicine is intrinsically bound to civilisation. A health system providing reasonable access, of reasonable quality and at reasonable cost is one of the great creations of civilisation. It is said that when Margaret Mead, an American social anthropologist was asked about when civilisation started her questioner was apparently expecting her to think it started with archaeological artifacts such as a fish hook or an earthenware cooking pot. Instead, Mead responded by saying she thought that civilisation started about 15,000 years ago because there were skeletons showing healed fractures of the femur (thigh bone) from that period. It may be an apocryphal story, but it fits with the sort of things that Mead did say and write about.

It takes at least six weeks of rest for a fractured femur to heal. The healing is evidence that another person has taken time to stay with the injured, has perhaps carried them to safety and has tended them through recovery, bringing them food and water. A healed femur indicates that someone has helped a fellow human, rather than abandoning them to save their own life. Helping someone else through difficulty is not a bad suggestion of where civilisation starts.

So 21st Century medicine has deep roots. [ix] [x] [xi] The ancient Egyptians and Babylonians introduced the concepts of physical examination, diagnosis, prognosis and remedies. Egyptian papyruses record a range of surgical and medical treatments, and even indicate that, based on constellations of symptoms and signs, what the prognosis was likely to be for patients. There were prescriptions for ointments to soothe, for example, haemorrhoids using herbs. There was plenty of opportunity for orthopaedics – there would not be much health and safety when slaves were building the pyramids – and one papyrus contains the cases studies of 40 patients in a format that is a familiar one to medical students today. For context, the pharaohs ruled Egypt for 3000 years; that is about three times as long as it is from William I defeating King Harold at the Battle of Hastings to today. The Egyptian doctors had plenty of time to work out empirically how to diagnose and treat people for many conditions, even if their knowledge of modern science was lacking.

Similarly, in India around 600BCE two ancient compendia, the Charakasamhita, and the Susrutasamhita both included details of the examination, diagnosis, treatment, and prognosis of numerous ailments. Over 1000 conditions are listed, and the Susrutasamhita also describes many readily recognisable surgical procedures.

Hippocrates is widely considered the father of Western medicine. Born around 460BCE on the Greek island of Kos, he and his followers left a legacy of 70 known medical textbooks. They categorised diseases into acute or chronic, and used the words endemic, epidemic, exacerbation, relapse, and convalescence. But around the same time, it was two other less well known Greek physicians, Herophilus and Erasistratus, who in Alexandria furthered the understanding of anatomy and physiology. Dissecting human bodies, they identified nerves and linked the nervous system to movement, as well as distinguishing arteries from veins and recognising the importance of the circulatory system.

Another Greek physician, Galen (129 - c216CE), working in Rome developed a theory of humours. Black bile, yellow bile, phlegm and blood were thought to be produced by various organs in the body and had to remain in balance of that person was to remain healthy. The balance could be achieved or maintained by diet, medicines and by bloodletting. Galen's texts were considered authoritative until well into the Middle Ages when better dissection techniques merged – all be it sometimes associated with what we now consider unsavoury practices such as dissecting executed criminals and body snatching. Science and scientific method were still a long way in the future, however. Bloodletting as a treatment continued well into the 19th Century and in an excessive form may have contributed to the death of the first President of the United States, George Washington in 1799.[xii]

Whilst the development of medicine in the West went into a decline after 400CE as the Greek and Roman empires declined, Islamic medicine developed the existing texts further. Knowledge of classical medical thinking from the time of Hippocrates and Galen was only regained by European physicians when they discovered Islamic medical authors in the renaissance of the 12th Century. In Persia, Muhammad ibn Zakariya al-Razi relied on the approaches set out by Galen but developed the concept of treating people as individuals and avoiding using multiple medicines when one was sufficient – ideas we shall return to when considering a rebalancing of 21st Century medicine. His book, Al-Hawi, was translated into Latin and used in European universities until the 17th Century. Abu-Ali al-Husayn ibn Abdullah ibn-Sina recognised the airbourne transmission of disease, the use of forceps for foetal distress, and described the usually self-limiting facial paralysis now known as Bell's palsy.

Medical schools began to become established in the West in the 12th Century as the first European universities became established. The study of human anatomy became central in both medicine and in art, as sketches by Michealangelo and Leonardo da Vinci testify. In the Renaissance of the 16th – 18th Centuries the pace of progress towards science as the basis for medical practice increased. Anatomical theatres were constructed for dissections of the human body. In 1628 William Harvey correctly described the circulatory system for the first time and in 1670 Antonie van Leeuwenhoek using a home-made microscope first observed bacteria.

In the 18th Century, in what became known as the Age of Enlightenment, a range of ideas came to the fore centred on reason as the primary source as authority, as opposed to truth being established through the power of an absolute monarchy and Church dogma. Whilst politically the American and French revolutions (beginning in 1765 and 1789 respectively) were the dramatic political events, there was a revolution in scientific

23

investigation and experimentation at the same time and at pace. New ideas were spread through the establishment of scientific societies, coffee house meetings and printed books and pamphlets. Lavoisier's discovery of oxygen in 1789 was readily accepted. Contrast this with Galileo being found guilty of heresy by the Roman Catholic Church in 1633 for suggesting the earth and other planets moved around the sun.

Yet even in the Age of Enlightenment, across Europe medical schools relied primarily on lectures and theoretical learning from books – there was little practical experience. The final year student would gain some clinical experience as an apprentice, following his teachers through the wards – an approach which continues as a key part of undergraduate medical studies to this day. The journey from novice to expert is also a required theme when considering rebalancing medicine.

Laboratory work was uncommon, as were anatomical dissections because of legal restrictions on cadavers. And physicians were comparatively rare. Care for most of the population was largely provided by a variety of self-trained or amateur healers, most with a little idiosyncratic training at best – barber surgeons, apothecaries, midwives, and a fair share of charlatans.

What became St Barts Hospital in London was founded in 1123 by Rahere, an Anglo-Norman priest and monk, and a favourite courtier of King Henry I. It was the first hospital in Britain to provide care for poor sick people. The innovation was slow to catch on. The London Dispensary did not open until 1696, Guy's Hospital in London was established in 1721, and small hospitals opened in Philadelphia in 1752, in New York in 1771, and the Massachusetts General Hospital in Boston in 1811. The forerunner of my own alma mater, the Leeds dispensary, opened in 1824.

Meanwhile, in the 19th Century rapid advances in science and medicine continued. Germ theory and bacteriology led to Joseph Lister establishing antiseptic techniques for surgery in 1865.[xiii]

24

Ignaz Semmelweis dramatically reduced the death rate of new mothers from puerperal fever in Vienna in 1847 by requiring physicians to clean their hands before attending childbirth.[xiv] He was, however, vilified by his colleagues and moved to Budapest – tragically dying in 1865 in an asylum from a gangrenous wound possibly after a beating and before his discovery was accepted by the medical establishment. Lister published his results from antisepsis in the Lancet just two years after the sad and untimely death of Semmelweiss.

It was a research group led by German physician Robert Koch who discovered the bacterium responsible for cholera in Alexandria in 1883. Koch beat a group led by Pasteur to that discovery, but it was Pasteur with Emile Roux who developed the first effective rabies vaccine just two years later in 1885. This was the first vaccine developed for almost a hundred years – since Edward Jenner had demonstrated vaccination against smallpox in 1796.

One of the most remarkable figures amongst many in 19th Century medicine is the English physician John Snow.[xv] In 1843 ether became available in Britain and Snow began to experiment with it as an anaesthetic. He also studied chloroform which had been introduced in 1847 by James Young Simpson a Scottish obstetrician. Snow was asked by Queen Victoria to administer chloroform during the delivery of her eighth child Leopold on the 7th April 1853, and he repeated the procedure for the delivery of her daughter Beatrice three years later.

However, at the same time as pioneering anaesthesia, Snow was also working on the causes of diseases such as cholera and bubonic plague. The dominant theory of the time was miasma – that a noxious form of "foul air" was responsible for such diseases. Snow published an essay refuting this in 1849, but it was his careful collection of data of cholera cases in London in 1854 which led to the local council removing the handle to the water pump and ending the outbreak. The following year Snow published his paper using dot maps to illustrate the cluster of cases near the pump together with statistics to illustrate the connection between the poor quality of the water source and cholera cases. It was the moment when the study of diseases using data from populations rather than individuals became a reality – the founding of epidemiology.

As a post-script, after the cholera epidemic had subsided the council officials replaced the pump handle. To accept Snow's theory would have mean they had to accept faeco-oral transmission of disease – and, just as with Semmelweiss, this was something too difficult for established thinking to readily accept. Louis Pasteur was demonstrating bacteria were responsible for fermentation in the 1860s, and his early cholera and anthrax vaccine experiments were another 20 years in the future. It took time for the revolutionary theory of bacterial causation of diseases to become accepted, both inside and outside of medicine. Sometimes human beings find it difficult to change their thinking, at least easily, in the face of new and very different data to the current, accepted norm – another topic to which we shall return.

But epidemiology had arrived in the form of Snow's dot maps, offering new insights into medicine, which by this stage was becoming dominated by science. Florence Nightingale, accompanied by 38 volunteer nurses, pioneered the analysis of large volumes of epidemiological data summarised in graphs and tables of the causes of mortality in the British army in the Crimea between 1854 and 1856.[xvi] The acceptance of her work can only have been helped by the fact that that she came from a rich, upper class and well-connected British family. She met the politician Sidney Herbert in Rome in 1847 and they became lifelong friends. Herbert was Secretary of War during the Crimean War, and with convincing epidemiological data showing that many times more soldiers died from disease than from battle, her work was instrumental in improving sanitation and the environment in hospitals.

Nightingale's work also established modern nursing. In 1843 Charles Dickens cartooned the nursing profession with the character of Sarah Gamp in the novel "Martin Chuzzelwit". Gamp was more interested in drinking gin than looking after her patients. It was barely a caricature. Before Nightingale nursing was undertaken by untrained former servants or widows who could find no other employment and were therefore forced to earn their living in some way in order to survive. In effect, before Nightingale there was no such profession as nursing. But with a fund of £45,000 (equivalent to about £3.4 million today) donated by the British public to recognise her work in the Crimea, in 1860 she was able to set up a school of nursing at St Thomas' hospital in London. Within a few decades many other nursing schools were established, nursing became attractive as a career largely for women at that time, and for women from all backgrounds. As a result, large hospitals were better served by a readily available, trained workforce committed to providing higher standards of care.

The Crimean War ended in 1856 and just five years later the American Civil War began. The United States Sanitary Commission operated in the North and raised $25million – the equivalent of $400million at today's values – to support sick and wounded soldiers. By late October 1861 there were more than 400 scientific reports collected at the Sanitary Commission's offices in Washington DC. When the Civil War ended in 1865 a young surgeon, John Shaw Billings, recognised the importance of data and data processing.[xvii] The problem now was the accumulating volume of evidence which needed compiling and categorising.

In 1865 Billings was appointed Director of the Surgeon General's Library and in the first eight years expanded it from 600 to more than 50,000 volumes. Initially housed in the Ford Theatre in Washington, which was no longer used for productions following the assassination of President Abraham Lincoln there in April 1865. Now the National Library of Medicine, from 1879 until December 2004 when an electronic database replaced it, it published the Index Medicus, a monthly book listing the research published in what became nearly five thousand medical journals.

During his thirty years as the Library's Director, Billings worked out how to analyse medical, demographic, and epidemiological data by turning information into numbers and punching the numbers onto cardboard cards that could be sorted and counted by machine. He supervised the 1880 and 1890 US Censuses, and his assistant Herman Hollerith invented the punch card and counter-sorter system that dominated statistical data manipulation until the 1970s. Hollerith's company became International Business Machines (IBM) in 1911.

As the end of the 19th Century approached, medicine had come a long way from a few dozen textbooks originating with Hippocrates and Galen but was still a long way from truly knowing what worked and what didn't work. Indeed, the whole professionalisation of medical education and practice still needed attention.

In 1910, Abraham Flexner published the *Flexner Report* which examined the state of medical education in the United States.[xviii] It led to far-reaching changes in the training of doctors and its effect was felt worldwide. Flexner was a Classics graduate from John Hopkins University who had founded his own experimental private school in his hometown of Louisville, Kentucky. Rebelling against rigid educational approaches, his school promoted small group learning and individual development. The school was a success and pupils began to be accepted in leading universities.

In 1908 he published a book critical of many aspects of American higher education. It seems it was this book that meant he came to the attention of Henry Pritchett, then President of the Carnegie Foundation who was looking for someone to lead a series of studies of professional education. The *Flexner Report* led to the closure of many small "proprietary" medical schools owned by one or more doctors, unaffiliated with a college or university, and run to make a profit. The regulation of the medical profession by state governments was minimal or non-existent and a degree was typically awarded after only two years of study. This was despite the American Medical Association at the time requiring two years studying anatomy and physiology, followed by a further two years of clinical studies involving patient care.

Flexner concluded that medical education is a form of education rather than a mysterious process of professional initiation or apprenticeship. He believed that admission to medical school should require a high school diploma and at least two years at college or university studying a basic science. It seems amazing today, but in 1910 only 16 out of 155 US and Canadian medical schools had this as an admission requirement. By 1920, 92% of US schools required this of applicants.

There is one more story to tell about Abraham Flexner. Between 1912 and 1925 he served on the Rockerfeller Foundation's General Education Board. He worked assiduously to improve medical education and implement the findings of his own report, working with a large number of private donors. He was approached in 1929 by the Bamburger family of New York who had made a fortune from the sale of their department store. They wished to endow a medical or dental school as an expression of gratitude to the State of New Jersey. Flexner persuaded the Bamburger family to instead create an institute for more abstract research, and they endowed the Institute for Advanced Study (IAS) in Princeton, New Jersey. Working with former Princeton mathematician Oswald Veblen, they found a building and land for expansion close to Princeton and set out to recruit the best mathematicians and physicists they could. The IAS became a key lifeline for Jewish scholars fleeing Europe; the faculty was joined in 1933 by Albert Einstein.

There are no degree programmes at the IAS, there are no tuition charges or fees, and research is never contracted or directed. Instead, each researcher is free to pursue their own goals. The institute is entirely supported by endowments, grants and gifts and is one of the eight US mathematics institutes funded by the National Science Foundation. Rooted in Flexner's original principles of self-directed enquiry which were first so successful at his private school in Louisville, the results are startling. The three major awards for outstanding mathematics research are the Field Medal, the Abel Prize and the Cole Prize. Forty-one out of 57 Field Medals have been awarded to Institute affiliates, 9 out of 16 Abel prizes have gone to Institute professors or visiting scholars, and 39 out of 56 Cole prizes have gone to academics associated with the IAS at some point in their career.

Pioneering work on the theory of the stored-program computer begun at Bletchley in the UK by Alan Turing to crack the Nazi Enigma code during World War II was developed further at the IAS by John von Neumann.[xix] The IAS machine built in the basement of the Fuld Hall from 1942 to 1951 under von Neumann's direction introduced the basic architecture of all modern digital computers. The IAS is now a leading centre of research in string theory – a broad subject that (as all viewers of the US TV comedy *The Big Bang Theory* will know) attempts to address a number of fundamental questions in gravity and particle physics and is a candidate for "the theory of everything".

As the sixth child of nine, born in 1866 in Kentucky to German Jewish immigrants, Abraham Flexner did many great things, but he was flawed. He regarded African Americans including doctors to be inherently inferior to whites. In the early 20th Century, he wasn't unique in taking that position, but it easily stops him being regarded as a great man of science. But Flexner did help embed science as the foundation of the practice of medicine.

Most European countries had recognised the need to improve the quality of medical education in the mid-19th century, some decades before the US *Flexner Report*. An ordered pattern of science-oriented teaching had become widely established in Europe as the Century progressed. But it was far from Flexner's self-directed learning. The approach was based upon teaching, where the student mostly listens to "experts" and was expected to follow exactly what the "expert" says or does, rather than learning, where the student is more investigative. The clinical component of a medical education was largely confined to hospitals, which were at the time still usually charitable institutions staffed by consultants working in an honorary (unpaid) capacity. This approach was confirmed in Britain by the passage of the 1858 Medical Act. It created the General Medical Council (GMC) which from that time has controlled admission to the medical register. The GMC continues to be legally responsible for medical education and the standards of professional practice and behaviour.

The establishment of the General Medical Council was not easy and followed more than twenty years of agitation. Thomas Wakely − a surgeon and founding editor of one of the world's leading medical journals *The Lancet*, can take much of the credit. Wakely campaigned against incompetence, privilege and nepotism in the medical profession throughout his life. He had an aggressive personality and was involved in several libel cases as he exposed poor surgical practice, but they only increased his influence. He called the Council of the Royal College of Surgeons "an antediluvian relic" and "an irresponsible, unreformed monstrosity in the midst of English institutions".[xx]

Tiring of the slow pace of reform within his own Royal College he stood as a radical candidate for Parliament and was returned for Finsbury in 1835, retaining his seat until 1852. His long campaign eventually led to the 1858 Medical Act. The second most famous Member of Parliament for Finchley is of course one Margaret Thatcher, who was first elected as MP for Finchley 107 years after Wakely stepped down.

Once it was established, the major professional organisations were represented on the GMC, and this made it easier to modify the curriculum. But the new trends were already well established; the time spent on basic studies of doubtful relevance was cut and the *Lancet* rejoiced that students no longer had to study, for example, the dentition of the mastodon (an extinct elephant-like creature). More time was left for clinical work but the *Lancet* frequently criticised aspects of the curriculum. There remained an emphasis on botany, influenced perhaps by the Apothecaries, and the *Lancet* challenged the General Medical Council in 1863 when it suggested that medical students need no longer be apprenticed to a general practitioner before beginning hospital work.

Above all, the *Lancet* supported science. In 1864 it delighted that "No case of illness is now admitted to a medical ward which does not demand the careful use of the stethoscope, microscope and test tube in its investigation." Nine years later the *Lancet* proposed the establishment in the teaching hospitals of special departments in orthopaedics, ophthalmology and ear, nose and throat disease to ensure that the students' education was complete. Above all, there was a thoroughness with which scientific and theoretical knowledge of the basic sciences were fused with clinical experience developed from the practical responsibility of taking care of human beings.

After his 1910 US report, Abraham Flexner came to Europe to report for the Carnegie Institute on the state of European medical education. Published in 1912, the report was complementary of the European approaches especially when compared to those he had found in the US. He found assessment tested "at the same time, theoretical knowledge, ability to think and technical skill", something we still strive to do today.

The *Flexner European Report* noted that the undergraduate courses in Europe were already five years long, and regarded the student already overburdened with the required volume of scientific knowledge. As the 20th century progressed, medical education slowly developed into four generally recognized stages: premedical, undergraduate, postgraduate, and continuing education. But it was a slow process. As late as the 1980s, after graduation from medical school and spending a single year under supervision in hospital posts in medicine and surgery, I could have become a general practitioner with no further postgraduate training being deemed necessary. There was no supervised requirement to undertake continuing professional education, and no assessment of ongoing competence.

What could possibly go wrong?

CHAPTER TWO

The Scientific Method

How did it happen that we now have a huge range of modern treatments that are proven to increase the probability of someone like Joan living longer and better than she might have done without modern medicine. Twenty years earlier her husband Herbert did not have the benefit of those newly developed medicines and died just a few years after developing heart disease. We could just stick with observing people – the hunter-gathers in 15,000BCE might have recognised that rest and time mended some broken thigh bones – but the problem is that observation and extrapolations can lead us astray. We don't now drill holes in the skulls of people with mental health problems or epilepsy to "let out the evil spirits". We have come to accept that a better understanding of how the human body works in health and disease means better approaches are possible in our search for treatments that are more likely to successfully treat such diseases.

For example, once we know what happens to diseased hearts – how they are working and not working, what controls the heart rate and its ability to continue to pump blood around the body even after a heart attack – all that knowledge and lots more means there can be a purposeful search for medicines to reduce the effects of the disease and increase the probability that people like Joan would live much longer and in pretty good health too. Even so, if that happened to Joan and people like her, it might have occurred just by chance. So we also need to work out how we *prove* that medicines help people, because someone might live longer just by good luck or because of some other factor – and not because of the medicine.

This is all science, and the ways in which knowledge is accumulated and assessed as representing "the truth" is the scientific method. If we are to think about where medicine has ended up and what is needed to rebalance it, we need to know quite a bit more about both of these things. Over the last three centuries they have come to dominate medicine and the way it is learned by those who provide healthcare.

Around the world medical schools only accept as students the brightest and the hardest working young people. Enormous efforts go into finding better ways in which universities might best select these from huge numbers who apply. This is because such undergraduate courses are relentless. The volume of science to be learnt, understood and then recalled when asked to do so either informally or in examinations is simply enormous and still growing. Only people who can absorb lots of information quickly, store it in their brains and apply it sensibly in the context of an ill person can survive the course. In recent years changes to the curriculum mean that medical students do devote some time, for example, to studying how have to have conversations with patients. But this is very limited, and surviving medical school requires learning and understanding science, science and more science.

The roots of modern scientific methods can be traced back to philosophers like Aristotle who emphasised the importance of observation and classification in understanding the world. Aristole, born in 384BCE, systematically gathered data, discovering patterns common to whole groups of animals, and inferring possible causal explanations from these observations. Among his correct inferences were that brood size decreases as body mass increases, so that an elephant has fewer young (usually one) per brood than a mouse, and that lifespan increases with gestation period and body mass. However, science based solely on observations does not normally carry the same level of certainty as experimental science. It can often only set out testable hypotheses.

After the fall of the ancient Greek and Roman civilisations, Persia became the focus of learning and science. Ibn al-Haytham, an Arab mathematician, physicist and astronomer[xxi] built upon a series of natural experiments performed by Aristole.[xxii] He noted that as soon as other observations are reported which are not in keeping with the inferred explanations then the theory needs to be adapted or a rejected and a new theory is constructed which fits with all the data. Born in Basra around 953CE, Ibn al-Haytham, also recognised that a hypothesis must be supported by experiments that could be repeated, and mathematical evidence was required. Most histories credit Galileo or Francis

Bacon at the beginning of the 17th Century with first developing what became the modern scientific method. But Ibn al-Haytham and other Arabic scholars were there fully five centuries before Renaissance scientists such as Galileo, Bacon and the French philosopher Rene Descartes. He also first correctly described the process of sight, linking his observations of a solar eclipse using a camera obscura with the anatomy and function of the eye. He deserved his place on the obverse of the Iraqi 10,000 dinar bank note.

Galileo was born in Pisa on 15th February 1564.xxiii His father, Vicenzo Galilei played the lute but was also a music theorist – it was Vicenzo who established that for a stretched string the pitch varies as the square root of the tension. It seems probable that Galileo was exposed to experimentation and associated mathematical or other forms of proof - as opposed to simple observation leading to theories or inferences - from a very early age. Galileo, aged 16, began studying medicine at the University of Pisa at the insistence of his father. Physicians were, after all, paid more than mathematicians. But after observing swinging chandeliers he set up an experiment at home and demonstrated that pendulums kept time together no matter how far the swing of the arc. He persuaded his father that he should switch from medicine to mathematics and natural philosophy (the term used then for what became "science"), and he flourished.

As we will see later, the modern approach to studying consultation skills in medicine only became possible due to technological innovations. Similarly, many of Galileo's most important discoveries were only possible because of a breakthrough in technology. In 1608 Hans Lippershey developed the first practical telescope in the Netherlands. Though he was unsuccessful in his patent application, word rapidly spread of the invention across Europe. Based only on descriptions, and by all accounts pretty sketchy descriptions, in 1609 Galileo made a telescope with about 3x magnification. On 25th August the same year he demonstrated to Venetian merchants a telescope with a magnification of 8 or 9, and on 30th November he was the first human being to identify lunar mountains and craters.

But it was on 7th January 1610 that Galileo observed "three fixed stars, totally invisible by their smallness", close to Jupiter, and lying on a straight line through it. On subsequent nights he observed the positions of these "stars" relative to Jupiter were changing in a way that would have been inexplicable if they had really been fixed stars. On 10th. January, Galileo noted that one of them had disappeared, an observation which he attributed to its being hidden behind Jupiter. Within a few days, he concluded that they were orbiting Jupiter, and on 13th January 1610 he identified what turned out to be the fourth of Jupiter's moons.

Conventional "truth" at that time, emanating from the Roman Catholic church, was that all heavenly bodies circle the Earth, and that was to give Galileo a problem. But he wasn't the first person to suggest that the earth and the other planets orbited the sun. Nicolaus Copernicus in 1512 began work on his heliocentric theory. Within two years he had completed an outline commentary which he circulated in manuscript form only to a few close friends and colleagues with whom he collaborated in observing eclipses.

By 1532 Copernicus had a complete hypothesis, but he resisted publishing, not wishing to risk the scorn "to which he would expose himself on account of the novelty and incomprehensibility of his theses." Despite his reticence, within a few years rumours about his theory had disseminated to other natural philosophers all over Europe. Still he hesitated to publish, perhaps from fear of the Church's reaction – and this may explain the subsequent dedication of his masterpiece to Pope Paul III.

In the 21st Century in many parts of the world an academic disagreement can get unpleasant, but it does not escalate to imprisonment, violence, or a tortured and slow execution. The 17th Century "natural philosophers" - as these early scientists were called - were well aware of the consequences if new theories were difficult for powerful religious leaders or monarchs to readily accept. Francis Bacon urged scepticism as a key principle which his fellow scientists should always employ. But he also made it clear that his investigations were to explain a world which God had created, and as a devout Anglican it seems certain that tenant did indeed truly form part of his core beliefs.

In science and medicine in the 21st Century, quite often new developments which challenge orthodox thinking are challenged and even dismissed - even when the evidence for the new thinking is very strong. But we do not face the consequences that are equivalent to a particularly unpleasant episode of "Game of Thrones". Learning things is hard. Unlearning things is even harder. Appreciating this important principle which drives much decision making in medicine is important, and it has not changed since the 17th Century. For the preceding 1000 years, the prevailing theory about how the Earth, the Sun and the other planets were positioned was the one that Ptolemy published in his book "Almagest" around 150 CE. Legend has it that Copernicus was presented with the printed version of his book setting out his findings that the earth circled the sun rather than the sun circling the earth on his deathbed aged 70 years on 24th May 1542, some 67 years before Galileo's observations of Jupiter's moons.

Again, the Persian's got there before Copernicus and Galileo. Ibn al-Haytham and several other Islamic astronomers questioned the Earth's apparent immobility, and centrality within the universe. In the 12th century, Nur ad-Din al-Bitruji described heliocentricity as an imaginary model, successful at predicting planetary positions, but describing reality. The Persian alternative explanation and model spread through most of Europe during the 13th century, with debates and refutations of their ideas continuing up the time of Copernicus and Galileo.

It seems possible that Copernicus was aware of these alternative models when developing his own. Aspects of his own models resemble closely those of the preceding Islamic scholars. This should not be seen as a criticism; it is still the norm that scientific discoveries build successively upon the work of many previous scientists. The notion of a sudden "breakthrough" transforming all previous understanding owes more to

Hollywood fiction than reality. As Isaac Newton wrote in 1675, "if I have seen further, it is by standing on the shoulders of giants".

It seems that Copernicus's theory was slow to catch on. Sixty years after his book's posthumous publication there were only a small number of European astronomers who publicly favoured his theories. Between 1543 and Galileo's 1610 discoveries, criticism and opposition to Copernicus mounted because it went against traditional Roman Catholic theology. This was in the context of ongoing religious upheaval for the best part of a hundred years. Martin Luther sent his Ninety-Five Theses on the Power and Efficacy of Indulgences to the Archbishop of Mainz on 31st October 1517. This is the event usually acknowledged as the start of the period known as the Reformation when the supremacy of the Pope and the Roman Catholic church was first seriously challenged. Defensiveness by the leaders of the Roman Catholic church may have played a part in what followed.

By 1615 Galileo's writings were submitted to the Roman Inquisition. This was a system of tribunals responsible for prosecuting individuals accused of a wide array of crimes relating to religious doctrine or alternative religious beliefs. Galileo, a devout Roman Catholic, went to Rome to defend his ideas. On 26th. February 1616 Galileo was ordered to abandon his theory and forbidden to hold, teach, or defend it in any way whatever, either orally or in writing. Copernicus's book and other heliocentric works were banned until correction.

Galileo worked on other matters for the next 15 years, but then returned to astronomy. In February 1633 he was brought before a Church inquisition in Rome. Galileo was found guilty of heresy for having held the opinions contrary to Holy Scripture. He was sentenced to formal imprisonment, but the following day this was commuted to house arrest. In 1634 he returned to his villa at Arcetri near Florence.

It was while Galileo was under house arrest that he dedicated himself to mechanics, the strength of materials, and the science of motion, including projectiles. It is almost certainly a myth that Galileo experimented by dropping different weighted balls from the Leaning Tower of Pisa. Much of the work involved inclined slopes and these, alongside a number of his telescopes can be viewed in the fascinating Museo Galilei in Florence.

When we consider Flexner's work on medical curricula at the beginning of the 20th Century and the development of European medical curricula 40 years earlier , it is clear that a reliance on scientific method in medicine had become the norm. This reflected the profound intellectual and social forces which had shaped science over the previous two centuries. They were about to further reshape medicine.

CHAPTER THREE

The First Clinical Trials

Gradually the scientific revolution began to impact on medicine. In 17th Century England, the thinking of natural philosophers Francis Bacon and Isaac Newton did not result in imprisonment and banning of their works. The gold standard approach began to shift from observation and study of individuals in health and disease to scientific experiment, data, scepticism and a need for mathematical proof. Gradually the notion took hold that whenever possible, the scientific method required trials of experimental and control groups to determine beyond reasonable doubt whether one treatment was superior to another.

Such trials appear sporadically in the historical record of different ancient civilisations around the globe. But as the scientific reasoning of the second half of the 17th century filtered into 18th Century medicine, reports of such experimental approaches began to appear – though they were still rare. One of the most famous is James Lind's investigations published in 1753 which demonstrated that citrus fruits prevented scurvy[xxiv]. However, once again, radical ideas even when accompanied by good data were not readily accepted. It was another 50 years before the Royal Navy made the provision of lime juice a requirement, and not until the Merchant Shipping Act of 1867 did the number of cases of scurvy fall to negligible levels. This sets a modern world record for time to implementation of evidence - 114 years from the scientific experiment until effective implementation of the results of that science. And it was even longer before the final piece in the jigsaw appeared. Vitamin C, the ingredient in citrus fruits responsible for health, was not discovered until 1912.

Whilst much of the remarkable improvement in life expectancy in the 20th Century can be attributed to improvements in public health – improved sanitation, clean water, and a better diet – there have been dramatic reductions in deaths due to infections. Biological and vaccine industries developed rapidly to confront the microorganisms identified towards the end of the 19th century as being responsible for many common and serious infections. With the chemical industry joining in as developers of treatments, they began to employ ever more sophisticated methods to demonstrate their treatments truly did work, and preferably worked best.

One of the most famous of these experiments is Johannes Fibiger's 1898 study of diphtheria toxin in 484 patients in Copenhagen.[xxv] Fibiger treated patients with diphtheria seen on one day with the experimental treatment and withheld the treatment on alternate days, and then compared the outcomes in those who received the experimental treatment and in those who did not. Eight out of 239 patients in the serum treated group and 30 out of 245 in the control group died. The results were regarded as convincing at the time, but to determine whether such results could have occurred by chance, formal statistical tests would be required. However, the appropriate statistical method – the Chi-squared test – was not developed by the English mathematician Karl Pearson until two years after Fibiger's paper was published. Applying that test to Fibiger's data retrospectively, his results could have occurred by chance only 3 times in 10,000. In modern medicine, if a statistical test shows that the results of an experiment could have occurred by chance less than 5 times in 100, the results are accepted as true.

In his investigation of diphtheria toxin, Fibiger had further developed much of the methodology of what would become commonplace in the second half of the 20th Century, the randomised clinical trial. Fibiger knew that diphtheria toxin seemed promising in some animal studies but trials conducted his head of department, Professor Sorenson, at Blegdamshospitalet in Copenhagen had not been convincing. What was obvious was the toxin had a significant side effect – serum sickness, and this side effect occurred in more than half the people who were given it. Fibiger was also aware of other trials of diphtheria toxin in Paris but knew that those results were based on the outcomes in one hospital where serum was used for all patients, versus the results in another hospital where serum was not used at all. The Paris results he rejected because of the risk that the results could have occurred due to other differences between the hospitals – for example, differences in isolation routines and hygiene.

He concluded that he had to have a large sample collected over a long study period (he suggested a year), allocated by chance into an experimental and controlled group. He knew he needed to measure mortality – an outcome that was not subject to measurement error by those conducting the experiment. He knew he needed to report in detail what happened to each patient including those who were admitted but not recruited into the experiment and the reasons why, and why some patients withdrew from the study as it progressed – for example, by refusing the diphtheria serum. And he considered the possibility that his results could have occurred by chance, although an appropriate statistical test could not be performed at the time.

Fibiger recognised the need to design the experiment carefully for any results to represent a true effect of the experimental treatment, rather than to have occurred by chance, or be due some other external factor. He had, for the modern era, identified the power of randomisation. By a process analogous to the tossing of a coin two groups of people in the experiment are created. Because of the random allocation into those groups, the groups should be identical apart from one group getting the experimental treatment and the other group control treatment. If that is the only difference between the groups and all appropriate care is taken to ensure that is the case, any difference in outcomes between the two groups ought to be truly due to the differences in treatment provided. Better outcomes in the experimental group compared to the control group, and it is likely that the difference is truly due to the treatment.

And yet Fibiger's methodological innovation had little immediate impact. It was better than James Lind's 114 years, but it was still 27 years before the requirement of randomisation in experimental design was formally stated by the English statistician and geneticist R. A. Fisher in his book *Statistical Methods for Research Workers*. Fisher, working on historic data from crop experiments, also recognised that randomisation eliminates bias and permits a valid test of significance. Disappointingly, like Flexner, Fisher was another scientist who held strong views on race; throughout his life he was a prominent supporter of eugenics.

After Fibiger, small numbers of controlled trials were published in the first half of the 20th century, most of them testing infectious disease treatments. Most of them did not use a true "coin toss" randomisation, and the number of trials was dwarfed many times over articles promoting therapies based on laboratory and physiological justifications, or simple narrative reports without any scientific approach at all. For many years there were no economic, regulatory, or social incentives to rigorously evaluate new medicines in controlled trials. The norm remained methods other than controlled trials or often no science at all – approaches that at that time were not challenged by scientists and society.

Slowly, as more experience was gained with trials using Fibiger's alternate allocation, critics identified deficiencies in the approach. In a number of instances, the data seemed to show that some choice may have been consciously or unconsciously exercised in selecting cases for treatment (or not) by those conducting the trial. Of course, this introduced a significant source of bias, when the whole purpose conducting the experiment was to reduce error and bias and hence arrive at a result which could be regarded as "the truth".

It was time for a new approach. And yet the storm clouds of the second World War were approaching.

CHAPTER FOUR

On Such Things Does History Turn

In 1901 a 20-year-old shipping clerk inherited some money following the death of an uncle. His elder brother, already qualified as a doctor, suggested he might use the money to support his studies at medical school. And so, in 1903 the shipping clerk enrolled at St Mary's Hospital Medical School in Paddington, London. His name was Alexander Fleming.[xxvi] [xxvii] [xxviii] [xxix] [xxx]

As a medical student, Fleming was a member of the medical school's rifle club. After he graduated, the captain of the rifle club wanted to retain Fleming in the team. He wanted Fleming to do postgraduate research at St. Mary's, and they found the post of assistant bacteriologist to Sir Almroth Wright, a pioneer in the development of a vaccine for typhoid, was available. On such things does history turn.

Wright had met the playwright George Bernard Shaw in 1905. The two men at one point debated what would happen if there was more demand from patients than could be satisfied. Wright apparently answered, "We should have to consider which life was worth saving."[xxxi]

GBS immortalised Almroth Wright as Sir Colenso Ridgeon in his play "The Doctor's Dilemma". The core theme of the play is that the newly knighted doctor has developed a revolutionary cure for tuberculosis. However, his private practice, with limited staff and resources, can only treat ten patients at any one time. From a group of fifty patients he selects ten he believes he can cure and he believes are most worthy of being saved. As if that were not bad enough, there is then a very attractive woman with a sick husband who begs for treatment. Then a friend and colleague finds he too needs treatment. The dilemma is that Sir Colenso must choose which patients he will save.

It seems that GBS may have been correct to be sceptical about Wright being deserving of his prominence within the medical establishment. Whilst he was undoubtedly academically decorated – a knighthood, five honorary doctorates, five honorary orders, six fellowships (two honorary), and so on – Wright held some controversial views. He argued that

47

microorganisms were vehicles of disease but not its cause, a theory that earned him the nicknames "Almroth Wrong" and "Sir Almost Wright" from his opponents. Hurtful, perhaps, but not "Games of Thrones" or Catholic inquisition territory.

But Wright was also opposed to women's suffrage, and argued that women's brains were not constituted to deal with social and public issues. Shaw dismissed Wright's views on the subject as absurd.

Despite a number of serious errors of judgement, Wright actually did a lot of good. In 1897 he developed a vaccine prepared from killed typhoid bacilli.[xxxii] Preliminary trials in the Indian army produced excellent results, and typhoid vaccination was adopted for the use of British troops serving in the South African War. Unfortunately, the method of administration was inadequately controlled, and the government sanctioned inoculations only for soldiers that "voluntarily presented themselves for this purpose prior to their embarkation for the seat of war." The result was that, according to the official records, only 14,626 men volunteered to be vaccinated out of a total strength of 328,244 who served during the three years of the war. Although later analysis showed that inoculation had had a beneficial effect, there were 57,684 cases of typhoid—approximately one in six of the British troops engaged—with 9,022 deaths. Vaccination is only effective if people are convinced it works and is safe, and therefore get vaccinated.

A bitter controversy over the merits of the typhoid vaccine followed, but immunisation was officially adopted by the army before the outbreak of World War I. In the South African War, the annual incidence of enteric infections (typhoid and paratyphoid) was 105 per 1,000 troops, and the annual death rate was 14.6 per 1,000. The comparable figures for World War I were 2.35 and 0.139, respectively. Even allowing for the better sanitary arrangements in the latter war, it is not surprising that Wright's typhoid vaccine placed him at the forefront of the British medical establishment. It seems unlikely he gave much thought to the decision when he gave Alexander Fleming the most junior of jobs in his department as a bacteriologist.

Fleming gained the necessary further postgraduate qualifications and worked as a lecturer at St Mary's until war came in 1914. He served throughout World War I as a captain in the Royal Army Medical Corps, and was mentioned in dispatches. Working in battlefield hospitals at the Western Front in France, he witnessed the death of many soldiers from sepsis resulting from infected wounds. Antiseptics, which were used at the time to treat infected wounds, often seemed to him to worsen the injuries.

Fleming published in the Lancet, arguing that antiseptics killed more soldiers than infection during World War I. Antiseptics worked well on the skin surface, but deep wounds harboured bacteria that thrived in the absence of oxygen.

After the war ended in 1918, at St Mary's Hospital Fleming continued his investigations into these mysterious "antibacterial substances". At the beginning of the 20th century, in Germany Paul Ehrlich had pioneered the search for a chemical that would kill a microorganism and leave the host unaltered - a "magic bullet." After extensive testing largely focussed on chemicals used as dyes, he found a drug with activity against the bacterium *Treponema pallidum*, which causes syphilis[xxxiii]. The introduction of this drug, arsphenamine (Salvarsan), and its chemical derivative neoarsphenamine (Neosalvarsan) in 1910 resulted in a transformation of syphilis therapy. They rapidly became the most frequently prescribed medicines in the world.

Many organisms, including many species of mould, naturally produce antibiotic substances. Ancient cultures, including those in Egypt, Greece and India, seemingly independently discovered their useful properties in treating infection. In England in 1640, the idea of using mould as a form of medical treatment was recorded by apothecaries such as John Parkinson, the King's Herbarian. In the 1870s there had been several reports published describing moulds inhibiting the growth of bacteria.

Testing mucous from a patient with a cold, Fleming found that it had an inhibitory effect on bacterial growth. One of his culture plates was covered with yellow colonies of a bacteria, but where the mucous had been the bacterial colonies had been destroyed. Fleming had discovered human lysozyme, one of the body's natural defences against infection. He found that lysozyme was present in many secretions including tears, saliva, and mucus. Fleming published his findings in 1922 and although he was able to obtain larger amounts of lysozyme from egg whites, the enzyme was only effective against small counts of harmless bacteria, and therefore had little therapeutic potential. But the discovery helped Fleming's career progress, and he became Professor of Bacteriology at St Mary's in 1928.

For the previous year Fleming had been studying the properties of a group of bacteria called *Staphylococci*. He went on holiday with his family in August 1928, and before leaving he had stacked all his cultures of staphylococci on a bench in a corner of his laboratory. On returning, Fleming noticed that one culture was contaminated with a fungus, and that the colonies of staphylococci immediately surrounding the fungus had been destroyed, whereas other staphylococci colonies farther away were normal. It was remarkably similar to how he had discovered lysozyme.

The fungus turned out to be *Penicillium notatum*, and the antibacterial molecule that it produced was of course penicillin. A particularly cool summer may have produced just the right temperatures for the fungus to grow. On such things does history turn. Fleming published his finding in 1929 in the Journal of Experimental Pathology, but the paper attracted little interest. Penicillium appeared to be difficult to culture, extract and purify. Despite working with two colleagues – Stuart Craddock and Frederick Ridley who were trained in biochemistry - they did not make significant progress on producing useable quantities of penicillin.

Fleming did manage to use some of his limited supply of penicillin - on Stuart Craddock. Craddock developed a severe sinus infection, and after surgery Fleming injected penicillin into the infected sinus on 9th January 1929 but without any apparent effect. In addition to doubts about the concentration and dose of penicillin administered, it is possible that the infection was with a bacteria called *Haemophilus influenzae*, subsequently found to not be susceptible to penicillin.

Fleming gave some of his original penicillin samples to surgeon Arthur Dickson Wright in 1928. Although Wright reportedly said that it "seemed to work satisfactorily," there are no records of its specific use. Cecil George Paine, a pathologist at the Royal Infirmary in Sheffield who was a former student of Fleming[xxxiv] also asked for a penicillin sample from Fleming. He initially attempted to treat infected beard follicles but was unsuccessful, and moved on to eye infections in new-born babies, Paine apparently achieved at least two cures in November 1930, but he did not publish his research. Given the limited data it seems unlikely that a journal would have accepted a paper submitted by Paine even if one had been written.

There was simply not enough penicillin to undertake more rigorously designed, scientific studies - even if the researchers considered them. Fleming continued to find that cultivating *Penicillium* was difficult; having with difficulty grown the mould it was then even more difficult to isolate, purify and concentrate the antibiotic agent. Fleming also became convinced that penicillin would not last long enough in the human body to kill bacteria effectively. He admitted that the problem was beyond him – he was a bacteriologist, not a biochemist.

While Fleming worked unsuccessfully on penicillin, Gerhard Domagk, another German bacteriologist who worked for the Bayer chemical company followed up Erlich's work on dyes. In the 1930s he developed sulphonamide from the dyes which were a major product of the chemical industry. Domagk found that sulphonamide had some activity against the bacteria streptococcus. In the pre-antibiotic era, any sepsis could be a threat to life. Domagk treated his own daughter with sulphonamide, apparently saving her the potential amputation of an arm. The hunt began to intensify for other medicines to treat infectious diseases which were more effective, and which had fewer and less severe side effects. Salvarsan, Neosalvarsan, and sulphonamide were the only effective chemotherapy for bacterial infections, and Fleming's penicillin seemed to be going nowhere.

Meanwhile, at Oxford University, Howard Flory had arrived in 1935 as Professor of Pathology.[xxxv] Flory was an Australian who graduated in medicine from Adelaide University in 1921. He came to Oxford as a Rhodes scholar based on a stellar academic record and being an excellent tennis player. His brilliant undergraduate career continued as a postgraduate with a PhD from Cambridge. After further academic posts in the United States and Cambridge where he gained wide experience in physiology, biochemistry, and pathology, he was appointed to the Joseph Hunter Chair of Pathology at Sheffield in 1931 at the astonishingly young age of 34. There seems to be no doubt that there was a conversation at some point between Florey and Cecil Paine about Paine's experience in treating patients with Fleming's penicillin. They did, after all, work in the same relatively small Department of Pathology. But given the difficulties with culturing Penicillium, it did not result in any further research at the time.

Flory was a brilliant scientist, but he was also expert at extracting research grants from the hands of controlling bureaucrats. To this day Heads of Departments at universities spend lots of time bidding for limited research funds. Being successful 30% of the time is considered an excellent success rate. No funds means no money to pay staff. No staff means no research. No research means no academic papers being published, and - even worse - other funding streams depend on the university's academic track record of published research. Florey's scientific and research grant-obtaining talents were recognised back in Oxford, and after only four years at Sheffield he was a candidate for the Chair of Pathology in Oxford.

Oxford had appointed its very first Professor of Pathology only in 1907, Georges Dreyer. A donation of £100,000 in 1922 changed things significantly in Oxford's Department of Pathology. The money was given by trustees of funds left by the Scottish trader Sir William Dunn, and it meant a brand-new pathology building could be built. The Dunn School with its stylish red brick frontage was one of the best equipped laboratories in the country. Dreyer, influenced by his work with the Royal Flying Corps in the war, had latterly concentrated on aviation medicine but had not been very successful in attracting research funding. He died in 1934 and Howard Florey arrived to find wonderful laboratories, but largely empty spaces, because research programmes were sorely in need of development funds.

It was lucky that Howard Florey was offered the chair. The appointment board had two influential external members – Sir Edward Mellanby, secretary of the Medical Research Council, and Sir Robert Muir, a Scottish pathologist. Mellanby preferred Florey but Muir had an older and more traditionally-minded candidate in mind. Mellanby's train meant he was late for the meeting that was to decide on the position. In his absence, the board decided to go for the safe pair of hands. But before the meeting ended, Mellanby finally arrived and persuaded them differently. On such things does history turn.

Florey set about recruiting an interdisciplinary group of scientists, an approach that reflected the multifaceted approaches to scientific research to which his education had exposed him. Interdisciplinary work was required to understand a broad range of the new scientific discoveries describing the causes of disease and ways in which they might be treated – and that team-based approach is still followed to this day. His team began to work on not just the pathological evidence of disease, but also the physiological processes which produced the symptoms and signs of disease, traced to molecular levels.

Among his first people he recruited was the biochemist Ernst Chain. Chain was of Jewish-Russian-German descent. When the Nazis came to power he realised he would not be safe in Germany

53

and had arrived in England in April 1933 with £10 in his pocket. His mother and sister remained in Germany and were subsequently killed in the Holocaust. Chain was recommended to Florey by Frederick Hopkins – who had been Flory's PhD supervisor at Cambridge.

Chain was charged with developing a biochemistry unit within the Dunn School. One of the early research projects was the crystallisation of lysozyme, the enzyme discovered by Alexander Fleming in 1921 - and the identification of the location on bacteria to which it attached in order to destroy the bacteria.

Chain was very self-confident and had an enthusiastic, volatile personality that was bound to clash with Florey's less flamboyant and sternly focussed approach. They were poorly matched in terms of personalities but in 1938, while the lysozyme research was concluding and during a rare period of camaraderie, Chain drew Florey's attention to Fleming's original 1929 paper on penicillin. With the likely prospect of a second world war approaching, the prize of more effective treatments for infections had become a priority. Rather than continue with their dye-based strand of research, a plan was laid for a systematic study of penicillin and other known, naturally occurring, antibacterial agents.

While Florey and Chain were assembling bids for research grants to fund themselves and their work, there was no time to waste. War clouds continued to gather, and they began work whilst still pursuing funding for their research. Chain, along with another biochemist, Edward Penley Abraham, worked on the problem that Fleming had not solved. They began working out a successful technique for purifying and concentrating penicillin. In this early process many gallons of mould broth were used to produce an amount just large enough to cover a fingernail. This trying and inefficient process was later improved on by Norman Heatley - another biochemist on the research team assembled by Florey.

In March 1940 Chain had two mice injected with a sample of the penicillin he and Abraham had extracted. The mice survived unharmed; the first toxicity test was apparently a success. On 25th May eight mice were injected with haemolytic streptococci - which among other diseases causes puerperal fever in new mothers - and four of these were subsequently injected with measured and timed doses of penicillin. Sixteen-and-a-half hours later the four mice that had received penicillin were alive, but their untreated fellows were dead. Understandably there was great excitement among the researchers.

On 24th August 1940, Florey and Chain reported their findings in the *Lancet*. The article electrified research groups around the world that were seeking cures for bacterial disease. The military importance of a more successful means of combating the diseases and infections that had decimated armies of the past was immediately recognised. Obtaining funds for research was no longer the problem.

In early January 1941 Florey was ready to test penicillin on humans. He needed a clinician with access to patients and was introduced to Charles Fletcher - a young doctor who had rowed in Cambridge's winning eight in the 1933 Boat Race.[xxxvi] Fletcher's father had been the Secretary of the Medical Research Council before Sir Edward Mellanby, the man who was responsible for bringing Florey to Oxford. Fletcher was just 29 years old, looking for research opportunities and meantime was doing clinical work at Oxford's Radcliffe Infirmary. He could hardly have expected that his research career would start with him giving the first intravenous injection of penicillin in the history of medicine.

The patient was Mrs Elva Akers, a 50-year-old woman with widespread breast cancer which was beyond treatment. This was to be a test of penicillin's toxicity. She showed little immediate reaction to the injection - but later she began trembling and developed a fever, which eventually settled. Abraham found that impurities in the drug, not the drug itself, had caused the adverse reaction. Further refinements were made to the production process in an attempt to remove the impurity.

At the time all large hospitals had a "Sepsis" ward in which valiant but often futile attempts were made to treat people with serious infections. It is hard now to imagine a pre-antibiotic era when there were no effective treatments for many infections. In February 1941, Albert Alexander, a seriously ill policeman, became the first patient with an infection to be treated with penicillin in the hope of achieving a cure.

Alexander had developed a small sore at the corner of his mouth, but staphylococcal and streptococcal infections set in. Some months later he had abscesses in his lungs and upper arm, a spreading infection across his face and head, and abscesses in his eyes - one eye had been removed surgically in the hope of relieving some of his pain.

The research team had no idea of the dosages and the length of treatment required to eliminate a bacterial infection. The policeman's condition at first improved with the penicillin therapy to the extent he was able to eat, but then the penicillin supply began to run out, and even retrieving penicillin from the man's own urine failed to save him. In retrospect Fletcher calculated that less that 250,000 units of penicillin were administered over five days – a tiny dose when compared with the later established doses required to treat patients. Twice that dose four times a day would quickly become the usual dose.

Administration of penicillin to several more cases of sepsis of varying severity in young children - because the doses required would be lower and supplies remained very limited - produced uneven results which nevertheless included some startlingly good clinical recoveries. The equivalent today would be to walk into a ward of terminally ill cancer patients, inject them with a new medicine, and within a few days observe some of the cancers melting away. Doctors from across the Radcliffe Infirmary would come and see the penicillin patients who recovered, and would regard them with wonder.

It was immediately obvious to the Oxford team that they were onto something important. Increasing production now became of overriding importance. Because *Penicillium* mould requires air to grow, it was first cultured in regular laboratory flasks. Soon all manner of vessels were being used, including hospital bedpans and hundreds of made-to-order ceramic pots. The operation quickly outgrew the space assigned to the Dunn labs, production workers were hired, and neighbouring facilities in Oxford were borrowed. There was a penicillin factory within the precincts of the ancient university.

Chain wanted a patent to be sought for penicillin, as was usual in German research institutes. Florey, influenced by the then head of the Medical Research Council Sir Henry Dale, refused to enter into such a commercial agreement for a discovery he presumed would benefit all mankind. The decision long rankled Chain, and with hindsight he had a point. When commercial production was subsequently established, it was American pharmaceutical companies who took out patents on novel aspects of the production process. Those patents made millions for the US companies after the war, and for the next 20 years Britain paid royalties on the drug that had been developed researched and developed in Britain.

Florey approached various British pharmaceutical firms to help with and improve production, but many were already committed to manufacturing other drugs needed for military and civilian populations. Other companies had had their facilities devastated by enemy bombardment. Seeking the assistance of the United States in increasing production, Florey and Heatley flew across the Atlantic in the beginning of July 1941.

Florey's previous American connections served him well. The two Oxford visitors spent the Independence Day weekend with a friend from his Rhodes year. Introductions were made at the U.S. Department of Agriculture's Northern Regional Research Laboratories (NRRL) in Peoria, Illinois, where large-scale fermentation processes for other purposes were already being worked on. Sparked by the high demand for use as flavouring agents in the newly popular carbonated beverages, moulds producing citric acid and lactic acid were being grown in the Midwest on a large scale. Alfred Newton Richards, Florey's old laboratory director when he had studied and worked at the University of Pennsylvania, was now chair of the Committee on Medical Research in the Office of Scientific Research and Development - an organisation established to support the Allies war effort. Richards agreed to unified action on penicillin after a single meeting.

The Penicillin Project had three main strands. The first was focused on improving the purification of penicillin and the second aimed to find more potent strains of *Penicillium*. Heatley worked closely with the US Department of Agriculture to characterise these strains. The last stream, headed by Florey and his American partners, set about finding pharmaceutical companies which would take on mass production of penicillin.

All three approaches quickly produced results. Within months several changes were made in the chemicals used in the purification process, increasing the yield substantially. A global search began for better penicillin producing strains, with soil samples being sent to the NRRL from around the world. But chance again played a huge part – this time in finding more potent strains of *Penicillium*. One hot summer day, a laboratory assistant at Peoria, Mary Hunt, arrived with a cantaloupe melon that she had picked up at the market and that was covered with "*a pretty, golden mould*". Serendipitously, the mould turned out to be the fungus *Penicillium chrysogeum*, and it yielded 200 times the amount of penicillin. With further enhancement induced by mutation-causing X-rays and filtration, it was ultimately producing 1,000 times as much penicillin as the first batches from *Penicillium notatum*.

Richards approached four drug firms that Florey indicated had shown some preliminary interest in the drug (Merck, Squibb, Lilly and Pfizer). Richards told them it was in the national interest if they undertook penicillin production, and that there might well be financial support from the federal government. A first meeting in Washington, D.C., on 8th October 1941, was held to exchange information on company and government research and to plan a collaborative research programme to expedite penicillin production. It was not a success. The second meeting, held in New York in December, was ten days after Pearl Harbor and the U.S. entry into the Second World War. Not surprisingly, the second discussions were more productive.

Apart from Pearl Harbor, it also helped having early, encouraging results from the changes to the purification process reported at the December meeting. It was agreed immediately that although the companies would pursue their research activities independently, they would keep Richards' team informed of developments, and the Committee could make the information more widely available (with the permission of the company involved) if that were deemed in the public interest. Some companies worked out collaborative arrangements of their own, and Heatley joined the Merck research staff for several months. By March 1942 enough penicillin had been produced under these arrangements to treat the first American patient - Mrs. Ann Miller, in New Haven, Connecticut. A further ten cases were treated by June 1942, all with penicillin supplied by Merck.

With more penicillin available, Florey, Heatley, and Chain conducted a series of further clinical studies.[xxxvii] Florey's wife, Ethel, was also his research colleague. But the supply penicillin remained so limited that the urine of patients who received it was still collected and returned to the laboratory for reprocessing and reuse. Ethel was among those who collected the patients' urine from the Radcliffe, and the story is she brought it back to the Dunn Institute on her bicycle. She and her husband were sole authors on the research paper published in the Lancet in 1943 - a description of the course of illnesses in several patients treated with penicillin for a wide range of infectious diseases, coupled with analyses of how penicillin was absorbed and distributed once in the human body.

One of the most dramatic of these early cases was in August 1942 when Fleming cured Harry Lambert of streptococcal meningitis. Lambert was a work associate of Robert, Fleming's brother. Robert had asked Fleming to help his colleague. Fleming asked Florey for a penicillin sample, which Fleming immediately used to inject into Lambert's spinal canal. Lambert showed signs of improvement the very next day, and was completely recovered within a week. Fleming wrote it up in the Lancet in 1943.

It seems that supplies of penicillin continued to preclude larger and more robust scientific experiments such as randomised trials. Indeed, given the apparent remarkable effect of penicillin, the notion of deliberately treating patients with control treatment in the context of a randomised trial may well have seemed inappropriate at the time, should it have been considered.

Careful observations of clinical use rather than randomised trials demonstrated the remarkable effect of penicillin in combating many bacterial infections - including battlefield injuries - without serious risks of toxic side effects. It was evident that penicillin would save the lives of many wounded soldiers. Once fatal bacterial infections, which took thousands of servicemen's lives during WWI, might actually became potentially curable thanks to penicillin.

And outside of the war effort, with most hospitals at that time having a ward full of terrible sepsis cases not much different from Albert Alexander, world-wide bacterial infections were one of the largest if not the largest cause of death and long term ill health. The prospect of being able to quickly, easily, and safely cure huge numbers of patients with serious infections - which up to that point were in effect untreatable - was mind boggling.

Collaboration between governments, industry, and British and American scientists led to sufficient supplies of penicillin being manufactured by D-Day in 1944, when Allied troops landed in France. From January to May in 1942, 400 million units of penicillin were manufactured. By the end of the war,

American pharmaceutical companies were producing 650 billion units a month. Medicine had entered the industrial age. By 1946, penicillin was widely available for general prescription.

But by then credit for the discovery of penicillin had become acrimonious. As early as 1942 the potential of penicillin was becoming clear and *The Times* ran a leader on penicillin on 27th August. Almroth Wright - Fleming's old boss at St Mary's - saw an opportunity to gain publicity for his organisation. He wrote a letter to *The Times* in response to the editorial that was published on 1st September. It suggested that the "*laurel wreath [for the discovery of penicillin] . . . should be decreed to Professor A Fleming.*" Oxford University were equally determined to get the due credit. Sir Robert Robinson, Professor of Chemistry at Oxford University, wrote to the Times a day later saying "*a bouquet at least and a handsome one, should be presented to Professor H W Florey*" for separating "therapeutic penicillin" from the complex mixture in which it was produced.

The first BBC radio broadcast dealing specifically with penicillin followed rapidly on 4th September. The broadcast explained what penicillin was, how it was produced, and its potency against bacterial pathogens. An internal BBC memo of 1st September, so written after *The Times* editorial and letters, said "*There is a good deal of disputed priority involved, the point being that Wright's nominee, Professor Fleming, made the discovery but never followed it up and the actual work has all been done by the Professor of Pathology at Oxford with the help and direction of the MRC* [Medical Research Council]".

Less than two months later there was a second BBC programme which was more controversial. This took the form of a re-enactment. Early in the script the actor playing Fleming exclaims "*I say, Jones, something's gone wrong with this culture. Just look at this Petri dish*". Then comes the critical moment: "*Just like Newton and his apple and James Watt and the lid of his mother's kettle, when world discoveries are hanging in the balance…*". The programme pointed out difficulties – penicillin was difficult to make and it "*kept badly,*" and according to the script for those reasons nothing more was

61

heard of it until war came. The scene then shifts to a committee meeting at the MRC, which eventually concluded that "*elaborate apparatus and a skilled team of biochemists*" would be required to "*investigate*" penicillin and that one "*can't expect a medical school to undertake this sort of work*". The chairman wants to know who could. The answer is "*I should suggest Oxford, sir*".

Florey wrote angrily to the BBC. Not unreasonably he questioned whether the BBC had considered whether it was in the public interest to "*call attention to a substance of therapeutic value which is unprocurable except in minute amounts*" and that this type of publicity had resulted in "*a flood of pathetic letters from as far away as Western Australia and Saskatchewan*" begging for supplies of penicillin. Later he says "*I am not concerned with the impersonation of Professor Fleming . . . But I wish to assure you that the whole passage about the MRC is a pure invention*".

Questions were demanded at the BBC. Apparently a Harley Street surgeon, Mr Johnstone Abraham, who was a friend of Fleming wrote the script. Fleming provided Abraham with the material and Fleming read the script and agreed to it being broadcast. This might be regarded as being at best naïve on Fleming's part. A week later Cecil Graves, the joint Director General of the BBC, wrote to Florey saying that "*it was felt that in dealing with the story of the discovery of penicillin we could safely rely on the authoritative guidance of Dr Fleming*".

Over a year later the BBC broadcast another programme on 20th December 1943 with Florey mentioning Fleming's "*important observation*". But he chose to commence his broadcast with reference to Pasteur who "*discovered more than 60 years ago that certain micro-organisms . . . can produce something that will stop the growth of other germs*". Florey makes specific mention in his broadcast to the fact that Fleming had unsuccessfully used dressings impregnated with crude penicillin.

Fleming himself made a radio broadcast on 7 April 1944. In May 1944 his portrait would appear on the front cover of *Time* magazine, and Florey and the group at Oxford did not receive a single mention. Instead, an abstract reference is made to the combined efforts of the mould and "the skilled chemist" in bringing penicillin to humanity.

How did all this come about? The dean of St Mary's, Charles Wilson (soon to be ennobled as Lord Moran), was also Churchill's physician and president of the Royal College of Physicians. When such a powerful medical figure said, "We [St Mary's] discovered it," it was difficult to challenge that. Then there was Lord Beaverbrook – a powerful press baron – who was a patron of St Mary's and was instrumental in setting the agenda in the press. And it may be that Florey did not help himself. It was understandable that he became exasperated with the media coverage focussing almost entirely on Fleming. However, his response was to refuse to speak to the press at all. That meant he lost the opportunity to put his and his team efforts in their rightful place.

Fleming's character is reliably described as modest and self-effacing, so it seems unlikely that that he was responsible for the imbalance in credit given for penicillin at the time. It seems more likely that academic power struggles orchestrated by those near the top of both St Mary's and Oxford accounts for the these unseemly parts of a wonderful story. Charles Fletcher interviewed Fleming for a BBC TV Panorama programme in 1954. It was the first time the two had met. Fletcher found Fleming to be self-effacing, and unprompted he gave the Oxford team all the credit they deserved.

The Nobel Prize committee did the right thing and Fleming, Florey and Chain jointly received the Nobel prize for their work in 1945. According to the rules no more than three people may share a Nobel Prize, and so unfortunately the contributions of Norman Heatley and Ernest Abraham were not included.

Heatley's contribution was finally recognised 45 years later; in 1990 that he was awarded the unusual distinction of an honorary Doctor of Medicine from Oxford University, the first awarded in Oxford University's 800-year history. Sir Henry Harris who succeeded Florey as Head of the Dunn School wrote in 1998, "Without Fleming, no Chain or Florey; without Florey, no Heatley; without Heatley, no penicillin." Heatley died at his home in Marston, Oxfordshire in 2004; the house now bears a commemorative plaque in his honour.

His obituary in *The Guardian* revealed one more twist in the tale of penicillin. When in the US working on pushing up the yields of penicillin, Heatley was working closely with an NRRL researcher, Andrew Moyer. Moyer suggested adding corn-steep liquor, a by-product of starch extraction, to the growth medium. Alongside other changes - using lactose in place of glucose, - they were able to push up yields of penicillin to 20 units per ml. But their cooperation fell apart too. Heatley noted *"Moyer had begun not telling me what he was doing"*.

Florey returned to Oxford in September 1941, but Heatley stayed on in the US and worked at Merck. In July 1942 he returned to Oxford and then found that Moyer had published their research results, but he had omitted Heatley's name from the paper. This was in spite of an original contract which stipulated that any publications should be jointly authored. Fifty years on, Heatley recalled that he was amused, rather than upset, by Moyer's duplicity.[xxxviii] I suspect that others might have not been so generous, especially at the time. It seems that financial greed led Moyer to claim all the credit for himself. To have acknowledged Heatley's part of the work would have made it difficult for Moyer to apply for patents with himself as sole inventor of the yield-increasing process, which is what he did.

Ernest Abraham's academic career continued to glitter in Oxford. With Ernst Chain he proposed a novel molecular structure for penicillin in October 1943; this was confirmed two years later by Dorothy Hodgkin using the new technique of X-ray crystallography for which she later received the Nobel Prize.

In 1948 he received samples of a *Cephalosporium acremonium* fungus with antibacterial properties from an Italian pharmacologist Giuseppe Brotzu. Abraham and another researcher, Guy Newton, purified the antibiotics from this fungus and found one, cephalosporin C, was able to cure infections caused by penicillin-resistant bacteria. They were able to establish its molecular structure, modify it to increase its potency, and then registered a patent on the compound. This resulted in the first commercially sold cephalosporin antibiotic, Cefalotin. There are now five generations of cephalosporin antibiotics. Through the registration of the patent on cephalosporin, Abraham and Newton were able to set up charitable trusts to support biomedical research. As of 2016 the combined endowment of these charities was over £194 million. He was knighted by Queen Elizabeth II in 1980.

Florey and Fleming were knighted in 1944, and in 1965 Florey became both Baron Florey and was awarded the Order of Merit. He became Chancellor of the Australian National University from 1965 until his death in 1968. Florey's portrait appeared on the Australian $50 note for 22 years. Sir Robert Menzies, Australia's longest-serving Prime Minister, said, *"In terms of world well-being, Florey was the most important man ever born in Australia"*.

Chain was keen to leave Oxford after the war. He and Florey were so different in character - Florey taciturn, blunt, and solely focused on getting the job done, and Chain naturally effervescent and bubbling with ideas. Contemporaneous accounts report they got on each other's nerves, and sadly after Chain left in 1948 for the Istituto Superiore di Sanità in Rome they rarely spoke. He returned to Britain in 1964 as founder and head of the biochemistry department at Imperial College London. He was knighted in 1969.

Charles Fletcher, the most junior of the Oxford team, also had a remarkable career. Sir Edward Mellanby, successor to Fletcher's father of course, had no hesitation in selecting him when the Medical Research Council sought a clinical scientist to head their newly established Pneumoconiosis Research Unit in Cardiff. Fletcher made it a huge success scientifically, in large part because he established excellent relationships with the trade unions and the community of miners in South Wales. As we shall see, he recruited some key people to work in the MRC Research Unit in Cardiff.

Tall and distinguished in appearance, Fletcher was a natural choice for television – which at the time was in its own pioneering age. It was he who from 1958 collaborated with the BBC's Richard Dimbleby in the first major television series that dealt with real-life medicine, *Your Life in Their Hands*. This was truly transformative - showing doctors at work including operations on TV was mind-boggling at the time. I remember watching the first series as a very young boy on a flickering black and white television. And it was Fletcher, with the support of Sir George Godber at the Department of Health, who persuaded the Royal College of Physicians to produce their epoch-making report in 1962 on the hazards of smoking. Fletcher himself was effectively the author of that report.

Fleming was feted across the world. In 1999, Time magazine named Fleming one of the 100 Most Important People of the 20th century. His discovery and the subsequent development process sparked a huge expansion of the pharmaceutical industry, and forming the basis for decades of new medicines – some of which also became "blockbusters". With some of those profits cyclically reinvested in the development of new medicines for a wide range of diseases, the pharmaceutical companies in turn sparked the therapeutic revolution that occurred in the second half of the 20th century that eventually benefitted many people, including Joan.

Fleming received a Knighthood, a Nobel Prize, fifteen honorary degrees, 140 other honours and decorations, and was granted five audiences with the Pope. His image was used on banknotes and stamps, buildings were named after him, and bullfighters in Spain subscribed for a statue to be erected outside the main bullring in Madrid because penicillin reduced the number of matador deaths. It is to his credit that he tolerated what must have been an intrusion into his academic career with charm and great good humour.

66

CHAPTER FIVE

The Medical Revolutions

The discovery and subsequent development of penicillin is perhaps the most remarkable of all science stories. There was huge jeopardy in the interplay of chance (Fleming's stacked Petri dishes when he went on holiday in an unusually cool summer), in insight (the recognition of the antibacterial properties of *Penicillium*), in the interactions of the big personalities and the multiple large organisations involved, and in the difficulties inherent in developing collaboration between new scientific disciplines - of chemistry, biochemistry, microbiology, and clinical medicine.

But perhaps the most dramatic change and the one which had the largest subsequent impact was the increase in the pace of development of the pharmaceutical industrial complex. The industrial scale of manufacturing medicines actually began long before penicillin, with many modern companies being founded in the second half of the 19th Century. For example, Bayer produced aspirin in the 1860s and diamorphine in 1898, Pfizer manufactured a successful parasitic in 1849 and it was their existing expertise in fermentation technology that was so useful to the penicillin project. Merck in the US was set up in 1891 and developed a commercial diphtheria toxin in 1925.

But the penicillin story does not stand alone. There were other remarkable stories involving the development of treatments for other conditions well before penicillin. Canadians Frederick Banting and Charles Best successfully extracted insulin in 1921, small scale production began later that year using pancreases from cows and pigs, and by January 1922 Banting successfully treated a 14 year-old boy - Leonard Thomson - with insulin.

At the time, the life expectancy of a young person who developed diabetes was somewhere between days to a few months. Unable to metabolise sugars, the body would instead begin to burn fats. This would eventually lead to a complex cascade of biochemical disorder within the body, followed by coma and death. The only known treatment was a starvation diet, in which the calorie intake was reduced to a level that the patient could tolerate without showing sugar in the urine. If the diet was followed, a person with diabetes could expect to live for perhaps two years before eventually succumbing – most commonly to an infectious disease due to their malnourished state.

Banting began his career training as a surgeon at the Hospital of Sick Children in Toronto, and then opened a surgical practice in London, Ontario.[xxxix][xl] His earnings from his practice were small, forcing him to take a part-time teaching position in the local medical school. Working as a part-time lecturer in pharmacology, Banting had his interest in the pancreas stimulated by the need to teach some students about it. His reading of unsuccessful attempts by others to extract insulin from the pancreas included a recent paper describing the effects of tying off the pancreatic duct. Banting realised that performing this procedure would mean insulin could then be successfully extracted.

This theory led him to approach JRR Macleod, professor of physiology at the University of Toronto, the university where Banting had been a student. Macleod was initially sceptical about Banting's theory, but eventually - despite Banting having almost no experience of physiology research - he relented. In May 1921, before leaving for his summer in Scotland, Macleod made available to Banting ten dogs for experimental work and two medical students, Charles Best and Clark Noble, as laboratory assistants.

Banting only needed one assistant at a time, so Best and Noble flipped a coin to see who would assist Banting first. Best won, and after that first day Banting decided to keep Best for the entire summer.

Banting's ligated the pancreatic duct of a dog and extracted whatever secretions were produced after the atrophy of the acini cells. These secretions enter the gastrointestinal tract to play a large part in digesting food. In 1901 Eugene Opie, an American pathologist at Johns Hopkins University, had made the association between the degeneration of the other type of cells in the pancreas, the dramatically named Islets of Langerhans, and the onset of diabetes.

Banting and Best began, only to find that it was difficult to keep duct-ligated, de-pancreatised dogs alive long enough to carry out any tests. After a summer of many unsuccessful attempts, by August they were keeping a severely diabetic dog alive with injections of an extract made from duct-ligated pancreas and prepared, following Macleod's instructions, in saline. This extract substantially lowered the blood sugar levels of diabetic experimental dogs.

On 30th December 1921, Banting presented their findings at the conference of the American Physiological Society, at Yale University. Banting was by training a young and not very successful surgeon, with relatively little academic experience. Out of understandable nervousness, he did a poor job delivering the paper and the audience was highly critical of the findings presented. Macleod was the chair of the session, and he joined the discussion to rescue Banting from the scathing commentary. After this fiasco Banting became convinced that Macleod had stepped in to steal the credit from him and Best, and relations between the two began to deteriorate.

Shortly before the Yale presentation, Macleod had invited James Bertram Collip, a biochemist, to help Banting and Best with purifying their extract. There are similarities here with Fleming making the initial discovery of penicillin but not able to turn it into a useful medicine, then Florey and his team were needed to make more progress, and finally many people from different backgrounds and from different organisations to make penicillin in sufficient quantities. Banting and Best needed large amounts of their extract, and Collip set to work purifying the extract for clinical testing in humans. Collip was quickly able to precipitate out the active ingredient insulin.

However, tension was rising as Banting became increasingly bitter toward Macleod, and pitted himself and Best against Collip in the race to purify the extract. At the end of January 1922,

Collip came to Banting and Best's laboratory and informed the two that although he had discovered a method to produce pure extract, he would share it only with Macleod. The story goes that it was Best who stopped Banting from attacking Collip. Fortunately for the future of insulin, an uneasy agreement made a few days later allowed them to continue to work together.

On 3rd May 1922, Macleod, representing the group, announced to the international medical community at a meeting of the Association of American Physicians that they had discovered insulin. Later that year one of Banting's early patients to have her life saved with insulin was Elizabeth Hughes Gosset, the 14-year-old daughter of the US Secretary of State.

The pharmaceutical company Eli Lilley developed large scale manufacturing capacity for insulin, whilst the patent was transferred to the British Medical Research Council to prevent exploitation. Banting and Macleod received the 1923 Nobel Prize in Physiology or Medicine. That the Nobel committee chose only Banting and Macleod for the award caused more animosity. Years later, the official history of the Nobel Committee admitted that Best should have been awarded a share of the prize.

By the end of 1923 insulin had been in commercial production for a year at the Eli Lilly and Company laboratories. Large numbers of people with diabetes who received insulin recovered from comas, resumed eating carbohydrates in moderation, and realised that science and the scientific method had saved them from a death sentence.

But a step change was coming in the way new treatments were tested. Penicillin and insulin made such dramatic differences to the natural course of diseases that was obvious to all that they worked, and it was also obvious when they did not work. Penicillin is ineffective against a range of bacteria and it was obvious to the early researchers that the natural course of diseases caused by those bacteria was not changed when an attempt was made to treat them with penicillin.

The reason for such certainty was not down to the characteristics of penicillin or insulin. Rather, it was the nature of the conditions they treated. The outcomes of diabetes and serious sepsis were so obvious in a short period of time, and the outcome was often death. One of the great ironies in medicine is that success is often best measured by how many people die. Further testing of penicillin and insulin in formal head-to-head trials against placebo treatments or usual treatment was unnecessary, and when judged by modern standards would almost certainly be regarded as unethical. This is because people with sepsis or diabetes, if allocated in a randomised controlled trial to placebo or usual treatment, would be harmed because participating in the trial would meant they would be denied treatment that could potentially save their life.

This is not the case for many other conditions and their emerging, potential treatments. Few people these days seem to know that a tuberculosis treatment would be a game-changer.

Tuberculosis was known to many ancient cultures and was described over 2000 years ago by Greek, Chinese and Indian physicians. There seems to be no question that tuberculosis became more common during the Middle Ages and the Renaissance peaking between the 18th and 19th century as rural populations moved to the cities looking for work. In 1808, William Woolcombe found that of the 1,571 deaths in Bristol between 1790 and 1796, 683 were due to tuberculosis. In London, 1 death in 7 was due to consumption at the dawn of the 18th century; by 1750 that proportion grew to almost 1 in 5, and to 1 in 4 by the start of the 19th century.[xli] The Industrial Revolution coupled with poverty and squalor created the optimal environment for the spread of the disease.

Tuberculosis typically progressed slowly. This allowed for a "good death" as sufferers could put their affairs in order. In the 19th Century an inappropriate romanticism became attached to the disease. Lord Byron wrote, "*I should like to die from consumption*", and the disease became the disease of artists. George Sand was besotted with her tuberculosis-infected lover, Frédéric Chopin.

Several novels depicted a grossly romanticised views of tuberculosis including Victor Hugo's *Les Miserables*, and these in turn inspired operatic depictions in Verdi's *La Traviata* and Puccini's *La Bohème*. Even after medical knowledge of the disease had accumulated, this bizarre, redemptive perspective of the disease remained popular.

There was scientific progress, all be it slow. René Laennec, who died from tuberculosis in 1826 at the age of 45, had invented the stethoscope in 1816. He spent those ten years corroborating his auscultatory findings and the respiratory symptoms seen in living patients with the pulmonary lesions found on the lungs of autopsied tuberculosis patients.

In 1869, Jean Antoine Villemin demonstrated that tuberculosis occurred in cows and in humans, was contagious, conducting an experiment in which tuberculous matter from human cadavers was injected into laboratory rabbits, which then became infected. On 24th March 1882, Robert Koch, a Prussian physician, gave a famous lecture at the Berlin Physiological Society in which he described his work which confirmed the disease was transmissible and moreover caused by a bacteria *Mycobacterium Tuberculosis*.[xlii]

Just three years later, Wilhelm Roentgen discovered the X-ray, which allowed physicians to diagnose and track the progression of the disease. It won him the first Nobel prize in physics. Roentgen refused to take out patents related to his discovery of X-rays, as he wanted all of society to benefit from the practical applications of his discovery.[xliii]

But at the beginning of the 20th century, despite establishment of sanatoria where bed rest and fresh air were prescribed, there was no active treatment. Tuberculosis was regarded as one of the most serious public health problems and in the UK a Royal Commission was set up in 1901. Its remit was to find out whether tuberculosis in animals and humans was the same disease, and whether animals and humans could infect each other. There were campaigns to stop spitting in public places, and

73

the infected poor were pressured to enter sanatoria that resembled prisons. In 1916, even under the best conditions and with death rates from TB starting to fall, 50% of those who entered sanatoria were dead within five years.[xliv]

Following the success of vaccination in preventing smallpox in the 18th century, it was hypothesised that infection with bovine (cow) tuberculosis might protect against infection with human tuberculosis. In the late 19th century, clinical trials using *Mycobacterium bovis* were conducted in Italy with disastrous results; *M. bovis* was found to be just as virulent as the human *M. tuberculosis*.

Albert Calmette, a French physician and bacteriologist, and his assistant and later colleague, Camille Guérin, a veterinarian, were working at the Institut Pasteur de Lille in 1908. They were working on virulent strains of the tuberculosis bacillus and testing different culture media. Again a chance finding was crucial. A glycerin-bile-potato mixture grew bacilli that seemed less virulent. They set about repeated subculturing, aiming to produce a strain that was weakened enough to be considered for use as a safe vaccine

Eventually the BCG (Bacille de Calmette et Guerin) strain was isolated after subculturing 239 times over a 13-year period. By 1919 the now avirulent bacilli were unable to cause tuberculosis disease in research animals. The BCG vaccine was first used in humans in 1921. Sadly Guerin's wife had died from TB in 1918. Public acceptance of vaccination was slow and was not helped by a disaster in 1930 in Lubeck in northern Germany. The BCG vaccine administered to 240 infants vaccinated in the first 10 days of life was contaminated with a virulent strain stored in the same refrigerator at the manufacturer. Almost all the babies developed TB and 72 died.

In the 1940s, tuberculosis was still regarded as a killer infectious disease. Early in its use, by 1941 at least, it was recognized that penicillin-the-wonder-drug was only clinically effective against some bacteria - those classified as gram-positive.

It was ineffective against gram-negative bacteria, and tuberculosis is gram negative. Research teams around the world were searching for the "magic bullet" which would work against TB.

In May 1942 Albert Schatz graduated from Rutgers University, New Jersey with a major in Soil Science. The next day he enrolled for his PhD degree in Professor Selman Abraham Waksman's department of soil biology, still at Rutgers. Waksman had spent a decade and more progressing soil microbiology as a science, and then for the previous five years had concentrated identifying antibacterial activity from moulds and actinomycetes (itself a bacteria, active in the production of compost) in soil samples. This research was of a very similar type to the work going on at the same time at Peoria, Illonois as that team searched for *Penicillium* species that would produce an increased yield of penicillin. Waksman's research team had already identified three potential antibiotics, but they were found to be too toxic for treating infections in humans. Nevertheless, Waksman had established working relationships with the pharmaceutical company Merck should the search identify medicines that would progress to the stage of manufacture on an industrial scale. Schatz had joined a team on a fast track when it came to antibiotic research.

After six short months of postgraduate research at Rutgers, Schatz had his plans interrupted. He was in the Air Force as a bacteriologist, stationed in army hospitals in Florida. This experience provided him with first-hand knowledge of the inability, at that time, to control many infectious diseases. He saw at first-hand the tragedy of uncontrollable gram-negative bacteria. They were killing wounded servicemen, some of whom had been flown back to the U.S. from the North African campaign. As he later wrote, *"I isolated and identified the deadly bacteria. That was the easy part. I often spent many hours at night with servicemen as they were dying. That was the hard part."* [xlv]

In his limited time off, Schatz isolated and tested moulds and actinomycetes from contaminated blood culture plates and from

75

Florida soils, swamps and coastal sea water. He sent Waksman cultures that he thought merited further testing which he could not do in army hospitals. In June 1943 Schatz was back at Rutgers. He was discharged from the military due to a back injury and returned determined to focus his doctoral research under Waksman on finding an antibiotic effective against gram-negative bacteria in general and specifically against TB.

Waksman funded Schatz with $40 a month. It was a pittance and Schatz lived rent-free in one of the Plant Physiology greenhouses at the university. In lieu of rent he prepared solutions for research on the hydroponic growth of plants, watered and fertilized other plants, swept the floor, maintained the proper temperature during winter months, and did other chores. He ate fruit, vegetables, and dairy products which he obtained free from the respective departments at the Agricultural Experiment Station. He was fascinated and intrigued by his research, and it became an obsession. He simply did not have the money for a social life so he would start work in his basement laboratory around 5am and often still be there at midnight.

I am reminded of "*Vaxxers*", Sarah Gilbert and Cath Green's account of their development of the Oxford – AstraZeneca coronavirus in 2022. Because of lockdown, they wrote, it wasn't such a burden starting work at 4am and working 18-hour days; there simply wasn't anything else to do. It probably helped that there was a worldwide pandemic and they were some of the few people on the planet who had the opportunity to really do something to end it. In the same way, Schatz was driven because of his experience with sepsis, by the emerging promise of antibiotics, and of course he simply did not have any money to do anything other than work.

Within a few months this frenetic pace of work coupled with an instinct for what direction to take the research began to pay dividends. Other research had already pointed the way to go, and Schatz grew many, many colonies of actinomycetes and then tested them against a range of bacteria that were known to cause a range of serious diseases. It wasn't systematic – Schatz could

76

later not describe why he would test one colony of actinomycetes and not a neighbouring one. But he knew he was in the numbers game. 99.99% of his experiments he knew were going to fail. Finding an actinomycetes with serious antibiotic properties was literally like looking for a needle in a haystack. Schatz knew the more and different actinomyces he grew, the more experiments he could run against disease-causing bacteria; the more experiments he ran the better the chance of a positive finding. With one positive finding he had a PhD thesis, potentially an academic career, and who knows what else. But if he ran 100,000 experiments and found nothing, he might not even get his PhD - that was how academia worked.

Against all the odds, after only three and a half months of admittedly dawn to beyond dusk workdays, on 19th October 1943 at about 2pm, in the words of Schatz's co-worker Doris Jones, "Al hit pay dirt". Schatz had found not one but two separate colonies of actinomyces with a wide range of antibiotic activity. Twenty-eight years previously Waksman had identified them and called them *Actinomyces griseus*, but only 6 months previously after further work Waksman had changed the name to *Actinomyces streptomyces*. The two separate strains had come from a patch of heavily manured soil at the Rutgers Agricultural Station and from a throat swab from one of the healthy chickens Doris Jones was using in her research. She had shared a discarded agar plate with Schatz, passing it through a window between the two laboratories.xlvi

Schatz was cautious, but one set of exciting experimental results followed another. And then he found startling activity against a relatively mild strain of tuberculosis. He had discovered what became streptomycin.

On 16th November 1943, exactly four weeks after Schwarz had first discovered the two actinomyces strains, Waksman was visited in his office on the third floor of the Soil Microbiology building by William H Feldman. Feldman was a vet working in animal research at the Mayo Clinic in Rochester, Minnesota - and his area of research was tuberculosis. After working on TB in cattle, he had collaborated on research into human TB for the past five years with a chest physician at the Mayo Clinic, Corwin Hinshaw. Together they had run some disappointing experiments with potential antibiotics against TB but had heard of the basic science work Waksman had been doing in identifying potential novel antibiotics. Feldman had come to propose a collaboration. Unaware of Schatz's work or his results, he offered the expertise of the Mayo clinic in evaluating any new, promising antibiotics against tuberculosis.

Feldman made one suggestion. He explained how vital he thought it was that early laboratory testing should take place with a virulent strain of human tuberculosis bacteria, rather than against the far less active strains routinely used in laboratory work. Waksman was immediately wary of having the powerful strains of TB bacteria in his building because of the risk of staff, including himself, contracting the disease. But he asked Feldman to send some samples over and was cautiously positive about a future collaboration.[xlvii]

Schatz's first paper describing his discovery of streptomycin was published on 1st January 1944 with the other authors being Elizabeth (Betty) Bugie and Waksman. As was required by established scientific protocol, Betty Bugie, another of Waksman's postgraduate students, had successfully replicated Schatz's results. The paper described results against a range of gram-negative organisms and there was only one line of results against the TB bacteria. Feldman and Hinshaw were in the process of drafting another request to Waksman when the invitation from Rutgers arrived suggesting a cooperative study of what became streptomycin.

Schatz now had enough data for his PhD now, but such were the implications of his research he drove himself again - this time he was back in laboratory to produce larger quantities of more concentrated streptomycin principally for Feldman and Hinshaw's next stage of toxicity and animal experiments. He made two small stills in the basement laboratory, and these ran 24 hours a day for weeks. Schatz lived, ate, and slept in the laboratory often for days at a time. He put a mark in pen on the stills and had the building's night watchman wake him when the level of the liquid boiled down to the mark. Schatz got up and added more liquid – several times a night.

Doris Jones at Rutgers published the first results of streptomycin in experimental animals in 1944. This paper was rapidly followed by two more papers - Schatz's tests against the virulent TB strain supplied by Feldman, and startling results from Feldman and Hinshaw's work on guinea pigs inoculated with TB which was then eradicated following treatment with Schatz's streptomycin. This was a moment very similar to the early Oxford experiment with mice surviving an otherwise fatal infection when given penicillin.

Waksman and Feldman met with Merck and work commenced on industrial manufacturing capacity, studies in humans, and the granting of a patent for streptomycin. This is still the process required when new medicines are developed to this day. Feldman and Hinshaw's early clinical studies with patients reported hopeful results, but these were in small numbers of people with no direct, matched, contemporaneous, comparator group. Given streptomycin's activity against a wide range of gram-negative infections and that World War II still raging, some of the early supplies from Merck went to treat wounded servicemen with other gram-negative infections.

One of those was a young second lieutenant in the US Army's 10th Mountain Division who had been badly wounded in his back and upper by machine gun fire. Fighting in Italy's Appenine mountains, the young man had been transported to the Percy Jones Army Hospital in Battle Creek Michigan. His recovery was slow, interrupted by blood clots and a life-threatening infection. After large doses of penicillin had not succeeded, by chance some early supplies of streptomycin were around, and he overcame the infection. That young soldier was one Bob Dole, who despite lifelong disabilities due to his wounds, thanks to streptomycin lived to have a distinguished career as a US Senator and be beaten by Bill Clinton in the 1996 Presidential election.[xlviii]

The natural course of tuberculosis is so variable and unpredictable – anything from a spontaneous disappearance of the disease without treatment to a rapid decline and death - that evidence of improvement or cure following the use of a new drug in a few cases could not be accepted of proof of the effect of that drug. In contrast to other dramatic discoveries, adequately controlled clinical trials would be required. In 1946 the UK Medical Research Council decided that the limited supply of the very expensive streptomycin allocated to it for evaluation should be undertaken in a rigorously planned study with concurrent controls. They began to plan what is now recognized as the first modern, randomised, controlled trial.

A special committee of the MRC was set up, chaired by Geoffrey Marshall, a senior chest physician at the Brompton Hospital, London. Also recruited to the committee was the epidemiologist and statistician Austin Bradford Hill. Bradford Hill had been a pilot in the First World War but was invalided out due to tuberculosis. He spent two years in hospital and two more years convalescing, and because of his poor health at the time took an economics degree by correspondence at London university.

Known to everyone as "Tony", AB Hill had needed to use "A Bradford Hill" in his early academic publications to distinguish himself from the then much better-known AV Hill – a British physiologist who had won the Nobel prize for his work on muscle physiology in 1922. Bradford Hill was aware of the limitations of the alternate allocation method used by Fibinger and many others as the then-standard approach to randomisation. He had been involved in evaluating pneumonia trials which used the method in the 1930s. As a result he published articles in the *Lancet* advocating a more rigorous, true randomisation approach which were quickly republished as a textbook *Principles of Medical Statistics* in 1937. It rapidly became a classic statistical text. The true randomisation approach was tested by the British Medical Research Council, in an approach designed by Philip D'Arcy Hart to assess the effect of patulin on common cold symptoms.

80

By 1946 Hart was well placed as chair of the MRC's Tuberculosis Research Unit. Marc Daniels from the MRC's scientific staff had experience of small, multi-centre trials, and with a highly efficient trial manager called Charlotte Agnew, a very powerful team was assembled to assess streptomycin.[xlix][1]

The committee decided that there was a need to recruit patients from several tuberculosis units throughout the UK. Understandably, the limited streptomycin studies so far had involved patients with the most serious forms of the disease – miliary and meningitic (both previously almost uniformly fatal), and very advanced pulmonary tuberculosis (with a high but not uniform mortality). But most patients with TB had less severe pulmonary TB, and by 1946 it was well-recognised that some patients did spontaneously recover from pulmonary tuberculosis - even from very advanced pulmonary disease.

Given the uncertain prognosis of pulmonary tuberculosis and the limited supplies of streptomycin, Bradford Hill proposed that it would be unethical not to assess what advantage streptomycin offered in this form of the disease compared with the current standard treatment which was bed rest. This view was accepted.

Only patients aged between 15 and 30 with "acute progressive bilateral pulmonary tuberculosis of presumably recent origin, bacteriologically proved and unsuitable for collapse therapy" were to be included in the trial. "Collapse therapy" was an approach involving the intentional creation of a pneumothorax (collapsed lung) to "rest" the diseased organ. Both the streptomycin and control group received the standard treatment of bed rest. If streptomycin worked these patients would receive it later, when supplies improved. Meanwhile, they would of course avoid any unknown ill effects of the new drug.

When a potentially eligible patient was identified, the patient's details were sent to Marc Daniels at the MRC. If the patient did indeed met the eligibility criteria, admission was arranged to the next available hospital bed in the nearest participating centre. The trial coordinator in each centre was allotted a numbered series of envelopes, bearing only the name of the hospital. Each envelope contained a card indicating 'S(treptomycin)' or 'C(ontrol)'. The numerical order of the envelopes was based on a series of random numbers. When a patient was approved for the trial the next envelope for that centre was opened. Streptomycin and control patients were usually admitted to different wards but otherwise treated identically.

Neither group of patients knew that they were in a trial – that approach would rapidly disappear as the ethical standards for such trials became established. Quite quickly (and quite rightly) it became standard practice that only informed volunteers for trials would be recruited. Remarkably, the streptomycin trial remained confidential and known only to the researchers throughout its 15-month duration. Progress was assessed with monthly chest X-rays, graded by three specialists who remained ignorant of (blind to) the identities of the allocation of patients to streptomycin with bed rest or bed rest alone. Any difference of opinion between the assessors was resolved by discussion. Monthly direct smear and culture of sputum was also reported by bacteriologists who also remained blind to the treatment group.

The results were published in the British Medical Journal on 30th October 1948. During the first six months after joining the study, there were 4 deaths among 55 patients who had been allocated streptomycin, compared with 15 among 52 patients allocated to bed rest alone, and this difference was reflected in radiological and other improvements. But during the next six months, the radiological and mortality differences were less marked - there were 8 more deaths in the streptomycin group and 9 more in the groups treated with bed rest alone. Although surviving patients in the control group deteriorated faster than those in the streptomycin group, deterioration occurred in the streptomycin group as well, and this coincided with the development of streptomycin resistance in the bacilli, especially after the fourth month of treatment. Up to this time the development of resistance to antibiotics was thought to be more theoretical than a practical reality – though it was not unexpected because it had been predicted by Fleming more than a decade before.

Nevertheless, after 12 months treatment there were 12 deaths out of 55 people in the streptomycin group (22%) and 24 deaths out of 52 people in the control group (46%). It is of note that the authors of the paper wrote "The difference in mortality is statistically significant", and that is the only reference in the paper to any testing directed to determining whether their results could have occurred by chance. It seems that the development of the randomised controlled trial was driven much more by a realisation that alternate allocation had the potential to introduce bias, rather than the development being driven in some way by better or more appropriate statistical tests.[li]

As with the penicillin story, there is a twist in the streptomycin tale. Schatz had made another discovery - a tall, cheerful young woman called Vivian Rosenfeld who studied at the New Jersey College for Women. She didn't seem to mind that Schatz had no money; most of their dates took place walking in the university grounds after a long day in his basement laboratory. They married in March 1945; the groom took his actinomycetes cultures on honeymoon.

But then, as word of the discovery spread, reporters flocked to Rutgers to record the amazing event. The university public relations office was in overdrive, but in telling and retelling the story, Waksman slowly began to drop Schatz's name and claim sole credit. Schatz learned about the results of Feldman's work at the Mayo Clinic from magazines and newspapers, who got all their information from Waksman. This echoes Flemming, Florey and the media mismanagement of the penicillin story. One newspaper article after another eulogised Waksman, and Schatz grew resentful. After completing his PhD, Schatz decided to leave Rutgers, bitter and penniless. In 1946, at Waksman's request, he had signed over his royalty rights from the streptomycin patent to the Rutgers Research and Endowment Foundation, on the understanding that neither Waksman nor the foundation would profit from the discovery. He was later asked to sign over all his foreign patent rights, too, and agreed because, as with Florey and penicillin, he felt that streptomycin was so important it should be made as readily available, and therefore as inexpensively, as possible.

Three years later he discovered that Waksman, contrary to his personal and very public assurance, had a secret agreement with the foundation, giving him 20% of all streptomycin royalties. This amounted to $350,000 – a sum which would be equivalent to around $3.5million today. Waksman channelled much of that money back into the university, creating the research institute that bears his name.

But as far as Schatz was concerned, this was the last straw. In March 1950, going against the academic establishment norms, the young scientist with a social conscience decided to sue Waksman and the Rutgers foundation, demanding both his share of the royalties and recognition as streptomycin's co-discoverer.

For Waksman, the lawsuit came as a shocking and unexpected blow. He came from the old European school, which considered graduate students as apprentices lucky to be given an opportunity to work alongside a master. From Waksman's perspective, the discovery of streptomycin was a natural step in the long-term research programme he had designed and coordinated, and Schatz had simply been in the right place at the right time.

The publicity of the lawsuit was deeply embarrassing to Waksman and Rutgers. Preparatory legal work uncovered inconsistencies and untruths in Waksman's evidence, the Rutgers lawyers got cold feet, and within a year they settled out of court. On 30th December 1950 Schatz was legally entitled to scientific credit as co-discoverer of streptomycin, and he received a lump sum of $120,000 for the foreign patent rights (40% of which went to Schatz's lawyer) and 3% of the royalties, which amounted to about $15,000 annually for several years.

It was a victory – of sorts. The scientific community closed ranks against Schatz. He applied for work to more than 50 universities and research institutions but was only offered a position at a small private agricultural college in Pennsylvania. Schatz was told many times "*Of course, you were justified in suing Waksman, but one doesn't do that sort of thing in academia.*" [lii]

Then in October 1952 came the news that Waksman alone would be awarded the Nobel prize for the discovery of streptomycin despite the lawsuit firmly establishing Schatz as co-discoverer. The vice-president of the agricultural college where Schatz worked wrote to the Nobel prize committee asking its members to reconsider, sending them substantiating facts and documents. He also asked Nobel laureates and other scientists to intercede in Schatz's favour. Only a few did.

The Swedish Karolinska Institute tried to defuse the tension by declaring that Waksman had been awarded the prize for his "ingenious, systematic and successful studies of the soil microbes that led to the discovery of streptomycin", instead of "for the discovery of streptomycin", as had first been announced. In his acceptance speech, Waksman did not once mention Schatz, using the royal "we" instead. And there is no reference to Schatz in Waksman's 1958 memoir - he is named only as "the graduate student".

After being awarded the Nobel, Waksman went on to oversee the development of several other antibiotics, co-authored almost 500 scientific papers and wrote or edited some 28 books. He died in 1973 at the age of 85, widely regarded as one of the "fathers" of antibiotics. Schatz never again worked in a first-class microbiology lab and spent the rest of his working life in academic obscurity.

Schatz's contribution to the field of antibiotics might have gone unnoticed altogether if it hadn't been for an English microbiologist Milton Wainwright. Researching the history of streptomycin, he went to Rutgers to investigate the archives. He was puzzled by what he found - why hadn't he heard of Albert Schatz? And quickly he realised Schatz had been the victim of a grave injustice. Wainwright's findings raised difficult questions at

Rutgers, but finally the faculty did the right thing. They lobbied for Schatz's rehabilitation and on 28th. April 1994, exactly 50 years and 160 days since he had discovered streptomycin, Albert Schatz, then aged 74, was awarded the Rutgers medal - the university's highest accolade. It wasn't the Nobel prize, but Schatz finally felt he had justice.[liii]

But it is tuberculosis that has the last word in the story of streptomycin. It soon became apparent that streptomycin caused serious side-effects, amongst them vertigo, nausea, and deafness, and that bacterial resistance to the drug developed at an alarming rate. Fortunately two other antibiotics - para-aminosalicyclic acid (PAS) which was discovered in Sweden in the same year as streptomycin but had its development delayed by the war, and isoniazid developed simultaneously by no less than three research groups in 1952 - when combined with streptomycin helped tip the balance in favour of winning the battle in western industrialised countries. It was a slow process. I vividly remember visiting my Uncle Bill on bed rest in a TB sanatorium in the 1960s. But with the help of improved diet and living standards, pasteurization of milk and the BCG vaccine, one by one the sanitaria closed and the terror that the diagnosis of tuberculosis induced has faded from memory.

But it is still a different story in less-developed countries. The complicated three-drug regime was and is a challenge for individuals and especially for resource-poor health systems. Multi-drug resistant TB bacteria have emerged and may now account for more than half of all cases in some countries. The battle against both TB and against antibiotic resistance continues.

Back in the 1950s, whilst many focussed on what the results of the streptomycin trial meant for TB, others applied some thought to the implications of the method of evaluation – the randomised controlled trial (RCT). The trial made a deep impression on those involved, and supported by MRC funding, Bradford Hill and his colleagues continued their research community with a slowly growing research stream of other randomised trials. British investigators were soon followed by U.S. and other researchers who embraced RCTs as urgently needed tools for separating the wheat from the chaff emanating from an ever-diversifying pharmaceutical industry.

As economies around the world recovered after the Second World War, the combination of a rapidly expanding, multi-faceted, well-funded, scientifically-based pharmaceutical industry meant that medicine could potentially treat many more diseases much more effectively than had hither-to been possible. The scientific revolution had eventually led to a medical revolution, but that revolution needed a revolution in the evaluation of the science. As an editorialist in the *New England Journal* wrote in 1956, "*Physicians should be particularly careful in accepting drugs purely on the basis of the manufacturer's evidence or on the basis of testimonials provided to the manufacturer. They should demand clear, unbiased, well studied and adequately controlled evidence produced and interpreted by reliable observers.*" [liv]

RCTs were simply the most recent development in a long history of attempts to adjudicate whether something really worked - thinking which had its roots in Aristotle, al-Razi and empiricism. RCT proponents increasingly won over detractors and were soon supported by crucial public funding and scientific regulatory infrastructures. RCTs became the expected study design for new medicines not only because they offered more sophisticated methods, but also because they served the critical social function of screening experimental therapies before they were broadly distributed. They clarified the actual effects and provided some safety data about new medicines, but despite being more widely used, randomised trials were not mandatory.

Tragically, that a more systematised approach was required, especially for safety, soon became all too obvious.

CHAPTER SIX

Thalidomide

The remarkable successes of, for example, insulin, penicillin, and triple-therapy for tuberculosis were accompanied by a boom in the basic scientific understanding of physiology, biochemistry and immunology. This meant that medicine was now in a new place. Abraham Flexner's scientific curriculum had no challengers, pharmaceutical companies had rapidly emerged as new, separate entities from their chemical company predecessors, and a different type of approach to developing new medicines began to be widely employed.

Developments in organic chemistry meant scientists were now beginning to be able to make small changes in the composition of active molecules by design. Both PAS and isoniazid were early examples of this approach. Teams of chemists could tweak the structure of an old molecule to produce a new potential medicine, and then test it with a scatter-gun approach using a range of healthy-tissue and diseased-related laboratory tests hoping to find that the potential new medicine would work to mitigate the effects of an often newly-discovered disordered physiological, biochemical or immunological mechanism causing a disease for which there was currently limited or no effective treatment.

Such was the ability of the chemists that large numbers of new molecules could be produced in a short period. Individuals working alone or with small teams to develop a new medicine following new intellectual insights on an idiosyncratic basis were being largely replaced by industrial scale, systematised innovation.

However, by the 1950s the regulation of medicines had not caught up with the industrialisation of medicines development and production. In the UK, the first modern attempt to create a process which would ensure efficacy and safety of medicines began before the First World War.

In 1909 in Frankfurt, Paul Erlich - working with Sahachiro Hata - had used a scatter-gun approach on hundreds of newly synthesised organic compounds. They discovered that one of the compounds – subsequently given the name Salvarsan – was toxic to the bacteria Treponema Pallidum which causes syphilis.[lv] [lvi] Salvarsan was rapidly manufactured in sufficient quantities by the company Hoechst AG and released onto the market in 1910. It was distributed as a crystalline powder which was highly unstable in air, so that it had to be stored in sealed vials in a nitrogen atmosphere to avoid oxidation. Before administration to a patient, the powder had to be dissolved in several hundred millilitres of sterile water with minimal exposure to the air.

When the First World War began, British manufacturing of Salvarsan began, and it was realised that toxic impurities were a problem - and that these could only be detected by biological testing. Potent biological substances, including the development of immunisation, had created new challenges. Ensuring proper quality control of such substances and the competence of the researchers and manufacturers were new problems.

As a result, in 1925 the UK Therapeutic Substances Act came into force. It created the modern framework of medicines safety, but it was limited both in scope and in its application.[lvii] There was in effect minimal obligation on drugs manufacturers - they could market almost any product, however inadequately tested, without having to satisfy any independent body as to its efficacy and safety. Crucially, although it had been known for some time that drugs taken in pregnancy could harm the unborn foetus in mammals, the medical world in general had paid little attention to this danger. At this time, it was assumed that the human placenta was impervious to any drugs the expectant mother ingested unless the was fatal to the mother. Drug companies did not routinely test new medicines for hazardous effects on the unborn baby. General warnings about avoiding the use of medicines in pregnancy whenever possible were circulated, but these were largely ignored.

In the US, at the beginning of the 20th Century the medicines market was dominated by a proliferating problem of patent medicines, many of which made unfounded claims for treating cancer, tuberculosis, and syphilis as well as a host of other illnesses - both serious and largely self-limiting. Several States began to hire their own chemists to certify the quality and purity of food and drugs sold. But there was little standardisation, and the laws usually punished retailers, leaving manufacturers untouched. Companies wielded substantial influence and it was only after investigative journalists exposed several fraudulent operations that momentum was established which resulted in the 1906 US Pure Food and Drugs Act.[lviii]

Important though it was, the 1906 Act had several shortcomings including the lack of factory inspections and no prior approval being required before the marketing of a medicine. There were disasters waiting to happen. In 1937 the S.E. Massengill Company in Bristol, Tennessee developed a liquid preparation of the first "wonder drug" sulfonamide, first developed by Gerhard Domagk and used to fight streptococcal infections. Sulfonamide was not patented, and many unregulated manufacturers had begun to produce it. The product was not tested in animals or humans prior to marketing. The solvent used to suspend the active drug, diethylene glycol, was poisonous to humans but this was not known to Harold Watkins, the company's chief chemist and pharmacist.

The company started selling its product in September 1937 and within a month the American Medical Association was receiving reports of deaths associated with its use. By the time the medicine had been removed from shelves and medicine cabinets around the country, 107 people had died including many children. President Roosevelt signed the Food, Drug and Cosmetic Act into law on 25th June 1938. It required that manufacturers had to prove to the Food and Drug Administration (FDA) that any new drug was safe before it could be marketed, authorised factory inspections, outlawed bogus therapeutic claims for drugs, and drugs had to bear adequate directions for safe use. A separate law brought drug advertising under the Federal Trade Commission's jurisdiction.[lix]

The Food, Drug and Cosmetic Act did not specify the kinds of tests that were required for approval but did allow FDA officials to block the marketing of a new drug or delay it by requiring additional data. The act also gave regulators limited powers of negotiation over scientific study and approval requirements with the pharmaceutical industry and the medical profession. After the Second World War, Bradford Hill at the UK Medical Research Council, and North American colleagues - including Harry Gold at the Cornell Medical School - began to map out general criteria for drug testing and specify stages through which drug development should proceed. As in the UK streptomycin trial, patients were to be selected through formal criteria and then randomly allocated into treatment and control groups. Trials were to be double blinded so that neither the patient nor their clinician and trial assessor knew whether they were receiving control or experimental treatment. Trials were required to use objective diagnostic technologies, drug doses were to be administered according to a fixed schedule, and patient observations were to be charted at uniform intervals.

Beginning in 1958, US Senate hearings chaired by Senator Estes Kefauver assessed progress with assuring quality medicines.[lx] He and his staff had obtained evidence documenting the high mark-ups and exorbitant profit margins that had become evident on prescription drugs, beginning with antibiotics. As popular with consumers as they proved unpopular with the pharmaceutical industry, these hearings generated important evidence documenting the frequently sorry state of drug testing and advertising, as well as the competitive pressures within the industry which supported such practices. Testimony was offered documenting many poor clinical studies done in support of the marketing of many mediocre drugs. Most new drug products, experts testified, were not improvements over old ones, and most were marketed before clinical studies were published. Many new drugs were combinations of older medicines, with or without modification, which gained extended patent life (and profitability) in combination. Adequately controlled comparisons of drugs were "almost impossible to find". In many circumstances, a physician from the company would go out in the community with some samples and say to a doctor, "I've got this new drug for so-and-so. Here's some samples. Try it out and let us know how you like it." And they would get back a letter from

him: "I tried it out on eight patients, and they all got along fine."
All this was about as far away from Bradford Hill's scientifically
robust approaches as could be imagined. A tragedy in the UK
and many other countries awaited. And yet in the United States,
it was largely avoided, thanks almost entirely to one woman.

Frances Kathleen Oldham was born a Canadian – in
Shawnigan Lake, British Columbia on 24th July 1914.[lxi] She
studied pharmacology at McGill University, obtaining a master's
degree in 1935. Encouraged by one of her professors, she wrote
to EMK Geiling, a well-known pharmacology researcher, to say
she was looking for a position where she could work and study for
her doctorate. Geiling, who had just been appointed as the first
professor at the newly established Department of Pharmacology
at the University of Chicago, presumed that Frances was a man
and offered her a position - which she accepted, starting in 1936.

Geiling was recruited to work on the sulfanilamide -
diethylene glycol catastrophe with Oldham as a junior assistant
in her second year. In 1938 Oldham received her PhD and joined
the University of Chicago faculty. Her post-doctorate work
focused on finding an effective treatment for malaria, and she
worked on drugs passing through the placental barrier to the
foetus. She also met Dr Freemont Kelsey and they were married
in 1943.

The new Dr Frances Kelsey graduated as a doctor from the
University of Chicago in 1950 and became a dual US-Canadian
citizen to continue to practice medicine in the US. In 1960 she
was hired by the FDA in Washington DC. At the time she was
one of only seven full time and four part time physicians
reviewing medicines.

Seven years earlier, in 1953 in the German pharmaceutical
company Chemie Grünenthal, pharmacologist Herbert Keller
recognised a newly synthesised chemical as an analogue of
glutethimide, a known sedative. In a post-war era when anxiety
and sleeplessness were prevalent, the medicinal chemistry work

93

quickly turned to improving the initial compound and creating a suitable drug. The resulting drug was called thalidomide.

The demand for sedatives was high in both Europe and the US, and the presumed safety of thalidomide, the only non-barbiturate sedative available at the time, gave the drug massive appeal. Barbiturates had many problems. People became tolerant to them and so needed larger doses. Those larger does risked suppression of breathing and accidental fatal overdoses were reported, especially if the barbiturate was mixed with alcohol. Researchers also found that thalidomide was a particularly effective treatment for morning sickness in pregnancy. In Germany it was first sold without prescription in pharmacies from October 1957, and in the UK it was licensed and marketed for insomnia and morning sickness in 1958.

Meanwhile in Washington, one of Frances Kelsey's first assignments was to review an application by the pharmaceutical company Richardson Merrell for thalidomide. Even though it had already been approved in the UK, Canada, and more than 20 other countries Kelsey refused approval and requested further studies. From 1960 there were some reports of patients developing peripheral neuritis[lxii], and despite pressure from Richardson Merrell, Kelsey - who by now was an experienced pharmacologist and physician - held firm.

In April 1961, Australian obstetrician William McBride noticed cases of a rare birth defect involving shortened or absent limbs in babies whose mothers had used thalidomide in pregnancy. His letter reporting his observations and asking if others had seen similar cases appeared in the Lancet and was just five sentences long. At about the same time, paediatrician Widukind Lenz noted many similar cases in Germany. No cases had been reported in the ten years between 1949 and 1959 in West Germany, but there were 477 cases in 1961 alone.

Thanks to Frances Kelsey the impact of thalidomide was greatly minimized in the US. The Washington Post made it a front page story with Kelsey as the star. She was given the

Presidents' Award for Distinguished Federal Civilian Service by President Kennedy in the White House in 1962. Kelsey publicly insisted that her assistants, Oyam Jiro and Lee Geismar, and the FDA management who had backed her strong stance, deserved credit as well. Although thalidomide was never approved for sale in the United States, over 2.5 million tablets had been distributed by the manufacturer to over 1,000 physicians during a "clinical testing program". It is estimated that nearly 20,000 patients, several hundred of whom were pregnant women, were given the drug to help alleviate morning sickness or as a sedative, and at least 17 children were consequently born in America with thalidomide-associated deformities.

Worldwide, the thalidomide scandal revolutionised the regulation of medicines. In the UK a Committee on Safety of Drugs (CSD) was established as a temporary measure until legislation could be enacted. This was an entirely voluntary arrangement under the chairmanship of Sir Derrick Dunlop and was official only in the sense that the Health Ministers provided the finance to run the committee. Despite the complete absence of legal sanctions, the pharmaceutical industry promised that their members would not perform a clinical trial or market a new drug against the advice of the Committee. The Committee advised solely on safety aspects and did not consider efficacy.

The CSD had three main functions: to scrutinise new drugs before clinical trials, before marketing, and then the surveillance of each drug after marketing so that adverse reactions not picked up in testing before licensing and marketing could be monitored, documented and, if necessary, warnings issued.

It was recognised that relatively small numbers of patients were required to be involved in randomised controlled trials to prove that a medicine worked. It was unusual for there to be more than 1500 patients in such trials, and most were much smaller. From a "does it work?" perspective this meant a smaller number of people only getting control treatment – a big ethical advantage if the experimental group received something which increased the probability of a good outcome. If the trial was larger and the new medicine turned out to work well, a larger control group meant more people not getting what turned out the be the better treatment. In addition, because a large trial would almost certainly take longer to complete, analyse and report that meant it cost more to run, and a longer period of time passing before patients could get prescriptions for the newly licensed medicine. It also meant a delay for the pharmaceutical company beginning to receive the financial benefits of their work.

Whilst some safety data would of course be collected and analysed in the randomised trials, a serious side effect occurring once in 10,000 patients might justify removal of the medicine from use. The maths was simple. A trial programme involving only 1500 participants or less would potentially not be big enough to detect a rare but serious side effect. The norm in the UK became established - trials to largely prove efficacy and provide initial safety data, and post-marketing surveillance for enhanced safety.

The Committee itself did not undertake testing of drugs but evaluated the manufacturers' submissions and other available evidence. In 1968 the Medicines Act became law, providing a licensing system for the marketing, manufacture, import, distribution, and clinical testing of medicinal products for human and veterinary use. The licensing authority was required to consider the safety, efficacy, and quality of medicinal products.

In the US, thalidomide resurrected Kefauver's bill to enhance drug regulation that had stalled in Congress, and the Kefauver-Harris Amendments became law on 10th October 1962. Manufacturers henceforth had to prove to FDA that their drugs were effective as well as safe before they could go on the market. Control over clinical investigations was placed on a firm statutory basis. The FDA received authority to regulate advertising of prescription drugs, establish good manufacturing practices to promote quality assurance, and access certain company control and production records to verify production procedures. The law required that all drugs introduced between 1938 and 1962 had to be effective. An FDA National Academy of Sciences collaborative study showed that nearly 40 percent of these products were not.

All this meant that almost overnight and around the world, the Bradford Hill vision was enacted. Each new medicine required several phases of study before it could be marketed by its manufacturer – first in animals, then in a small number of healthy volunteers, and finally in patients. At last, scientific method in the form of the randomised controlled clinical trial had made it to prime time. And the availability of lots more randomised trials was itself to have wider consequences for the practice of medicine.

Meanwhile Frances Kathleen Oldham Kelsey continued to work at the FDA, evaluating new medicines. In 1995 at the age of 81 she was appointed deputy for scientific and medical affairs. Aged 87 she was inducted into the US National Women's Hall of fame, and she retired at the age of 90. Just after her hundredth birthday, in the autumn of 2014, she moved from Washington DC to live with her daughter in London, Ontario. Kelsey died there the following summer at the age of 101, less than 24 hours after Ontario's Lieutenant-Governor visited her home to present her with the insignia of Member of the Order of Canada for her role in reducing the toll of the thalidomide tragedy.

CHAPTER SEVEN

Effectiveness, Efficiency And Evidence

98

In 1909 in Galashiels, Scotland, Archie Cochrane was born. His father was a successful tweed maker who was killed in the first World War, when Archie was only eight years old. Then his youngest brother Walter died at the age of two due to tuberculous pneumonia, while another brother, Robert, died after a motorcycle accident at the age of 21. It was no wonder that he treasured his sister, Helen.[lxiii] [lxiv] [lxv]

The young Archie was offered a scholarship for Uppingham School in Rutland, England. Here he excelled, both academically and at a range of sports. In 1927, he gained a second scholarship, this time to King's College in Cambridge where he read Natural Sciences and graduated with a First.

A small inheritance enabled him to stay on at Cambridge doing postgraduate tissue culture research in Cambridge for about a year, but he soon became restless. He had become concerned about his sexual development. He received little help from the British doctors he consulted but found that doctors at the Kaiser Wilhelm Institute in Berlin were willing to consider his problem. Between 1931 and 1934 he underwent psychoanalysis with Freud's leading lay analyst, Theodor Reik, initially in Berlin, but then in Vienna and the Hague as Reik fled from Hitler. In those three, formative years in Europe Archie became fluent in several languages including German, developed a hatred of fascism, and adopted a sceptical attitude towards all theories which had not been tested in scientific experiments, including psychoanalysis.

He was right to be sceptical. It was years later that the possible cause of Archie's symptoms was discovered. Archie's beloved sister Helen had been admitted to a psychiatric hospital with a diagnosis of dementia. Typically, Archie challenged it. Further investigation led to the discovery that she - and Archie - both had chronic porphyria, an inherited disease. Because he was concerned that other members of the family scattered around the world might unknowingly have the condition, he requested urinary and faecal samples from 153 relatives and received specimens from 152 of them. Completeness of data collection was a feature of Archie's approach.

After returning to Britain from Germany in 1934, Archie enrolled as a medical student at University College Hospital, London. He abandoned his studies two years later to serve as a volunteer during the Spanish Civil War in a Field Ambulance Unit. He resumed his medical studies in 1937 and qualified as a doctor in 1938. At the start of the second World War, he quickly became a captain in the Royal Army Medical Corps, serving first in Egypt as a hospital medical officer, then as a medical officer in a commando unit. He saw action when the German forces invaded Crete – a battle which ended disastrously for the British forces, and he became a Prisoner of War. He said later that the reason he was captured was because "he found himself unable to swim to Egypt" - over 1000 kilometres. From 1941 until the end of the war he was as a prisoner of war a medical officer in Salonica, and then later in several camps in Germany.

His ability to speak German was of course a huge advantage. But one remarkable act amongst, no doubt, many was that he carried out what he described as his "first, worst, and most successful" clinical trial. And of course, controlled trials were far from the normal approach in those days - the MRC streptomycin trial took place after the war ended - and Archie had only practiced as a doctor for a few months before the war started. Just knowing how and why to undertake a controlled trial at that time is an indication that Archie Cochrane, even at such an early stage of his career, was a remarkable man.

What led him to conduct the trial was the high incidence of severe leg oedema of unknown origin in his fellow prisoners. Cochrane himself, developed oedema to above the knee. His theory was that the underlying cause was vitamin deficiency resulting in "wet beri-beri"; the prisoners were eating a very limited diet of 400–500 calories per day. He expressed his concerns to the Germans who initially refused to help in any way. To test his hypothesis, he bought yeast and vitamin C supplements from the black market in the camp, selected a

100

sample of 20 prisoners, and divided them into two groups of 10. The subjects in the first group received daily portions of yeast, while those in the other group were given vitamin C supplements.

After 4 days, Cochrane found that the prisoners in the yeast-eating group had improved; the ankle oedema had subsided, and the subjects felt better. There was no change in the health of prisoners in the other group. He carefully wrote down the results of this primitive clinical trial - which almost certainly had too few subjects for the results to be truly considered to be a meaningful, as well as a dubious approach to both recruitment and randomisation - and presented them to the Germans. Fortunately, his German guards knew little to nothing about the design intricacies of randomised controlled trials. As a result, the camp prisoners were then provided with yeast. Cases of wet beri-beri among the general population of prisoners in the camp subsequently dropped dramatically.

Cochrane himself knew this trial to be of poor quality. Ten patients in two groups meant any results were very open to the play of chance distorting the results - an element of luck was a great contributor to its success.[lxvi] But after the end of the war Cochrane continued with postgraduate studies at the London School of Hygiene and Tropical Medicine, where one of his teachers was Austin Bradford Hill. Bradford Hill's teaching on randomised controlled trials and epidemiology mesmerized Cochrane, who acknowledged Hill's influence on him for the rest of his life.

In 1947 Cochrane won a third scholarship - this time a Rockefeller Scholarship in which enabled him to spend some time at the Henry Phipps Clinic in Philadelphia. There Cochrane reviewed the reporting of chest X-rays by doctors when diagnosing and estimating the prognosis of pulmonary tuberculosis. He found observer errors - differences in interpretation of the same X-ray between different doctors.[lxvii] And if doctors are asked to report on a stack of X-rays twice, with the X-rays shuffled into a different order before the second reading, in a minority of cases the doctors report on the same X-ray differently – in effect disagreeing with themselves.

His scepticism about the lack of scientific evidence substantiating some medical interventions grew and made him question even those treatments that were well established and widely accepted. The requirement for experimental evidence and a general approach requiring "proof" begun by Bacon, Galileo and Descartes was not yet being played everywhere by everybody at a high volume in medicine - but it was for Archie Cochrane.

Returning from America, in 1948 Cochrane was recruited by Charles Fletcher who, having played his part in the penicillin story, had been appointed Director of the Medical Research Council's Pneumoconiosis Research Unit in South Wales. Cochrane began with studies of dust levels in the many coal mines in the area, and two years later he launched a study to investigate the causes of progressive massive pulmonary fibrosis. His interest in this field continued for the rest of his life, and he completed 20- and 30-year follow-up studies of the population of the Rhondda Fach. He recruited a team of disabled miners to help maximise survey follow-up rates. This was an unusual approach, but Archie's miner assistants - despite their lack for prior training in research methodology - drew in their colleagues and helped to overcome resistance to taking part in the research.

Such was the quality of his research, in 1960 Archie became Professor of Tuberculosis and Chest Diseases at the Welsh National School of Medicine, and the Medical Research Council invited him to establish and direct a new epidemiology unit there. Under Cochrane's direction, the MRC Epidemiology Unit quickly established an international reputation for the quality of its surveys and studies of the natural history and aetiology of a wide range of common diseases, including anaemia, glaucoma, asthma, and gallbladder disease. This work, its quality, and his natural scepticism then led to an interest in the validation of screening strategies within the National Health Service.

Although the quality of his epidemiological studies set new standards for the specialty, they were observational studies - they described the natural history of conditions or explored the causes of disease. His scepticism about medical interventions meant he would return to randomised controlled trials, and the MRC Epidemiology Unit provided him with the opportunity to put that into practice. His unit coordinated an increasing number of randomised trials; many of those now viewed as most important were led by Archie's colleague Peter Elwood, who succeeded him as director in 1974. These studies included the first to establish that aspirin could reduce the incidence of cardiovascular diseases.

Throughout the 1960s there were quietly voiced concerns about both the lack of evidence from trials about effectiveness, and about the over- and under-implementation of medical treatments. All this was, of course, in the context of a post-war explosion in technical interventions. There were lots of new medicines being developed by the expanding pharmaceutical industry, but also new surgical techniques, and ever more complex surgical and diagnostic equipment. The costs of health care were becoming a live issue - more treatments becoming available led to increased demand for those treatments by both doctors and their patients. An invitation from the Nuffield Provincial Hospitals Trusts to prepare the 1971 Rock Carling Lecture provided Archie with an opportunity to develop these themes - and the book based on his lecture *Effectiveness and Efficiency: Random Reflections on Health Services* - promptly became a classic and a best seller.

This little book covered not only the lack of evidence for the effectiveness of many treatments - making the case for more randomised controlled trials - but also the inefficiencies in the ways treatments were used. Evidence of inefficiencies, including variation in the use of health care resources, was emerging - for example the length of time patients spent in hospital after an illness or treatment was inexplicably very different in different parts of the country. Way ahead of its time was a discussion about assessing the costs of the options available when deciding what medicines to make available within the British National Health

103

Service. Cochrane believed that decisions should be made on the basis of a cost: benefit analysis.

And Archie Cochrane was not a lone voice. Just as Archie Cochrane published *Effectiveness and Efficiency*, a young health researcher called Iain Chalmers arrived to work in Cardiff. Chalmers had qualified as a doctor in the mid-1960s and began to work in obstetrics. He recalls being woken in the middle of the night to attend to a young woman who had gone into premature labour. Premature labour is an obstetric emergency - being born well before the normal length of a pregnancy of 40 weeks carries significant risk of harm to the baby. Like many young doctors in most specialties, Chalmers had learnt that the first question to ask was "Who is this patient's consultant?" - because very often treatment of the same condition was determined by the preferences of the individual specialist and not by the evidence of what worked.

Before arriving at Cardiff, Chalmers worked for a few years in a United Nations Camp in the Gaza. Much of his undergraduate course he felt had consisted of a huge volume of so-called scientific facts which he was required to remember and regurgitate in examinations. In Gaza his discomfiture increased as he discovered that some things he had been told as absolute truths by his professors and committed to memory were in fact quite wrong. Further, he found that evidence had already been published demonstrating that what he had been told was wrong, but it was not easily available to him. When he arrived in Cardiff and met Archie Cochrane it was if he had found a way forward - and he set about constructing a repository of the evidence of effective care in pregnancy and childbirth.

And it was not just Cochrane and Chalmers who were sceptics. A few years earlier a young doctor called David Sackett was invited by John Evans, a cardiologist and the founding dean of McMaster University Medical School in Ontario, to join a new and different kind of medical school. Evans had been appointed at the age of 35; Sackett was just 32 years old. Years later Sackett recalled his own conversion to what became evidence-based medicine - as opposed to expert-based medicine.[lxviii] His story vividly describes the change in thinking common to Cochrane, Chalmers, and Sackett.

In 1959 Sackett was at the end of his undergraduate studies and a teenager with infectious hepatitis (now called Hepatitis A) was admitted. "He had the classical constellation of symptoms and clinical signs - severe malaise, an enlarged and tender liver, and a colorful demonstration of deranged bilirubin metabolism including significant clinical jaundice. However, after a few days of total bed rest his spirits and energy returned and he asked me to let him get up and around.

"In the 1950s, everybody "knew" that such patients, if they were to avoid permanent liver damage, must be kept on bed rest until their enlarged liver receded and their bilirubin and enzymes returned to normal. And if, after getting up and around, their enzymes rose again, back to bed they went. This conventional wisdom formed the basis for daily confrontations between an increasingly restless and resentful patient and an increasingly adamant and doom-predicting clinician."

Sackett wanted to understand how letting the patient out of bed would exacerbate his disease. After exhausting several unhelpful texts, he found a citation in the *Journal of Clinical Investigation* for *"The treatment of acute infectious hepatitis. Controlled studies of the effects of diet, rest, and physical reconditioning on the acute course of the disease and on the incidence of relapses and residual abnormalities."*[lxix]

The paper's lead author was Tom Chalmers (no relation to Iain), who was an avid fan of randomised controlled trials and influenced many people as evidence-based medicine took shape. Tom had been a US Army gastroenterologist in the Korean War and had become involved in a major outbreak of infectious hepatitis among American recruits. The application of conventional wisdom on enforced bed rest was keeping affected soldiers in hospital for about two months and requiring another month's convalescence. Tom wrote *"This drain on military manpower, along with more recent [short-term metabolic] observations suggesting that strict bed rest might not be as essential as heretofore thought, emphasized the need for a controlled study to determine the safety of a more liberal regimen of rest and less prolonged hospitalization."*

In order to answer this question, Tom and his colleagues allocated soldiers who met pre-defined hepatitis criteria at random either to bed rest (continuously in bed, save for one trip daily to the bathroom and one trip to the shower weekly), or to be up and about as much as the patients wanted (with no effort made to control their activity save 1-hour rests after meals) throughout their hospital stay. The time to recovery (as judged by liver function testing) was indistinguishable between the comparison groups, and no recurrent jaundice was observed.

Armed with this evidence, Sackett convinced his supervisors to let the patient be up and about as much as he wished, and his clinical recovery was uneventful. The case made a big impression on Sackett.

After initial training in internal medicine and nephrology, Sackett's career was shaped by the 1962 Cuban missile crisis. Suddenly he was conscripted into the US Public Health Service and was posted to learn epidemiology at Buffalo. Continuing with some medicine at the bedside, he became interested in whether the application of some of the methods used in classical epidemiology (which was Cochrane's early work in Cardiff) would help with more accurate diagnosis in individual patients – an approach called clinical epidemiology. Sackett spent a year at Harvard studying a wide variety of public health methodological courses, including an elective course in designing clinical epidemiology courses for health professionals. He had only been back at Buffalo a short time working on how to teach clinical epidemiology when he got the letter from John Evans 70 miles across the border in Canada.

Sackett's radical ideas matched those of Evans, who planned to teach undergraduate medicine using a "problem-based learning" approach. Students would learn from the problems of patients as opposed the orthodoxy of learning basic science subjects for the first two years, and then attempting to apply that to patients. Epidemiology and statistics would be taught completely integrated with the clinical disciplines.

No longer was the mainstay of undergraduate teaching in medicine a formal lecture or bedside teaching from an expert, with the students expected to learn the stated facts and emulate the recommended treatment without questioning it. The Flexner "scientific" model using laboratory data and theoretical mechanisms of action to determine real patient care had not been abandoned, but the approach to teaching and learning the science underpinning medicine had been radically modified.

The students, working in small groups, would be faced with a clinical problem and would themselves identify what they needed to know, and then spend time finding as much of that as possible themselves. In order to do that they needed to explore themselves the basic sciences, how the body works (anatomy, physiology and biochemistry) and how it goes wrong, and then - especially when having to work out what were the treatment options that might work - they would have to explore the published evidence which described what really did work (or not) in real patients, preferably with evidence from randomised controlled trials.

Such problem-based learning was no less rigorous for the students than a traditional curriculum - a cycle of a single problem dominating learning and teaching each week would be followed by a different problem the next week, and the next, and the next, and so on throughout the year. Students worked together, learning from each other, and their teachers were facilitators and coaches rather than experts placed on an academic pedestal and beyond questioning.

After a decade of the McMaster programme, Sackett and his colleagues decided that they wanted to share what they were teaching and wrote a series of articles about what they then called "critical appraisal". The first article appeared in the *Canadian*

107

Medical Association Journal in 1981.[lxx] The first paragraph is worthy of reproducing here:-

"This series of Clinical Epidemiology Rounds has been prepared for those clinicians who are behind in their clinical reading. As nearly as we can tell from several informal polls, this includes all of us. And well it should. To keep up with the 10 leading journals in internal medicine a clinician must read 200 articles and 70 editorials per month. There are now over 20000 different biomedical journals published (up from 14000 10 years ago); to "read up" on viral hepatitis requires selection from among 16000 citations published on this topic in English alone in the last 10 years."

In 1971 Archie Cochrane was concerned about how little research there was about what was truly an effective treatment and what was not. Move forward a decade to the Sackett paper from 1981 and it was a completely different problem. Medical developments were coming on stream at pace and in in large numbers. These were a product of the pace of the post-war scientific explosion. And whilst there were still lots of gaps in the evidence, evidence was now increasingly in the form of randomised controlled trials.

In 1959, the year that the hepatitis study by Tom Chalmers and his colleagues was published, there were only 347 reports of randomised trials. Half a century later, about 50,000 reports of randomised trials were being published every year, with the total number of trial reports by then exceeding half a million. Even by 1981 the problems had become finding the evidence and managing information overload, determining what amongst the published research was high quality and what was not, and incorporating the best evidence into it into clinical practice quickly and everywhere - and in doing so reducing unwarranted variation in care provided.

Sackett and colleagues called their approach "critical thinking" – and immediately ran into problems with established clinicians who took offence at the implication that their current approach to diagnosis and treatment did not involve thinking critically. It wasn't a "Game of Thrones" episode or even a

Catholic Inquisition in Rome, but it was a pretty sharp response from the medical establishment. The name quickly got changed to "critical appraisal", reflecting one of their initial developments which were checklists to sift high quality research - which should inform patient care - from poor quality, unreliable data, which should not.

The innovative approach at McMaster attracted like-minded people, eager to press on with adding more science to the art of practicing medicine. Many of them had a moment in their education when they realised that eminence had to give way to evidence. Brian Haynes was a timid second-year medical student and remembers attending a psychiatry lecture on Freud. At the end of the lecture, he asked whether there was any evidence that Freud's theories were true. The lecturer admitted there was no evidence, and that he himself did not believe in Freud's ideas, but the head of the department did, and it was he who had asked the lecturer to deliver the session. Haynes, now a quiet, diligent, highly intelligent, and still active researcher and teacher with a wicked and very dry sense of humour, worked his way around several Canadian universities asking difficult questions until he found his natural home at McMaster.

Gordon Guyatt arrived at McMaster as a general physician and became fascinated by the work of Sackett and Haynes. Guyatt was to go on and write more than 1,300 scientific papers and is now 14th in Google Scholar's all-time list of researchers whose work has been cited by other researchers. Haynes and Archie Cochrane no doubt both look at that list quizzically; the top position is occupied by Sigmund Freud.[lxxi]

Together McMaster had a formidable team. With rheumatologist Peter Tugwell, Sackett, Haynes and Guyatt developed their thinking and published their classic textbook *Clinical Epidemiology: A basic science for clinical medicine*. By the time of the second edition was published in 1991 they had devised new ways of looking at diagnosis, prognosis, and treatments. They outlined using numbers and sums to interpret research-derived data to produce probabilities of, for example, having or not having a certain disease, or the chances of an individual patient benefiting from a treatment. They also continued to work away at the thorny problem of how to efficiently find evidence and identify the best of evidence.

Guyatt oversaw specialist postgraduate training in medicine at McMaster. Sackett had started taking critical appraisal to the patient's bedside, seeking to find the best evidence for an individual in real time, and Guyatt rightly assessed that their training programme was groundbreaking. Initially he called the approach "Scientific Medicine" – and that term also evoked howls of protest from established clinicians who professed to having "been scientists all along, thank you very much, Dr. Guyatt". His second attempt at an all-encompassing term was "evidence-based medicine", and that stuck. With 30 other authors, on 4th November 1992 Guyatt published a paper in the Journal of the American Medical Association.[lxxii] Its title was "Evidence-Based Medicine: A New Approach to Teaching the Practice of Medicine", and it began:-

"A new paradigm for medical practice is emerging. Evidence-based medicine de-emphasizes intuition, unsystematic clinical experience, and pathophysiologic rationale as sufficient grounds for clinical decision making and stresses the examination of evidence from clinical research. Evidence-based medicine requires new skills of the physician, including efficient literature searching and the application of formal rules of evidence evaluating the clinical literature".

Francis Bacon, Galileo Galilei and Rene Descartes would have approved. By the end of the 1980s, scientific developments had led to medical innovations of the kind that would have been difficult to imagine when David Florey and his team at Oxford were developing the first batches of penicillin some 40 years earlier. And the evaluation of those treatments had changed out of all recognition too. This was in part driven by Bradford Hill's and Archie Cochrane's devotion to the randomised trial, but also by the realisation that proof that something worked and was safe was obligatory - the thalidomide tragedy had been a real watershed too.

110

CHAPTER EIGHT

Numbers And Sums

As the scientific and medical revolutions progressed, understanding numbers – not just having the numbers - started to become part of the requirement. For example, in the paper describing the results of 1948 streptomycin trial there were 4 deaths among 55 patients who had been allocated streptomycin, compared with 15 among 52 patients allocated to bed rest alone. Just looking at those numbers without any further work being done on them, it looks obvious that streptomycin was better than not having streptomycin. But how could we best express "how much better", and could that result have occurred due to a play of chance? If that seems unlikely and the benefit is likely to be a true one, let us remember that only the probability of a good outcome is only improved by treatment. Lots of people – 37 out of 52 –survived without streptomycin; with treatment death was less likely but survival was not guaranteed. And in a worst-case scenario, it would be perfectly possible for an individual to get no benefit from streptomycin, but suffer a serious side effect such as permanent deafness.

Ideally, treatment of patients in the real world outside of randomised trials would involve a fortune teller - someone able to reliably predict the future – except there is no such thing as a real fortune teller. If there was, it would be possible to identify those individuals who would recover naturally without any medical treatment, and those who would definitely benefit from a treatment. But that is, of course, a pipe dream.

Two separate, but linked, approaches developed in order to make better sense of uncertainty and probability. Statistics and probability are words that most human beings intuitively shy away from. Even working with any numbers is tricky for many human beings. There is anthropological work on several continents showing some groups of people in remote areas do not have an extensive numerical vocabulary. Whilst it is over simplistic to say their numbering systems are limited to "One, two and many", it does make sense that since our human brains spent hundreds of thousands of their development years as hunter-gatherers when even the number of other humans would be in very small numbers, it is not surprising that many human beings find numbers and sums difficult. Our brains are more suited to hunter gathering than we realise. A lack of effort at mathematics at school on our part and the limitations of our teachers might be simple but wrong explanations.

There is even a well described state of "statistics anxiety" which describes the apprehension that occurs when even a well-trained, hardworking human being with some pre-existing ability with numbers is exposed to statistics.[lxxiii] It is, however, perfectly possible to appreciate the role of statistics and probability theory and use that information in making decisions about health and healthcare without being a PhD-level mathematician. Of course, there are a few numbers to work with and some simple sums, but nothing needing more than a simple electronic calculator, or even a pencil and a piece of paper.

At a basic level, statistics can just be the collecting of data and describing it. In the 17th Century John Graunt analysed births, deaths, and causes of deaths in London.[lxxiv] These were listed weekly in "The Bills of Mortality". This data started being collected in 1592 and was consistently released from 1603. The Sexton of each church would be visited by the data collector - termed the Searcher. The Searcher would record the cause of death and make a weekly report to the Parish Clerk. On each Wednesday the data would be tallied and printed and published on each Thursday. Graunt critiqued the Searchers who determined cause of death of the corpses, suggesting that many causes of death were misrepresented. Nevertheless, by comparing years in the Bills of Mortality, he was able to make estimates about the size of the population of London and England, birth rates and mortality rates of males and females, and the rise and spread of certain diseases.

He knew that there were around 13,000 funerals per year in London and that three people died per eleven families per year. He estimated from the parish records that the average family size was eight, and was able to calculate that the population of London was about 384,000. Such estimates became useful to governments, not least in estimating the revenue from different taxation strategies used to fund military campaigns and explorations - one of the first instances of the application of descriptive statistics in decision making. He produced the first life table, giving probabilities of survival to each age, and his work laid the basis for modern census methods, demography, and epidemiology.

Initially restricted to sets of collected information, statistics began to be extended into analytical work which calculated future probabilities - for example population growth - and then taking data from a small sample of the population and using it to calculate the effects across the entire population. This analytical work – called statistical inference – has come to be central to the way medicine is now practiced. Treating the entire population with a condition in a randomised trial is not ethical, feasible, safe, necessary, or affordable. There is a need to estimate what the results would be in the entire population when we test a treatment in a sample of the population, and determine if the trial result is likely to have occurred by chance. For example, the mortality data in the streptomycin randomised trial was tested to determine whether the benefit seen was real and due to the streptomycin, or whether it could have occurred by chance. Strictly speaking, the analysis undertaken is whether, given the results in the trial population, what are the chances of there being no difference with the treatment? Conventionally, given the results of this experiment, if the chances of there being no difference is less than 5 times in 100, then we accept that the difference detected in the trial is true. Such inferential work using statistical tests is the norm as evidence has become a requirement across medicine, and indeed across other sciences.

But descriptive statistics and statistical inference go back long before John Gaunt. Early civilisations often took censuses of their population or recorded the trade in various commodities. Early astronomers such as Tycho Brache in Denmark in the 16th Century used the average of several astronomical readings - in modern terms "the mean" - to increase the accuracy of their observations. In a 9th-century Arabic book entitled Manuscript on Deciphering Cryptographic Messages by Al-Kindi (801–

114

873CE), there is a detailed description of how to use statistics and frequency analysis to decipher encrypted messages. For example, the letter E is used in 11% of commonly used words in the English language, the letter A in 8.5%, the letter R in 7.6%, and so on. The most used words are "the", "be", "to", "of", and "and". In simple codes, the most commonly appearing letters or words will be the same in the original language and in the code. Frequency analysis remained an important technique in code breaking in the second World War.

The modern approach to estimating how likely something was to happen in the future - probability - has its roots in attempts to analyse games of chance. Geralmo Cardano graduated with a medical degree from the University of Padua in 1525. Always interested in mathematics, he practiced medicine and taught mathematics simultaneously in Milan. Cardano was always notoriously short of money and kept himself solvent by being an accomplished gambler and chess player. His book about games of chance was published in 1563, and he used the game of throwing dice to understand the basic concepts of probability – something that around 450 years later I have often done in my own teaching. Including a section on effective cheating methods, he demonstrated the usefulness of defining odds as the ratio of favourable to unfavourable outcomes.

Applying this approach to a randomised trial, streptomycin offers better odds of a favourable outcome if a patient has TB, than treatment without streptomycin. Four deaths among 55 patients who had been allocated streptomycin gives an odds of death of 4:51 in that group; $4/51 = 0.078$. Fifteen deaths among 52 patients allocated to bed rest alone gives an odds of death of 15:37 in that group; $15/37 = 0.405$. If we then compare the odds of death on streptomycin with the odds of death without it we have $0.078/0.405 = 0.19$. If streptomycin made no difference, then the odds in both groups would be the same, and when we compare the odds in the two groups the fraction would be 1. When we compare the odds in a ratio and get 0.19 that tells us there is a very big benefit of streptomycin.

We could also compare the risks of dying instead of considering the odds. With streptomycin the risk of dying is 4/55 = 0.072; without streptomycin the risk of dying is 15/52 = 0.288. The risk ratio is 0.072/0.288 = 0.25. Again if the rates had been the same in both group the ratio of rates would be 1. A risk ratio of 0.25 means a relative reduction in risk of 0.75, and we often express that as a percentage. "75% fewer deaths with streptomycin" we can instantly grasp, and that is because it is a way of expressing the differences between the two groups with which we are very familiar. If we go shopping and we see a coat with a price tag that says "75% off" we know that is a bargain. Note that does not mean everybody should buy the coat. There are other factors to consider – we might not like the style or the colour, we might have an alternative coat already, or we might not have the money to pay for the coat even at the reduced price. The decision to buy to coat is an individual one, not a decision that should be for everyone.

Probability is also one approach to more accurate diagnoses. Chest pain and sweating occur more frequently in people having a heart attack than in people with appendicitis. With sufficient examples from people with confirmed diagnoses, is possible to work out the probabilities of various potential diagnoses in new patients based on their constellation of symptoms and examination findings.

It works like this. Imagine that John, your neighbour, excitedly tells you he's won the lottery. Does this irrefutably mean he's won the lottery? Well, no. Because he is well known to you as someone who likes to joke around. You have some doubts. But then the next day a Rolls Royce car appears in his driveway. Is it more probable that he's won the lottery? Yes, but he's still a joker. Then a few weeks on he's no longer your neighbour because he's moved to a big house in the country with a tennis court and swimming pool. Now you are starting to think he really might have won the lottery – maybe he truly did have that condition and you are starting to feel a bit bad that you didn't believe him from the start.

In medicine, a patient presents with chest pain. Are they having a heart attack? Well, perhaps, but there are many other causes of chest pain. The patient is sweating. Now it's a bit more probable, because a good proportion of people who have chest pain and who sweat are found to have had a heart attack. If you weren't taking it seriously from the start, this consultation now has your full attention. Then the patient says the pain has spread from the chest and is now also in the left arm and the jaw. At this point you're starting to instigate emergency management – for sure, it could be another condition, but the probability is high enough to initiate action targeted at the heart.

Yet your initial assessment could still be wrong – in both instances. It is still possible that a few months after John moves to the country you hear that the police have arrested him on suspicion of defrauding his employers. And it's possible that having instigated emergency treatment for a heart attack that subsequent heart tests prove to be entirely normal, and the patient's pain is found to be due to an inflamed oesophagus – a condition well known to be one of the great cardiac mimics in terms of symptoms.

Understanding probability is at the core of medicine, and its importance is often poorly appreciated. Compared to acquiring scientific knowledge, it does not feature significantly in undergraduate or postgraduate teaching, and almost all human beings are just not very good at understanding risk without some instruction and practice. We tend to think something is very worrying or very likely or both, or not at all worrying and very unlikely or both. The reality is that most things fall somewhere in between.

Every time we leave the house, we are taking risks. Even sitting in the house is risky. I could be sitting on the sofa and a large meteorite destroy not only my house but the entire street. The impact of the event would be severe, but it is very unlikely, and also I cannot do much myself to mitigate the meteorite risk other than pay my taxes and hope the government is collaborating with other governments in scanning the solar system. So, I do not spend much time on the sofa worrying about that risk, nor can I go through life computing a formal risk appraisal for that event incorporating "how likely" and "how severe" and making decisions based on a conscious, formal decision making process.

However, humans do tend to overestimate risks that are rare but dramatic. On the increasingly rare occasions I get on a plane I still get a frisson of anxiety. That is common to many people, yet most of us get in a car without any real anxiety. Travel is statistically much safer by air than by car, but we have all seen media coverage of plane crashes where large numbers of people are killed dramatically. Emotion can trump rationality very easily.

Sometimes we can mitigate risks. Some people chose not to fly at all, either because of safety fears or increasingly because they factor in the risks of climate change to their decision making. If it snows or there is fog, many people choose not to drive and postpone their journey. If I am weeding the strawberry plants on our allotment, I now wear trousers, not shorts. Sometimes in the past when doing that job in shorts I've been stung on my knees by ants. It does not happen every time, but it has happened enough for me to do something very simple to mitigate the risk of a few days of sore and itchy knees. So sometimes we can assess probabilities, can do so without too much difficulty, and can do a reasonable job – all without the aid of a fortune teller.

In the lottery winning scenario the initial scepticism was reasonable, and turned out to be justified even though the initial grounds for the scepticism were not correct. John was not a lottery winner, but in this instance he was not just acting the fool. Decisions in healthcare can be trickier, with unresolvable uncertainty about what the outcome might be. With streptomycin, if you prescribe it for someone with pulmonary TB and they die 11 months later is that going to be considered an error? The probability of that happening was, according to the trial data, always four times out of 52, or around 8%. The outcome of the decisions to prescribe streptomycin for that individual was poor. However, at the population level, giving streptomycin was the right thing to do because it increased the probability of a good outcome. It follows that to analyse whether an error was made we must look at the process of how decisions were made, and not just the outcome of the decision.

Sir William Osler knew a few things about probability.[lxxv] Born in Ontario in 1849, he was the first Physician-in Chief of the new John Hopkins Hospital in Baltimore. At John Hopkins, Osler was quickly recognised as an outstanding clinician, humanitarian, and teacher. In 1905, he crossed the Atlantic and was appointed the Regius Professor of Medicine at Oxford, which he held until his death in 1919. When it comes to probability, Sir William Osler knew how even if decisions are made using an optimal process, it is still possible that there will be an undesirable outcome. *"Medicine is a science of uncertainty and an art of probability. Errors in judgement must occur in the practice of an art which consists largely of balancing probabilities."*

The beginning of the development of modern probability theory was in 1654, when two of the most well-known mathematicians of the time, Blaise Pascal and Pierre de Fermat, began a correspondence discussing the subject. The problem was one of dividing the stakes in a theoretical two-player card game in which a prize must be divided between the players due to external circumstances halting the game. Eventually the solution posed was that the division of the stakes in the card game that finishes early is based on the ratio between the size of the lead and the length of the game. In a game of 100 hands of cards, it divides the stakes in the same way for a 65–55 lead as for a 99–89 lead. The former is still a relatively open game whereas in the latter situation victory for the leading player is almost certain. This was a philosophical watershed. Firstly, what had happened in the past was no help in determining the future - whether this was in successive hands of a card game or a treatment for a disease. And secondly, in some circumstances, it was impossible for all parties to be satisfied.

Consider three treatments for three conditions:-

For condition A, without treatment 89% of people survive the illness. With treatment 99% of people survive.

For condition B, without treatment 1% of people survive the illness. With treatment 11% of people survive.

For condition C, without treatment, 45% of people survive the illness. With treatment, 55% survive the illness.

Which of these treatments should be the highest priority for a health system to provide? Of course, all of them increase the number of people surviving in absolute terms by 10%, or 10 people in every hundred, compared to no treatment. But some people might think the highest priority is treatment for condition A, because it shifts a disease with a more than 10 in 100 death rate to one with only 1 in 100 death rate – almost everybody can be cured. Other people might prioritise treatment for condition C on the grounds that a disease which only 1 person in 100 survives becomes, with treatment, a condition that more than 10 people in 100 survive. An almost certain death sentence is transformed by treatment into one with some hope. And yet, in terms of population benefit, Treatment B is just as valuable as A and C, even though some might view the survival as still being as "about half". Pascal and Fermat were right - convincing everyone of the "correct" answer might indeed be difficult.

Pascal and Fermat reasoned in the middle of the 16th Century, that the division should not depend so much on the history of the part of the interrupted game, as on the possible ways the game might have continued, were it not interrupted. A player with a 7–5 lead in a game to 10 has the same chance of eventually winning as a player with a 17–15 lead in a game to 20. Pascal and Fermat therefore thought that interruption in either of the two situations ought to lead to the same division of the stakes. In other words, what is important is not the number of rounds each player has won so far, but the number of rounds each player still needs to win to achieve overall victory.

Fermat was able to create a table for all the possible permutations of future games and counting how many of them would lead to one or the other player winning. He could therefore compute the odds for each player to win. Fermat proposed it fair to divide the stakes in proportion to those odds.

Fermat's solution was improved by Pascal in two ways. First, Pascal produced a more elaborate argument why the resulting division should be considered fair. Second, he showed how to calculate the correct division more efficiently than Fermat's tabular method. Instead of just considering the probability of winning the entire remaining game, Pascal devised a principle of smaller steps incorporating the expected outcome of each succeeding game.

In the wake of these pioneers came Jacob Bernoulli. Born in 1655 in Basel, Switzerland, he was appointed professor of mathematics at the University of Basel in 1687. As a result of his travels he established lengthy correspondences with many leading mathematicians and scientists of his era, which he maintained throughout his life. Bernoulli made an important distinction between "*a priori*" and "*a posteriori*" probabilities. These Latin labels mean "from theory" and "after observation". For example, if we know that an urn contains 100 identical white balls and 300 black, then the *a priori* probability of pulling white at random from the urn is 1/4. In contrast, if we don't know the fraction of white in the urn, then we can only estimate it by looking at *a posteriori* evidence we collect after doing the experiment of pulling balls sequentially from the urn and estimating the true proportions of the whole from the available sample which is progressively observed. These are the beginnings being able to make assumptions about treatments for the general population from seeing the *a posteriori* evidence from a randomised trial.

It has become routine to calculate the "sample size" for a trial - how many people are needed to be recruited to participate given the expected difference in outcomes between the experimental and control groups and the degree of certainty required. Too few people in the trial and there is the risk of not finding a difference between treatments when one truly exists. Too many people in the trial, as discussed earlier, and the trial both takes longer, so the results are delayed more than they should be, and some people in the control group are denied effective treatment because they are included in the trial rather than being given the active treatment following the publication of the smaller, more efficient trial results. There is something rather wonderful about those principles being developed in the mid-1700s, and something quite disappointing about them not being utilised in medicine until the middle of the 20th Century.

Whilst the origins of statistical theory lie in these 18th-century advances in thinking about probability, the modern field of statistics really only emerged in the late-19th and early-20th century. The first wave, at the turn of the century, was led by the work of Francis Galton and Karl Pearson. Pearson founded the world's first university department of statistics at University College, London, in 1911. He transformed statistics into a rigorous mathematical discipline used for analysis, not just in science, but also in industry and politics. Unfortunately, the legacy of Galton and Pearson is tainted by their belief in eugenics; it is to the credit of University College that in 2020 they renamed two buildings formerly named after Pearson because of this connection.

Further developments by Ronald Fisher involved the development of better design of experiments, models, hypothesis testing and techniques for use with small data samples such as those in randomised trials. Educated at Harrow School, he won a scholarship to study mathematics at Gonville and Caius College, Cambridge, graduating with a First in 1912. Lifelong poor eyesight saved him from military service in the First World War, and after a time working as a statistician in the City of London, in 1919 he began working at the Rothamsted Experimental Station in Hertfordshire, where he would remain for 14 years. There he investigated the possibility of analysing the vast amount of crop data accumulated since 1842 from the "Classical Field Experiments", and as a result he pioneered the use of randomised trials in agriculture.

In 1925 he published *Statistical Methods for Research Workers*, one of the 20th century's most influential books on statistical methods. This was followed in 1935 with *The Design of Experiments* which was equally well received, and further promoted statistical technique and application. There is no doubt that his work led directly to the wider use of randomised trials, their better design, and their better analysis and reporting. One of his many thought experiments – loosely based on a real life experience – involved "The Lady Tasting Tea". The lady in question claimed to be able to tell whether the tea or the milk was added first to a cup. Fisher proposed to give her eight cups, four of each variety, in random order. One could then ask what the probability was for her getting the specific number of cups she identified correct, but just by chance. The statistical calculation – using Fisher's exact test, now widely used as a statistical method – showed that the chances of getting all 8 cups correct by chance was 1 in 70.

Developments is statistical approaches meant that it gradually became the norm to test the results of scientific studies and experiments to see whether those results could be considered "true", or whether any differences detected could have been due to chance. Creating this as the new norm in medical research was one of the larger pieces in the jigsaw leading to evidence-based medicine.

Finally, whilst Fisher's great legacy in statistics and in relations to randomised trial design is undoubted - he was knighted in 1952 - his legacy is also badly tainted. It is to their credit that finally in 2020 Gonville and Caius College, Cambridge - where he was Professor of Genetics until 1956 - announced that a 1989 stained-glass window commemorating Fisher's work would be removed because of his connection with eugenics. In the same year Rothamsted Research released a statement condemning Fisher's involvement with eugenics, and an accommodation building, only built in 2018 and named after him, was subsequently renamed.

CHAPTER NINE

Janet Elizabeth Lane-Claypon

Ronald Fisher's pioneering work using randomised controlled trials in agriculture preceded Austin Bradford Hill and the streptomycin trial only by a few years. But there were two other types of study that science needed to shed light on the causes of disease and to point the way to better treatment. Their story begins almost 70 years before the streptomycin trial.

Janet Elizabeth Lane-Claypon was born in 1877 into an affluent family, in Boston, Lincolnshire.[lxxvi] [lxxvii] [lxxviii] She was privately educated and entered the London School of Medicine for Women in 1898. This medical school had been established in 1874 by an association of pioneering women physicians including Elizabeth Garrett Anderson, for whom the London hospital was later named. The UK Medical Act of 1876 had allowed for the first time the medical authorities to license all qualified applicants irrespective of gender. In 1877 an agreement was reached with the Royal Free Hospital that allowed students at the London School of Medicine for Women to complete their clinical studies there. Lane-Claypon was a pioneer; she won numerous undergraduate prizes, and as a medical student in 1902 and 1903 she held a British Medical Society research scholarship - the first ever awarded to a woman.

Graduating with first class honours in 1902, after several hospital appointments at the Royal Free, she - and this too is remarkable for the era - gained her postgraduate doctor of philosophy in 1905 and a doctorate in medicine in 1910. Her initial research consisted of laboratory studies of reproductive physiology and the bacteriology and chemistry of milk. Between 1907 and 1912, Lane-Claypon was one of just two women working at the Lister Institute of Preventative Medicine in London, and she travelled extensively in Europe as a Jenner Research Fellow funded by the Institute between 1909 and 1911. By the start of 1912 she had already published ten scientific papers, and she was then awarded a research grant by the Local Government Board, a forerunner of the Medical Research Council.

Her brief was to investigate the effects of feeding infants breast milk or boiled cows' milk. Bacteria, especially TB, in cows' milk coupled with high infant mortality had let to a general approach to boiling it before giving it to infants when it was used as an alternative to breast milk. An effect on infant mortality was not obvious. Why had boiling the milk not saved babies' lives? Theories abounded - for example, that boiling destroyed some or all of the goodness in the milk. Lane-Claypon's brief was to shed some scientific light on the question.

Reviewing the data on the effect of boiling cow's milk when it was given to calves fulfilled the requirements of the current scientific culture, which was still dominated by the investigation of scientific and biological mechanisms rather than experiments to determine whether people lived longer or better. However, a sceptic would quickly recognise that human beings are not cows. Therefore alongside the animal data, Lane-Claypon proposed to analyse clinical data on the effect of the two milks on human infants. She wanted to compare babies of "known or as far as possible the same social environment" who were fed on raw or boiled cows' milk with a control group of babies who were breast fed. She knew there should be such data collected on babies at "Infant Consultations", the forerunner of Well Baby Clinics. However, she found the data samples in the UK to be too small or incomplete, and so she used the contacts she had made in Europe and settled on an excellent dataset from Berlin. The resultant study population was the babies attending for checks in Berlin, and in that population there were 204 infants whose primary milk source was boiled cows' milk and 300 infants whose primary milk source was the breast. Those babies had been followed up during their early life and there was now data available to determine, for example, the weights of the babies with different at set periods.

The basic analyses consisted of calculating the mean weights of the babies in the two series for each 8-day period for a year. The cow's milk babies weighed more for the first 8 days of life, but after that the breast-fed babies leapt ahead until about the 7 months of age when the difference disappeared. Lane-Claypon went on to test statistically whether she had inadvertently worked with a biased sample which was atypical of the general population and found that not to be the case. She then checked her data for alternative explanations for the differences she had found. Could they, for example, be due to differences in available household income? Again, that was not found to be the case.

Finally, she addressed the crossover of the weights for the two series of babies during the first 8 days of life. The higher average weight of the babies fed on boiled cows' milk was based on 10 observations, and the breast fed babies average weight was based on 24. Was this difference an error caused by the extremely small number of observations available, especially for the cows' milk series. To deal with this possibility, Lane-Claypon took advantage of a statistical approach that had first been reported only four years before.

William Sealey Gosset had been recruited into the brewing industry after graduating from Oxford. Claude Guinness, the owner of the company, aimed to recruit the best graduates from Oxford and Cambridge to apply biochemistry and statistics to Guinness's industrial processes. Gosset devised a new statistical test as an economical way to monitor the quality of stout in repeated batches. Were any differences due to, say, a new barley, or were those differences due to chance or other factors?

Gosset studied the issue and made progress by personal study, trial and error, cooperating with others, and by spending two terms of study leave from Guinness in 1906–1907 in the laboratory of Karl Pearson at University College, London. Pearson helped Gosset with the mathematics of his papers. The Guinness Board of Directors allowed its scientists to publish research on condition that they do not mention beer, Guinness, or their own surname. Gossett published his paper in 1908 using the pseudonym "Student", and in modern statistics. Student's T-test is still used and known by that name.

Pearson and Gosset got on well, but Pearson apparently had little appreciation of the importance of Gosset's work. The papers

127

addressed the brewer's concern with small samples; bio-statisticians like Pearson, typically had hundreds of observations and saw no urgency in developing small-sample methods. It was Ronald Fisher who quickly appreciated the importance of Gosset's small-sample work and its application to the smaller data samples usual in randomised trials, and as in Lane-Claypon's case, other study designs.

As for Lane-Claypon's use of the Student T-test, she received help from a colleague and statistician at the Lister Institute, Major Greenwood. "Major" was simply his forename, not a military rank. Early in his career he worked for the physiologist Leonard Hill, father of the future statistician and streptomycin trial pioneer Austin Bradford Hill. Leonard Hill recognized Greenwood's talent and appointed him as his assistant at the London Hospital Medical College. He studied with Karl Pearson before being appointed statistician at the Lister Institute in 1910. It seems from Lane-Claypon's report of her research into infant feeding that Greenwood, through his association with Pearson, was aware of Gosset's new statistical test and it was he who helped Lane-Claypon with it.

Janet Lane-Claypon had designed, carried out, and published the first, modern cohort study. The babies in Berlin were her cohort, and she looked back in time at the weights of the babies, measuring the weights of groups of babies according to which type of milk they were fed on. It would be possible to do the same study on babies born today if their data was recorded as part of a cohort dataset and the cohort data contained the information on both feeding and weight. In addition, she had undertaken a search for other causes of her findings, and against the mainstream medical culture at the time had used medical statistics to determine that her results were unlikely to be flawed due to biases or her findings due to the play of chance. The whole approach was as important to epidemiology as the Bills of Mortality and Fisher's development of randomised trials in agriculture. Whilst similar types of studies were only undertaken sporadically over the next 40 years, Lane-Claypon's first modern cohort study remains an important foundation stone for what followed. But she was not finished with her pioneering.

In 1917 Lane-Claypon became the Dean of the Household and Social Sciences Department at King's College for Women. It seems she had no appetite for departmental politics (not a bad trait in my experience) and in 1923 she returned to research. Neville Chamberlain, then the Minister of Health, appointed a Committee on Cancer "*to consider available information with regard to the causation, prevalence and treatment of cancer.*" Having decided to first study cancer of the breast, the Committee hired Lane-Claypon to work in the Department of Health and review the relevant literature. It then commissioned her to "*investigate a sufficient and suitable series of cases of cancer of the breast in regard to specified antecedent conditions, and at the same time a parallel and equally representative series of control cases, i.e., women whose conditions of life were broadly comparable to the cancer series but who had no sign of cancer*".[lxxix]

Lane-Claypon embarked on the first, modern, scientific, case-control study. To enrol a sufficient number of cases and controls, Lane-Claypon enlisted the participation of other physicians she knew, mostly women. Eventually more than 1000 breast cancer cases and control patients were recruited from eight hospitals in London and three in Glasgow. About 80% of the controls were surgical or medical in-patients who were free of cancer. Most were between 45 and 70 years of age, and the rest of the controls were outpatients of similar age.

Lane-Claypon developed a detailed, structured questionnaire that the cases and controls filled in with details with their age of menarche, age of marriage, age of completed pregnancies, whether they had breast fed, and so on. She was conscious of the potential for recall bias, noting that cases with breast cancer might be psychologically disposed to remember symptoms or events that they related to their breasts, whereas controls might well have forgotten them.

The first step in the data analysis was to ascertain whether the characteristics of the populations of cases and controls were similar enough to be suitable for comparison. They were, apart from more single women among cases and married women among controls. Given the known increased risk of cancer of the breast among single women this difference was perhaps to be anticipated. Lane-Claypon then investigated the influence of various features of reproductive life on breast cancer risk. She was the first to demonstrate that age at marriage of cases was significantly higher than for controls. Taking age at marriage as a surrogate for age at first birth, this was the first demonstration of the well-known fact that early pregnancy lowers breast cancer risk.

Lane-Claypon then proceeded to establish, again for the first time, the strong relationship between fertility and risk. She was not content, however, until she had accounted for the potential confounding effects of age at and duration of marriage. Major Greenwood again contributed, constructing a statistical equation to predict the number of children expected among married case women as a function of marital age and duration, and similarly for control women. When the equation for the case series was applied to the controls, 3.89 children per women were predicted whereas an average of 5.34 were observed. Conversely, applying the control equation to the cases, an average of 4.72 children were expected, whereas the observed number was 3.48. Both differences were highly statistically significant. Having children has a protective effect against breast cancer.

Lane-Claypon also investigated age at menarche. She observed that 20% of control women reported menarche before 13 years versus 13.3% for the breast cancer cases. The percentages for onset of menarche over 15 years were 25.7% and 22.4%, respectively. A reanalysis of her data in 2010 using modern statistical methods showed the observed differences would indeed be regarded as significant by current statistical standards.[lxxx] Her findings have been subsequently replicated in several other studies.

Janet Elizabeth Lane-Claypon's work remains under-recognised to this day. A comprehensive review of early cohort

130

studies cites a 1933 study of familial acquisition of tuberculosis in the Black population of Kingsport, Tennessee, as the first published example[lxxxi]. Bradford Hill used a retrospective cohort design in his study of nickel refinery workers, which was not, however, reported publicly until he described it in the eighth edition of his textbook in 1966. Whilst cohort and case-control study designs were only sporadically used over the next 30 years, key researchers such as Bradford Hill were aware of them and the situations in which they could provide useful evidence. More foundations of evidence-based medicine had again been laid.

Her research was remarkable, but Lane-Claypon herself gained something more personal from her time at the Department of Health. In 1929, at the age of 52, she married the Deputy Head of the Health Department, Sir Edward Rodolf Forber, becoming his second wife. Such were the constraints of the time that married women were not allowed to work in the civil service and she resigned from the Department. In the 1930s she co-authored a report into stillbirths and neonatal deaths with the President of the Royal College of Obstetricians and Gynaecologists, Sir Eardley Holland, but otherwise she seems to have lived quietly in the countryside in Kent. She died in 1967 at the age of 90, and her obituary in the British Medical Journal says nothing about her pioneering work on study designs. The University of Lincoln, the closest university geographically to her place of birth, named its Science Centre after her in 2018 - but otherwise she remains little known outside the small world of academic clinical epidemiology.

CHAPTER TEN

Smoking, Cohorts, and a President's Death

William Richard Shaboe Doll was born in Hampton, Middlesex on 28th October 1912, the son of a general practitioner, and was educated at Westminster School. He wanted to read mathematics at Cambridge, but did badly on the entrance paper having drunk too much of the Trinity College beer the night before. The admissions tutor rang his father and said he could have an exhibition but not a scholarship, so in pique Doll studied biology quickly and a year later was accepted at St Thomas' Hospital Medical School, London.[lxxxii] He is one more example of a doctor whose interest in mathematics coupled with a natural scepticism and curiosity was of enormous value throughout his career.

As a medical student he published a paper demonstrating that many of the studies underpinning current medical practice were too small to be relied on because the results could have occurred by chance.[lxxxiii] Doll showed he had the talent for a stellar career, and he wanted to undertake research after qualifying. However, in 1937 when he graduated a research career was an impossible dream without either a private income or becoming a consultant and earning enough to do it in one's spare time. He spent six months as casualty officer and anaesthetist, and six months as a house physician, still at St Thomas', for which he received free beer and free laundry, but no pay.

He then wanted to be a house physician at the Royal Postgraduate Medical School in Hammersmith, attracted by the research possibilities and the £100-a-year salary. Someone else had just been appointed for six months, but he was told he could have the job after that. To fill in time he took a night job as resident medical officer at the London Clinic, which needed someone because they advertised that there was always a doctor on the premises, day and night. The last thing any of the consultants wanted was for anyone else to see their fee-paying patients (this was of course before the creation of the NHS), and he was called from his bed three times in six months. "This," he later reported, "suited me very well."

War broke out a month after he finally took up his post at the Hammersmith, and he was called up. He was in the army from 1939 to 1945, being a battalion medical officer in a remarkable retreat to Dunkirk. Late in life he told the story in five parts in the British Medical Journal; scavenging for food and alcohol in the chaotic retreat of the British Expeditionary Force featured prominently.[lxxxiv][lxxxv][lxxxvi][lxxxvii][lxxxviii] After that he served in Egypt, where he ran a ward for serious infectious diseases - diphtheria, typhoid, typhus, polio, and smallpox. Later he was posted to a hospital ship in the Mediterranean and took part in the invasion of Sicily.

Doll contracted renal tuberculosis in the middle of 1944 and was discharged early in 1945 after having a kidney removed. He then worked as a psychiatrist in an army hospital for six months but returned to St Thomas' as a junior medical assistant. There he got on badly with the young doctors who assumed that he knew nothing about medicine after five years in the army, and he railed against the pyramidal structure and the power of the medical establishment. Jobs were hard to come by and the dream of research seemed far away.

In 1946 his friend Dr Joan Faulkner, who later became his wife, was working at the Medical Research Council's headquarters. Doll took a course on medical statistics at the London School of Hygiene and Tropical Medicine where Austin Bradford Hill worked and taught. Bradford Hill was impressed by Doll, and Doll soon went to work for him. The research dream was, at last, a reality.

Doll started work with Bradford Hill at the Medical Research Council in January 1948. He was straight into the deep end. A phenomenal increase in the annual number of deaths attributed to lung cancer had been causing concern for some time. For example, in 1922 only 612 deaths from lung cancer were recorded in the UK. In 1947 the number was 9,287 − roughly a fifteenfold increase. Similar patterns had been reported from Switzerland, Denmark, the United States, Canada, Turkey, Japan, and Australia.

134

At the time smoking seemed a normal and harmless habit. Eighty per cent of men smoked. Doll and Bradford Hill both thought the most likely cause would prove to be pollution - coal fires and heavy industry were prevalent and there were more cars, more tarring of roads, and more exhaust fumes. There was a known association of pipe smoking with lip cancer, but that was thought to be caused mainly by the heat of the pipe stem. Could the increase in lung cancer be due to improved standards of diagnosis? Yet there were big variations in the rate of cases between different, large, English cities which made it unlikely to be an issue of diagnostic standards.

But early work investigating smoking as a factor was concerning. A 1939 German study found only 3 out of 86 male lung cancer patients were non-smokers, whilst 56 were heavy smokers. In contrast, among 86 healthy men matched for age there were 14 non-smokers and only 31 heavy smokers. Small scale research of this nature could never provide conclusive evidence and the Medical Research Council commissioned Bradford Hill and Doll to undertake larger studies.

They first used a case control study. A short questionnaire was administered to 650 male patients in London hospitals. The interviewees were newly admitted patients with suspected lung, liver, or bowel cancers. To reduce bias, the interviewing researchers were not told the suspected diagnosis. And for every lung cancer patient, they interviewed a control patient – a patient in hospital with a non-cancer diagnosis.

The findings were, at the time, unexpected. There were many more smokers in the lung cancer group, there appeared to be a greater proportion of heavy smokers in the lung cancer group, and though the number of women with lung cancer was smaller the findings were the same in men and women. These results were so compelling that Doll and Hill took the results to the MRC head Sir Harold Himsworth, who advised them that the results might be peculiar to London, and suggested that they repeat the study in other cities. So they studied 750 similar patients in Bristol, Cambridge, Leeds, and Newcastle.[lxxxix]

While they were doing this, they were beaten to publication.[xc] Ernst Wynder was a medical student at the Washington University School of Medicine and Barnes Hospital, St. Louis. He witnessed at post mortem the blackened lungs of a man with lung cancer and later learned that he was a heavy smoker. Wynder sought the assistance of Evarts Graham, a thoracic surgeon, and head of the department. Although Graham did not believe in the increased risk of lung cancer from smoking, perhaps in part because he was like many doctors at the time a heavy smoker himself, he enabled Wynder to conduct a case-control study by providing subjects with lung cancer to interview. They eventually ended up with nearly 700 cases matched to controls and found that 97% of lung cancer patients were moderate to heavy smokers for an extended period.

Hill and Doll went to the BMJ's then editor, Hugh Clegg, and the BMJ published their paper quickly.[xci] At the time it seemed a shame to be beaten to publication but Doll said later, "*It was a principle that I have adhered to ever since: namely, that if you find something that is unexpected and is going to be of social significance you have a responsibility to be sure that you're right before you publicise your results to the rest of the world. This does at least require repeating some of your observations.*"

The 1950 BMJ paper on smoking and lung cancer was largely ignored by the public. It was the same story in the United States following Wynder and Graham's paper in the Journal of the American Medical Association. The UK Department of Health's cancer committee was not convinced by the findings and thought that urging people to quit could start a mass panic. For humans, whilst learning stuff is hard, unlearning stuff is even harder.

Some were convinced that the only reasonable explanation was that smoking was a factor in the production of the disease. Others considered the association to be simply that - in other words that smoking caused lung cancer had not been shown, and alternative explanations were possible. The major limitation was that the studies were necessarily all case control in design, and therefore relied upon the memories of the participants in recalling, for example how much they had smoked and when, what age they had started smoking, and so on. It was the same potential recall-bias problem Lane-Claypon recognised in her breast cancer study in 1926.

And yet it was hardly feasible and unethical to set up an experiment - a randomised controlled trial in which half of a large number of volunteers would be allocated to a potentially harmful intervention of smoking, say, 20 cigarettes a day for the next 20 years, whilst the other volunteers had to avoid smoking.

And of course, the tobacco industry was active. Years later Doll said that "*if there was a report of it in the newspaper or on the radio, the reporter would always be careful to mention a doctor so-and-so - who had been put up to it by the tobacco industry - saying the research was controversial and the link wasn't proved.*" Journalists smoked - even television presenters did while discussing the report on camera - and newspapers earned huge amounts of money from tobacco advertising.

But there was another type of study that could overcome the reliance on individual memories. Doll and Hill recognised that additional case control studies would not advance knowledge materially. Instead, they set out to undertake the alternative observational study design – a prospective cohort study. If there were an undetected flaw in the retrospective evidence, then it should be exposed by the alternative approach.

It was not just Janet Lane-Claypon who understood the utility of a cohort study when the research question required that design. In 1919 Sir James Mackenzie, a general practitioner recently returned to St Andrews from a glittering cardiovascular research career in London, recognised that studying the occurrence and development of disease, especially cardiovascular disease, would require collecting data from a defined population. By following and periodically collecting data from that

137

population over many years it would be possible to look at people with heart attacks and strokes and compare, for example, their blood pressure to the blood pressure of people who had not had a heart attack or stroke. The simple act of collecting data in advance of the development of disease avoided many of the limitations of the retrospective approaches; it was more difficult to refute the findings when data was collected prospectively.

In his early career Mackenzie did not have the time or enough research assistants to complete his project - he was simply too busy clinically to be able to manage collecting lots of data from many people. Because the occurrence of disease, even relatively common diseases, occurs slowly over many years, prospective cohort studies need to recruit large numbers of people to detect results that can be shown to not be the result of chance. But he returned to St Andrews after the First World War ended, and at the age of 64 he brought together all the general practitioners working in the town to encourage the systematic recording of diseases.[xcii]

Toss a fair, two-sided coin with a head and a tail on the two sides four times and by chance it may come down heads every time, leading to the false conclusions that the coin can only come down heads or that it has heads on both sides. Toss the same fair coin 100 times and it is highly improbable that it will come down heads every time; indeed, it is highly likely that the number of heads and tails will be about equal. So, more people in the study means more new cases of the disease, and the larger number of those events means that differences are less likely to be due to chance. Cohort studies could potentially recruit big numbers of people quickly, and whilst there is inevitably a period after recruitment before sufficient numbers of new cases occur for the cohort design to begin to produce useful data, even big cohort studies were comparatively simple and comparatively low cost to undertake. And if they are well conducted they can produce evidence that is difficult to refute.

It was the 1940s before Mackenzie's concept of a large prospective cohort study would really come to life. In Japan, after the dropping of the atom bombs on Hiroshima and Nagasaki in 1946, by far the greatest proportion of the approximately 180,000 deaths were as a direct result of blast and heat. Several thousand of the immediate survivors died shortly afterwards because of acute radiation sickness, and thousands more experienced acute symptoms and recovered. What might happen to those who recovered was unclear. It was recognised that knowledge of the long-term effects of substantial amounts of whole-body irradiation was incomplete and the joint commission of the US Army and Navy, which visited Japan shortly after the war, recommended a long-term study of the survivors to find out what they were. Large prospective cohort studies were consequently initiated in January 1948 into the effects of radiation, with the survivors of the two explosions as the study participants.[xciii]

But it was not just lung cancer that was rapidly increasing as a cause of death. Cardiovascular disease had become the number one cause of mortality among Americans, accounting for more than 1 in 3 deaths, and the same was true in some other higher-income countries. Prevention and treatment were so poorly understood that most accepted the possibility of early death from heart disease as unavoidable.

The President was no exception. Franklin Delano Roosevelt, the United States' war-time President from 1933 to 1945, had what would now be considered high blood pressure when he took office (140/100 mm Hg). Between 1935 to 1941, the President experienced a gradual rise in blood pressure to 188/105 mm Hg. Despite the rising blood pressure, his personal physician insisted that the President was healthy, and his blood pressure was "no more than normal for a man of his age." But when British Prime Minister Winston Churchill visited the White House in May 1943, he asked his own physician Lord Moran whether he too had noticed that the President was "a very tired man?"

On 27th March 1944, as planning for the Allied landing at Normandy was at its height, daughter Anna Roosevelt insisted on a second opinion, and the President was admitted to Bethesda

Naval Hospital for shortness of breath on exertion, and abdominal distension. The President's high blood pressure had damaged his heart and it was unable to pump blood with sufficient force to maintain health. Whilst the diagnosis was now established, his doctor had few useful treatments – they would not be developed for a few more decades - and Roosevelt had little time left.

In 1945, two months before his death, Roosevelt attended the Yalta Conference with Churchill and Soviet Premier Joseph Stalin to negotiate the anticipated post-war administration of Germany, and a future United Nations. Lord Moran wrote in his diary *"the President appears a very sick man. He has all the symptoms of hardening of the arteries…"* and *"I give him only a few months to live."* As Moran predicted, President Roosevelt died a few weeks later on 12th April 1945, at the age of 63, from cerebral haemorrhage with a blood pressure of 300/190 mmHg. Like countless other Americans, he had succumbed to the national epidemic of cardiovascular disease.[xciv]

On June 16, 1948, President Harry Truman signed into law the National Heart Act. The law allocated a $500,000 seed grant for a twenty-year prospective cohort study to investigate the then unknown causes of the cardiovascular disease epidemic. There was enthusiasm for the project at Harvard Medical School and Massachusetts General Hospital, and the small town of Framingham about twenty miles outside Boston was selected. The one-time farming community was by 1947 a factory town of 28,000 residents. The town had been a site for a tuberculosis study 20 years previously.

The way the study was planned was that from all the people of Framingham who were willing, all sorts of information and many measurements would be collected at regular intervals. These might be how old they were, their gender, whether they smoked tobacco, how much tobacco, blood pressure and how high it was, whether they had diabetes and how well it was controlled, and so on. After a period, the rate of heart attacks and strokes could be measured in people with, say, higher blood pressure and compared with the rate of heart attacks and strokes in people with lower blood pressure. If there were more heart attacks and strokes in the higher blood pressure group, then evidence would have been obtained showing that high blood pressure was likely to be one of the causes of the cardiovascular epidemic.

The original cohort was recruited between 1948 and 1952 and consisted of 5209 residents aged 28 to 62 years. The first major study findings were published in 1957, almost a decade after the initial participant was examined.[xcv] Defining high blood pressure as 160/95 mmHg, they found a nearly four-fold increase in coronary heart disease in people among people with a blood pressure higher than that level. A few years later they found that stroke was also a major consequence of high blood pressure.

Back in the UK, Doll and Hill – faced with the need to produce additional evidence on smoking – made a smart decision on the formation of their cohort. They set about recruiting doctors.

In October 1951 Doll and Hill sent a questionnaire about smoking habits to all the doctors resident in the UK and registered with the General Medical Council (GMC). Out of almost 60,000, more than two-thirds replied. The choice of this cohort was brilliant. Follow-up of UK doctors is easy since they must update their names with the GMC to continue to work. Moreover, the collection of data on the causes of death could not have been easier in this group of subjects, all of whom had routine access to high quality medical care.

Data from subjects younger than 35 years old and from women were excluded since lung cancer was rare in these cohorts and in those days the number of women doctors were few. Therefore, they collected 34,440 questionnaires from male doctors and in only 29 months they had enough data to show an increased rate of lung cancer and heart attacks which increased proportionately with increasing consumption of tobacco. Although there were only 36 lung cancer deaths in the first 29

141

months of the study, after four years there were 200, almost all of them in heavy smokers.

Not long afterwards Doll and Hill were visited by the chairman of Imperial Tobacco and his statistician. Five years later the statistician told his employers that unless they accepted that tobacco smoking caused cancer, he could not work for them any longer. They didn't, and so he resigned. The last act of the statistician as their employee was for him to take Doll and his wife out to a very expensive dinner on his company expense account.

As early as 1952, Ian Macleod, the Minister of Health announced that Richard Doll had proved the link between smoking and lung cancer. He did so at a press conference throughout which he chain-smoked. Charles Fletcher wrote his influential Royal College of Physicians report on smoking and its harmful effects in 1962. The tobacco manufacturers, of course, used every possible device to question, deny, undermine, and oppose both the evidence and any worthwhile action.

But gradually the evidence triumphed. When Doll and Hill began their work 80% of men and 40% of women smoked. In the UK today 9% of adults smoke. The development of study designs and the accumulation of evidence has combined to reduce the burden of tobacco-related premature disease and mortality, but not yet to abolish it.

Richard Doll became the world's most distinguished medical epidemiologist. He went on to show smoking caused bladder and other cancers, and cardiovascular disease. He did seminal work with Richard Peto on the health of doctors and their families, demonstrating an increased incidence of suicide and liver disease. He also carried out major research on the risks and benefits of the contraceptive pill, the risks of asbestos, on low level radiation, and the dietary treatment of gastric ulcers.

He was made a Fellow of the Royal Society (FRS) in 1966, knighted in 1971, and in 1996 he was made a Companion of Honour for services of national importance. Having become

Regius Professor of Medicine at Oxford University in 1969, he founded Green College there in 1979. He died on 24th July 2005, at the John Radcliffe Hospital in Oxford at the age of 92 after a short illness.

Austin Bradford Hill was President of the Royal Statistical Society between 1950 and 1952, was awarded a CBE in 1954, became a Fellow of the Royal Society in 1954 with Ronald Fisher as one of his proposers, and was knighted by the Queen in 1961. He died in 1991 and Richard Doll wrote his obituary. He described him as the greatest statistician of the 20th Century - even though he held no specialist qualification in either medicine or statistics. He taught an innumerate profession to begin to think quantitatively, persuaded it to adopt the principle of randomisation in its assessment of the efficacy of therapy, and laid the basis for the explosive development of epidemiology by showing how that old science could be refurbished as a tool to discover the causes of non-infectious disease.

CHAPTER ELEVEN

Overload

Whilst the scientific revolution of the 17th Century spread ideas of rationalism and experimentation, the industrial revolution of the late 18th and early 19th centuries transformed the production of goods. Marrying the two concepts in medicine to produce the vast range of treatments available today started at the end of the 19th and continued throughout the 20th centuries, accelerating greatly after the Second World War. Basic understanding of disease processes was a necessary precursor to the development of effective treatments. For example, whilst notions of diseases spreading from person to person have featured in medicine since ancient times, it was not until the work of Louis Pasteur in the 1850s and Robert Koch in the 1880s that there was general acceptance of germ theory. Once basic understanding of mechanisms of disease improved, a search could be undertaken for more effective treatments.

The roots of modern medicines go back to apothecaries and pharmacies making their own traditional remedies as far back as the Middle Ages. It was bringing this empirical knowledge together with industrial processes, particularly those involving dyes in the late 19th Century that began the process of modernising medicines development and production. Dyes began to be used to stain tissue specimens for examination under the microscope. A tiny guillotine-like apparatus called a microtome which could slice tissues thin enough to be examined under a microscope was developed in 1848. The Gram stain to identify bacteria under the microscope was developed in 1875, the Giemsa stain to identify different cells in a smear of blood in 1891, the Ziehl-Nielsen stain to show tuberculosis bacteria in 1883. It was not so big a step from using dyes to identify diseased tissues under a microscope to attempt to use them and their derivatives to treat diseases.

Many of the large pharmaceutical companies with names that are now familiar worldwide had their origins in traditional pharmacy, or early industrial chemical processes or both. Merck in Germany was a family pharmacy founded in Damstadt in 1668. In 1816, Emanuel Merck, a descendant of the original founder, took over the pharmacy. He isolated several different alkaloids in the pharmacy's laboratory including morphine, codeine, and cocaine. He began the manufacture of these substances in bulk in 1827 and gradually built up a chemical-pharmaceutical factory that produced raw materials for an increasing range of early, modern medicines.

In the USA, Pfizer was founded in 1849 by two immigrants from Germany, initially as a chemicals business. During the American civil war as demand for painkillers and antiseptics rocketed it grew rapidly. At the same time a young cavalry commander named Colonel Eli Lilly was serving in the Union army. A trained pharmaceutical chemist, after his military service Lilly set up a pharmaceutical business in 1876. He was one of the first to focus on scientific research and development of new medicines as well as manufacturing.

Edward Robinson Squibb was a naval doctor during the Mexican-American war of 1846–1848 and apparently threw the drugs he was supplied with overboard due to their low quality. He set up a laboratory in 1858, like Pfizer supplying Union armies in the civil war, and laying the basis for the huge organisation that decades later became Bristol Myers Squibb. Switzerland also rapidly developed a pharmaceutical industry in the second half of the 19th century. Previously a centre of the trade in textiles and dyes, Swiss manufacturers gradually began to realise their dyestuffs had antiseptic and other properties and began to market them as pharmaceuticals. Companies such as Sandoz, CIBA-Geigy, and Roche all had their roots in this Swiss boom.

Back in Germany, Bayer was founded in 1863 as a dye maker in Wuppertal. It later moved into medicines, commercialising aspirin around the turn of the 20th century, one of the most successful pharmaceuticals ever at that point.

The unregulated nature of the trade in medicines during this period ensured there was a far less strict delineation between 'pharmaceutical' and 'chemical' industries than we now have. These companies focused on products such as cod liver oil, toothpaste, citric acid for soft drinks, hair gel, and selling products like heroin as an over-the-counter medicine marketed as suitable for teething babies.

The disruption to Germany's position as the leader in pharmaceuticals in the early 20th century by the first World War meant that others, particularly in the US, could take relative advantage. The beginnings of the globalisation of the industry were seen both before and after the war - in the UK, tax advantages incentivised many foreign companies such as Wyeth, Sandoz, CIBA, Eli Lilly and MSD to set up subsidiaries in Britain.

As we have seen, the period between the two World Wars was marked by the two breakthroughs of insulin and penicillin. Both required the new pharmaceutical companies - for their scientific expertise, for their scalable production facilities, and for their storage chains and distribution skills. Banting and colleagues could sufficiently purify their pancreatic extract and industrially produce and distribute insulin as an effective medicine only in collaboration with the scientists at Eli Lilly. And for penicillin, the government-supported international collaboration including Merck, Pfizer and Squibb was required to turn laboratory work into mass production. The immense scale and sophistication of the penicillin development effort marked a new era for the way the pharmaceutical industry developed drugs. The war also stimulated research into everything from new painkillers to medicines for typhus.

Attempts to alleviate the pain of disease, injury, or simple surgical procedures by producing unconsciousness are almost as old as civilisation. However, ether, the first anaesthetic agent to be successfully demonstrated in public, was originally synthesised (by the action of sulphuric acid on ethanol) in the thirteenth century. There are early reports of it producing both pain relief and loss of consciousness, but such observations were not applied clinically for centuries.

147

During the Enlightenment the gases carbon dioxide (Joseph Black, 1754), oxygen (Joseph Priestley, 1771), and nitrous oxide (Priestly again, 1772) were discovered. As with other scientific developments, the therapeutic possibilities were explored. Thomas Beddoes, once Black's student, established a Pneumatic Institute near Bristol in 1798 to allow objective studies, and appointed the young Humphrey Davy to perform them.

Davy's 'research on nitrous oxide was published in 1799. It described two major effects of its inhalation: euphoria (he coined the term 'laughing gas') and analgesia (it eased the pain of his erupting wisdom tooth). Davy suggested inhalation of nitrous oxide during surgical operations, but this was not acted upon.

Davy went on to work at the Royal Institution in London, giving demonstrations of nitrous oxide and other discoveries of the age. In 1813, another scientist famous in later life, Michael Faraday, joined him as assistant and studied the inhalation of ether. He published his findings in 1818, and these included soporific and analgesic effects. However, one subject had taken over 24 hours to recover full consciousness. Whilst the medical establishment ignored the medical implications of inhaling nitrous oxide and ether, their potential for "recreational" use was very much taken up. "Laughing gas parties" and "ether frolics" were all the rage.[xcvi]

Then on 10th December 1844 in Hartford, Connecticut, Gardner Quincy Colton, a travelling showman, gave a demonstration including the effects of inhalation of nitrous oxide. In the audience was Horace Wells, a local dentist who was already using new materials to make dentures, and had sought ways of easing the pain of first removing the patient's own rotten teeth. The following morning Wells had one of his own teeth removed by a colleague, John Riggs, after Colton administered the gas. Wells learned how to make nitrous oxide and used it in his practice until he felt confident enough to demonstrate the technique at the nearest major medical centre, Boston. He gave a talk to a class of the Harvard Medical School and then administered the gas to one of them who, unfortunately

148

for Wells, cried out when a tooth was removed. Even though the student remembered nothing, Wells was dismissed as a charlatan.

It fell to William Morton, who had previously been Wells's student and had helped with the demonstration, to take the next steps.[xcvii] He was by then a medical student at Harvard and consulted, among others, his chemistry teacher, Charles Jackson. What part Jackson played in Morton's decision to use ether by inhalation became the subject of great controversy, but there is no doubt that it was Morton who studied it, tested it in animals and then tried it in his patients. Having been successful with these trials he offered to demonstrate his method to John Warren, surgeon at the Massachusetts General Hospital, and was invited to do so on 16th. October 1846. Before a large audience, Morton administered ether vapour to Gilbert Abbott before Warren removed a tumour from Abbott's neck without any sign of distress. A new era had dawned.

There is evidence that ether inhalation was used for surgery elsewhere in the USA as early as 1842, but those practitioners did nothing to communicate the news to others, making the events in Boston definitive. But scientific credit for the first modern use of ether was hotly disputed by Morton and Jackson and the argument raged for so long that the "Ether Monument", commemorating these events in Boston, bears no name.

News spread at the time at the rate a ship could travel, and so the first modern anaesthetics in the United Kingdom were given on 19th December 1846, one "probably" in Dumfries, though there is no contemporary record, and the other at 24 Gower Street, London.

Francis Boott, an expatriate American, learning of Morton's success through a letter from Boston, arranged for a Miss Lonsdale to have a tooth removed by James Robinson before a group which included Robert Liston. Liston, then London's leading surgeon, was so impressed that he arranged to perform an amputation under ether on 21st. December at University College Hospital. At the time, James Young Simpson, Professor of Midwifery in Edinburgh was on his annual visit to London to learn of the latest advances, and he became an enthusiastic advocate of anaesthesia.[xcviii] He pioneered inhalational analgesia for women in labour, was a major force in countering objections (both religious and medical) regarding its safety and use, and sought a better agent – discovering the anaesthetic properties of chloroform in 1847.

Objections to anaesthesia were to continue for some time, though they were apparently not very commonly made by patients in need of surgery. No one knew how these new agents worked, there was no substantial and documented experience to draw on to guide safe practice, and little understanding of normal physiology, let alone the potential adverse effects of anaesthesia. All these problems were often compounded by the delegation of administration of the anaesthetic to one of the more junior members of the surgical team. A few individuals developed a special interest, and - as mentioned earlier - John Snow, a London physician, published some of the earliest instructional literature. In 1853 he administered chloroform to Queen Victoria for the birth of Prince Leopold, and Princess Beatrice in 1857. This royal patronage silenced the last objections to anaesthesia.

The introduction of anaesthesia made surgery more bearable, but attempts to extend the scope of surgical techniques ran into another problem - infection. Operations were brief, and mostly minor, until antisepsis and later asepsis were developed. The challenges of managing servicemen injured in the two world wars made major contributions to the advancement of both surgery and anaesthetics.

Another challenge was that to perform surgery in the chest or abdominal cavities, relaxation of the muscles of the body wall and diaphragm was required. This could be achieved with difficulty using high concentrations of a general anaesthetic but the consequence was marked depression of circulation and respiration, usually with very delayed recovery of consciousness. Once again, the solution had been recorded years before; the

South American arrow poison 'curare' produces neuromuscular blockade and the required muscle relaxation. Introduced into mainstream use in 1942, its availability meant the amount of anaesthetic need only be enough to maintain unconsciousness. The method required anaesthetists to learn to insert tubes into the trachea to better allow mechanical ventilation of the lung to preserve gas exchange and, consequently, to 'control' breathing. In turn this led to the development of modern Intensive Care Units, and by about 1950 all the elements of modern anaesthesia were in place. Very few of the anaesthetics and medicines used in anaesthesia at that time are still in use, but their successors use the same principles.

With blood transfusion beginning in 1914, and the widespread availability of anaesthesia the route to ever more technically complex surgical procedures was at last open. New Zealander Harold Gillies pioneered modern plastic surgery for wounded British World War one soldiers. The first metallic hip replacement was performed in 1940, although outcomes would only improve radically with John Charnley's technical improvements at Wrightington Hospital just outside Wigan in the 1960s. Open heart surgery began to become, if not routine, at least possible in the late 1940s, and the first kidney transplant was 1954. When South African Christiaan Barnard performed the first heart transplant on 3rd December 1967 on the 54-year-old Louis Washkansky there was worldwide publicity, general astonishment, and anything seemed possible. I remember going to hear Christian Barnard lecture at the Leeds General Infirmary in about 1973 and his reception was more popstar than academic doctor.

As for medicines, after the second World War, the arrival of healthcare systems such as the National Health Service (NHS) and other insurance-based schemes in Europe created a much more structured system, both for the prescription of medicines and their reimbursement. In 1957, the NHS brought in the Pharmaceutical Price Regulation Scheme to allow reasonable return on investment for drug manufacturers, solidifying the incentive to invest in new medicines whilst allowing control of prices for those medicines until their patents expired.

The US pharmaceutical industry boomed after 1946, thanks to being part of the world's biggest and most dynamic post-war economy. Its growth was also helped by generous funding from the government, with the National Institutes of Health seeing its federal funding rise to nearly $100 million by 1956. This investment helped to fuel the development of many new medicines over the coming decades.

Meanwhile, as the industry grew wealthy thanks to its growing portfolio of products, the potential ethical conflicts of making money from selling healthcare products became increasingly apparent. George Merck addressed this question directly in 1950, proclaiming that: "*We try never to forget that medicine is for the people. It is not for the profits. The profits follow, and if we have remembered that, they have never failed to appear. The better we remember it, the larger they have been.*" In the second half of the 20th Century, as we shall see, these words were sometimes forgotten.

This still new industry required greater oversight, and following the thalidomide tragedy government regulations on medicines increased on both sides of the Atlantic. The 1964 Declaration of Helsinki put greater ethical structures onto clinical research, cementing the difference between production of scientific prescription medicines and other chemicals.[xcix]

But with new methods of mass production and increasing understanding of biology and chemistry, drug candidates began to be chosen systematically rather than discovered serendipitously. This "golden age" of drug development took place in the broader landscape of the post-war boom, a general context of massive improvements in standards of living and technological optimism that characterised the period from the 1950s to the 1980s, as well as the science-boosting competition of the Cold War with Russia. The processes of internationalisation begun before the second World War continued - in 1951 alone Pfizer opened subsidiaries in nine new countries.[c]

152

The list of novel drugs from the post-war era speaks for itself. The contraceptive pill, introduced in 1960, had an impact on society almost as massive as that of penicillin, enabling women to effectively control their fertility and beginning a trend towards sexual equality.

Valium (diazepam) was brought to the market by Roche in 1963, followed by the introduction of the monoamine oxidase inhibitor (MAOI) class of anti-depressants and the antipsychotic haloperidol. These medicines ushered in a new era in psychiatry with chemical treatments largely supplanting psychoanalytic approaches. The 1970s provided a first wave of cancer drugs – initially very blunt instruments with many serious side effects, but followed with an increasingly targeted process that continues to this day and which has significantly contributed to a doubling of cancer survival rates since the early 1970s, and with chemotherapy that is generally much better tolerated.

At the end of the Second World War the causes of the cardiovascular epidemic were unknown. The Framingham project and other cohort studies rapidly exposed the contributions of high blood pressure, smoking, and cholesterol. A whole range of cardiovascular medicines were developed, not just to treat the survivors of heart attacks and strokes, but also to be prescribed as prevention – medicines taken by well people who were deemed to be at risk of developing disease in the future. Even drugs as ubiquitous today as paracetamol and ibuprofen were only developed in 1956 and 1969 respectively.

As the 1970s ended, a shift began in the way the pharmaceutical industry focused its energies. In 1977, Tagamet, an ulcer medication, became a "modern blockbuster" drug, earning its manufacturers more than a billion US dollars a year and Sir James Black, a Scottish physician and pharmacologist, the Nobel Prize. This marked a new departure as companies competed to be the developer of the next big blockbuster, and many achieved great success. Eli Lilly released the first selective serotonin reuptake inhibitor (SSRI), Prozac, in 1987, another step-change in mental health. The first statin – a class of medicines which for the first time effectively lower cholesterol - was also approved in 1987, manufactured by Merck (MSD).

Medicine could do so much more, but there emerged many challenges. First among them was the sheer volume of scientific evidence now being produced. Before 1945, randomised controlled trials were rare. By 1962 they were a requirement of the US Food and Drug Administration for licensing of a medicine. But all types of research were increasing - a total of 8.1 million journal articles were indexed by the US National Library of Medicine between 1978 and 2001. Between 1978 to 1985 and 1994 to 2001, the annual number of articles increased 46%, from an average of 272,344 to 442,756 per year, and the total number of pages increased from 1.88 million pages per year during 1978 to 1985 to 2.79 million pages per year between 1994 to 2001.[ci]

The growth in the literature was particularly concentrated in clinical research. The volume of advancements in basic science reporting was overtaken with the application of science to humans - clinical care and public health. The proportion of all research published which was randomised clinical trials tripled from 1.9% between 1978 and 1985 to 6.2% between 1994 and 2001. This combination of increasing numbers of articles and increasing proportion of randomised trials resulted in a dramatic increase in the absolute number of randomised controlled trials over the three eras, from 5,174 RCTs per year during the first 8 years to an astonishing 24,724 trials per year by 2001. No wonder David Sackett was sceptical about how up to date practicing doctors could be.

Not surprisingly evidence emerged of the gap between the published evidence and the knowledge of that evidence by practicing clinicians. In 1985 clinicians said they needed evidence twice a week (for example, the accuracy of diagnostic tests, the ability of clinical symptoms, signs, or tests to accurately predict the course of a disease, or the comparative effectiveness and safety of interventions). They tended to get it from textbooks, journals, and colleagues.[cii] But when clinicians were directly observed and their actions dissected by interviewers after consultations, researchers found that important clinical questions arose twice for every three outpatients and five times for every inpatient.[ciii] The clinicians were working their way through their consultations with patients despite lots of uncertainty. Traditional sources of information were inadequate. They were either out-of-date textbooks,[civ] frequently wrong experts,[cv] or ineffective didactic continuing medical education.[cvi] Even if clinicians were motivated to look for the best available evidence for themselves, the best evidence was most likely hidden amongst a plethora of journal articles, which were too overwhelming in number and described research which was variable in the quality of its design, conduct and reporting to be of practical clinical use.[cvii]

Unsurprisingly, research then uncovered wide variability in clinical practice - variations in the care that was provided in different localities was produced and analysed in the US by Jack Wennberg and colleagues at Dartmouth College, New Hampshire. Variation in clinical practice wasn't new. In 1938 a British doctor, J. Alison Glover was the first to understand the significance of medical opinion in influencing the rate of surgery. He uncovered a more than four-fold variation in the rates of tonsillectomy in British school districts.[cviii]

Wennberg's work was initially funded by a grant from President Lyndon Johnson in 1967, and he and his colleagues then spent four decades exploring variations in care. Their work revealed alarming discrepancies in the incidence of medical and especially surgical procedures in the US which were institutional as well as regional. As Wennberg described,[cix]

"The situation in Boston and New Haven is an example. Residents of these two communities receive most of their care from physicians who are faculty members of some of the nation's most prestigious medical schools. One might assume that because of these credentials, the care received by these two populations would be of the highest quality. Yet how different the quality: for some operations the risk of surgery was much higher in New Haven than in Boston; for others, Bostonians were much more likely to undergo surgery. During the 1980s, the risk for a hysterectomy (to treat symptoms of

menopause) and for bypass surgery (to treat coronary artery disease) was nearly twice as high for New Haven residents as for Bostonians; while for carotid artery surgery (to prevent stroke) and hip replacement operations (for arthritis), the risk was 2.4 and 1.6 times greater, respectively, for residents of Boston.

"The common cause was traced to Glover's medical opinion—theories strongly held by small groups of physicians concerning medical efficacy or value. I learned through interviews with physicians in both communities that the differences in carotid endarterectomy rates could be attributed to a group of sceptical neurologists who simply didn't believe in the procedure, preferring aspirin to surgery for any New Haven patient that came to them for advice. By contrast (although relative to many other parts of the country the rates were low) the physicians in Boston had, on average, greater 'faith' in carotid artery surgery. The conservative medical management of coronary artery disease and symptoms of menopause was more popular in Boston, while clinicians in New Haven more often preferred surgical management. On the other hand, New Haven physicians were more conservative in the management of arthritis of the hip".

Wennberg's data was shocking and fascinating at the same time. As we shall see, the root cause lies in the vagaries of the ways humans make decisions. At the time the data ran completely counter to what conventional wisdom said they would be. If there was variation, everyone expected to see underservice in the rural hospital service areas remote from academic medical centres. But when they looked at the data, they found tremendous variation in every aspect of healthcare delivery, even among communities served by academic medical centres. Variation was not rare. It was everywhere and in all aspects of care. The basic premise - that medicine was driven by science and by physicians capable of making clinical decisions based on well-established fact and theory was simply incompatible with the data.

In other words, the doctors' decisions were different in one practice than in another, and in one locality to another. The decisions of the clinicians shaped the health care provided. This operated alongside the needs of the population they served, but the variation indicated that aspects were driven by the doctors and not solely by the needs of the population. Wennberg's research agreed with Archie Cochrane - neither money nor health care was being distributed wisely, effectively, or efficiently.

The extent of the variation raised serious quality issues, and variation in provided care became something to be remedied. The variation of provided care meant that not only did the quality of clinical care become to be seriously questioned, but it provided a lever to debate the costs of care. After the second World War, with all aspects of healthcare growing dramatically, except for the United States, national health insurance systems were established or significantly extended. Hospitals everywhere were expanded and modernised.

But despite the rapidly escalating costs of care, in both the United States and Europe, medical decisions before the 1980s were usually left to doctors. The exception was public health. From the start of the 20th Century, to prevent and treat infectious diseases doctors were constrained in a variety of ways - through standardised forms to provide public health data that were both uniform and comparable, and in the requirements to standardise the handling of technologies which carried potential dangers to patients, doctors or both, for example X-rays.

But steadily the new managed care organisations in the United States and the national health insurance systems in Europe all recognized they needed to try and slow or stem rising costs. The new generations of medicines and the massive expansion in surgical and other specialties were, and are, expensive. In the late 1980s and early 1990s some new medicines in particular and health care in general led to a situation where they came to be considered unaffordable by the publicly funded health systems. In the US the cost pressures were an increasing cause of bankruptcy to those who unfortunately developed serious illness when they were not covered by medical insurance.

This meant that the technical advancements in medical practice moved from being something to wonder at, to being a polarising topic in the public and political arenas. Medicine and its costs was transformed into an object of intense media scrutiny. Public accountability became an increasing issue. Archie Cochrane's messages about the lack of evidence for effectiveness and efficiency were finally taken to heart as costs and quality of care became a real concern. The difference now was that thanks to randomised controlled trials, the evidence about what worked and what did not work was now increasingly available. But that had not solved the problem. There were now new difficulties. Even when the evidence was available, clinical practice did not always follow the evidence. And as the boundaries of science were pushed, so the knowledge limits of doctors were under as much strain as the health care systems' finances.

There was overload.

CHAPTER TWELVE

Evidence and Measurement

Health care in the late 1980s and early 1990s had entered the best of times and the worst of times. Centuries of scientific and technical development had led to an explosion in understanding how the human body operated in health and disease. New ways of studying the causes of disease – Janet Elizabeth Lane-Claypon's cohort and case control studies – and new ways of demonstrating whether technical advances in diagnosis and treatment really were an advance – Austin Bradford Hill and Ronald Fisher's randomised controlled trials – were everywhere and were transforming medicine. And the knowledge explosion had been exponential in the four decades that followed the end of the Second World War.

Life expectancy in England in 1920 was 56 years for men and 59 years for women.[cx] By 1990 it was 73 years for men and 79 years for women. Much of this was down to public health measures – clean water and sanitation, immunisation, and improving nutrition. The under-5 mortality rate in London decreased from 74.5% (in 1730–1749) to 31.8% (in 1810 –1829) - all this long before the science and technology of modern medicine could make any impact.

But the science and the technology did begin to play their part - notably in improving mortality rates in infancy and childhood from infections. More and better vaccines, and then later antibiotics, removed the dread fear of losing one or more children in early life. Better general education, better employment prospects, and better and more widely available methods of contraception meant that the crude birth rate (per 1000 people) fell in the UK from 18 in 1960 to 12 in 1977.[cxi]

Better access to health care began in the UK with Lloyd George's National Insurance Act of 1911. Lloyd George emulated similar schemes in Germany; he wanted Britain to compete with Germany in matters other than armaments. Behind the scheme was the notion that access to health care would mean a fitter male workforce, which in turn would be better for the economy. Dependents of working men were

160

initially not covered by the schemes. But between the First and Second World Wars a patchwork of local services developed.[cxii] For example, local authorities ran midwifery and child health services, the school health service and TB sanatoria. Charitable hospitals provided some care too. But it was of course 1948 until there was universal access to health care in the UK.

As health care grew, especially after the creation of the NHS, the research sector grew significantly as well - especially in the more prosperous post-war United States where government funding for research rose to unprecedented levels. Total research spending in American medical schools, adjusted for inflation, grew almost fifty-fold between 1946 and 1993, with the federal government providing about 75 percent of the funds through the National Institutes of Health (NIH).[cxiii] Pharmaceutical companies contributed additional funding, with an expectation of a significant financial return on that investment, that eventually surpassed the NIH's.

With the rising costs of healthcare, there was a constant debate about where the additional funding was to come from, and whether the NHS was providing value for money, or even providing the best possible care consistently and everywhere. These were questions across health systems internationally, of course, and not unique to the United Kingdom or the NHS.

In many ways medicine was playing catch up. Whilst there was now lots of evidence published it was incomplete, of variable quality, and was scattered across multiple, densely written scientific publications. Usual medical practice remained more heavily influenced by what seemed to work in practice and especially what a body of respected medical colleagues would do in similar circumstances.

Indeed, since 1954 in the UK doing what other doctors would do had been a key defence against medical negligence. According to the Bolam principle, legally a doctor would not be guilty of negligence if s/he acted in accordance with a practice accepted as proper by a responsible body of medical wo/men

161

skilled in that particular art.[cxiv] Putting it the other way round, a doctor would not be negligent, if s/he acted in accordance with such a practice, merely because there is a body of opinion that takes a contrary view.

But the practice of medicine based upon this John Wayne-esque mantra of *"a doctor's gotta do what a doctor's gotta do"* was crumbling. The evidence of practice variation was inconvertible and began the undermining of the notion of an entirely self-regulated profession. Pharmaceutical companies had grown rich and large, and spent millions on selling their latest wares to the people who held the keys to healthcare spending – the doctors. In some ways it is understandable that they would use marketing techniques which included partial representations of their data which favoured their product in such marketing. It was a pharmaceutical Wild West as companies sought to outdo their rivals' sales' trajectories in the pursuit of promoting their latest "blockbuster" medicine.

Many health care systems lacked basic management information about what was spent and on what and how much good it did for the health of the population. Whilst variation in provided care was now obvious when it was measured, it was less obvious what was warranted variation (due, say, to real differences in the health needs of the population) and what was unwarranted variation (and apparently due to differences in provided treatments that did not actually benefit the population health).

Therefore, the rise of evidence-based medicine in the early 1990s was well-timed. In part it was due to a technological development. The landscape of the medical literature being hidden away in thousands of different scientific paper journals was transformed by computing and the Internet. Since 1879 and George Billings, the US National Library of Medicine (NLM) had published *Index Medicus*, a monthly guide to medical articles in thousands of journals. The huge volume of bibliographic citations was manually compiled. In 1957 the staff of the NLM started to plan the mechanisation of the *Index Medicus*, and by the end of 1964 *Index Medicus* was computerised. In late 1971, an online version called Medline became available for online searching from remote medical libraries. This early system covered 239 journals and boasted that it could support "as many as 25 simultaneous online users" remotely logged-in from distant medical libraries at one time. This system remained primarily in the hands of libraries and librarians, with researchers able to submit pre-programmed search tasks and obtain results on printouts, but rarely able to interact with the NLM computer output in real-time.[cxv]

The availability of personal computers and especially the development of the Internet and world wide web meant that after the evidence had been collated, it was possible for anyone to access the best available evidence from anywhere with a computer and a modem. The change from largely books and paper journals holding the reference material to it becoming electronic happened very quickly. Sir Tim Berners-Lee had the first web-page in 1991. Within a few years websites were ubiquitous for all public sector organisations and private companies, and in June 1997 a free public version of Medline called PUBMED became available – switched on in a public ceremony by US Vice President Al Gore. Adoption was rapid. By 1999 I was home working, sending critically appraised summaries of the best available evidence in Word documents from North Yorkshire to the British Medical Journal in London.

There had been more developments in methods which could compile existing evidence now that there was evidence to compile. Summarising results from different but similar studies eventually became the formalised technique referred to today as systematic review and meta-analysis.

Karl Pearson appears to have been the first to apply methods to combine observations from different clinical studies. He was asked to analyse data comparing infection and mortality among soldiers who had volunteered for inoculation against typhoid fever in various places across the British Empire with that of other soldiers who had not volunteered. In 1904 he published the

163

results in the *British Medical Journal* with a table in which each study was assigned its own line showing its measure of effect, together with a measure of the within-study uncertainty. The last line gives a pooled estimate of the effect when all the studies were combined — his "meta-analysis".

It was largely the failure to use clinical trials to evaluate clinical treatments which was responsible for there being no further need for meta-analysis within medicine for around 70 years. But as the number of trials and other types of studies increased, finding all the existing research on the topic of interest, identifying the well-done research (the "systematic review"), and then adding the results of all the similar studies together (the "meta-analysis") slowly became to be recognised as a very useful technique in what was to become evidence-based medicine.

Conceptually it enabled advocates of evidence-based medicine to acknowledge all the previous high-quality research on a clinical topic. That gave them ammunition to resist the arguments of their critics who decried evidence-based medicine on the basis that it failed to acknowledge previous research and researchers. There were two stark choices – ignore all previous research on the assumption that it had not been conducted to modern standards and undertake a new randomised controlled trial, or alternatively identify all previous research with a systematic review, and then use the research which had been well designed, well-conducted and well-reported to construct a meta-analysis. The systematic review and meta-analysis won hands down as long as the quality of the historic research passed muster. This was not least on ethical grounds - if previous research had shown that a particular treatment was superior to other treatment, usual care, or placebo then it would have been unethical to conduct a controlled trial which randomised patients to a control group.

Two meta-analyses were particularly influential in establishing it as a worthwhile technique. The first followed the randomised trial conducted by Peter Elwood, Archie Cochrane and their Cardiff colleagues to assess whether aspirin reduced recurrences of heart attack. The results were suggestive of a beneficial effect but were not statistically convincing. Additional trials reported in the next few years, and each individual study showed marginal benefits for aspirin, which could still be attributed to chance. Elwood and Cochrane assembled and synthesised their results in collaboration with the British medical statistician Richard Peto. The meta-analysis left no doubt that aspirin could reduce the risk of a recurrence of a heart attack, and the results were published in 1980 in an anonymous *Lancet* editorial.[cxvi]

The second influential meta-analysis was performed by Tom Chalmers, Elliot Antman and colleagues and it was published in the Journal of the American Medical Association on 8th July 1992.[cxvii] This was, of course was a mere 33 years since Tom Chalmers had published his trial of hepatitis which subsequently inspired David Sackett. The 1992 paper introduced cumulative meta-analysis - performing a new meta-analysis every time the results of a new, topic relevant clinical trial is published. The meta-analysis therefore showed sequentially the results of all the previous trials up to a point in time, and then how this changed as more trial data was published. Chalmers, Antman and colleagues compared those results with the recommendations of the experts for various treatments for myocardial infarction. They found huge time-lags between the meta-analytic results of proven effectiveness in the randomised trials and the recommendations of experts writing textbooks. Review articles often failed to mention important advances or exhibited delays in recommending effective preventive measures. In some cases, treatments that had no effect on mortality or were potentially harmful had continued to be recommended in apparently gold-standard textbooks written by clinical experts. It was a situation that nobody could reasonably defend any longer.

Inspired by Archie Cochrane's call for up-to-date collections of all relevant randomised controlled trials in the field of healthcare in the 1970s, Iain Chalmers set out to make it a reality. In 1978 he set up the National Perinatal Epidemiology Unit in Oxford. Initially staying close to his clinical specialty of obstetrics,

Chalmers led the construction of the Oxford Database of Perinatal Trials and in 1989 published the two volumes of the groundbreaking *Effective Care in Pregnancy in Childbirth* which summarized the evidence in that area.

Cochrane died in 1988 but a few years later in 1993 Chalmers, on the back of universal praise for *Effective Care in Pregnancy in Childbirth*, obtained research funding from the NHS Research and Development programme to establish a "Cochrane Centre". The aims were to collaborate with others, in the UK and elsewhere, to facilitate systematic reviews of randomised controlled trials across all areas of healthcare. The Cochrane Collaboration, of which Iain Chalmers was the first Director, grew rapidly - such was the enthusiasm for evidence-based medicine in general and for systematic reviews in particular. Over 30,000 people in many countries and specialties - many of them volunteers - are now involved in preparing and maintaining systematic reviews and meta-analyses of randomised trials and other evidence within an international, non-profit organization covering all areas of clinical medicine. At the last count there were 53 reviews groups covering different specialisms within medicine and more than 8,000 Cochrane Reviews published. It should be a matter of national shame that in 2024 the UK Cochrane Centre closed due to the withdrawal of government funding.

Immediately the new problem is obvious. Even when the evidence is collected together, and the best of it identified and summarised, doctors would still end up with more information than they can possibly read, remember and recall just at the time that they and their patient needs it.

But such thoughts were for the future as evidence-based medicine gathered pace in the early 1990s. Sackett and colleagues wrote their famous BMJ editorial in 1996 that *"The practice of evidence based medicine means integrating individual clinical expertise with the best available external clinical evidence from systematic research"* and that *"Increased expertise is reflected in many ways, but especially in more effective and efficient diagnosis and in the more thoughtful identification and compassionate use of individual patients' predicaments, rights, and preferences in making clinical decisions about their care."* Deservedly that single editorial is now cited in hundreds of thousands of other research papers.[cxviii]

Enthusiasts for evidence-based medicine (EBM), me included, saw it as necessary for delivering high quality care for individual patients, and also as a tool for addressing unwarranted variation within medicine. The practice of EBM was defined early on and involves a process of lifelong, self-directed learning in which caring for patients creates the need for important information about clinical and other health care issues. EBM recognises that the research literature is constantly changing – new research findings may mean that the best treatment today may change next month or next year. The task of staying current, although never easy, was envisaged as being made much simpler by teaching doctors to track down and critically appraise evidence and incorporate it into every-day clinical practice.

The practice of EBM traditionally involves five steps:-
1.   Converting information needs about an individual patient into answerable questions.
2.   Finding the best evidence with which to answer the questions.
3.   Critically appraising the evidence for its validity and usefulness
4.   Applying the results of the appraisal into clinical practice
5.   Evaluating performance - checking that the appraisal results were now a part of routine care for patients with the relevant condition.

As an example, imagine a four-month-old baby admitted to hospital with viral bronchiolitis. Bronchiolitis is a common lower respiratory tract infection caused by the respiratory syncytial virus (RSV) that affects babies and young children under 2 years old. Around 1 in 3 children in the UK will develop bronchiolitis during their first year of life and it most commonly affects babies between 3 and 6 months of age. Vaccination programmes against RSV are likely in the near future.

167

The early symptoms of bronchiolitis are like those of a common cold, such as a runny nose and a cough. Most cases are mild and clear up within two to three weeks without the need for treatment, although some children have severe symptoms and need hospital treatment. A high temperature, a dry and persistent cough, rapid and noisy breathing with wheezing and difficulty feeding may be reasons for admission to hospital.

The child's symptoms get progressively worse and the child's parents, knowing a little about asthma wonder whether giving corticosteroids might help their baby. As their doctor, in your training you have always been told not to prescribe corticosteroids for bronchiolitis - but being an advocate for EBM, you decide to investigate the matter for yourself.

Step 1: The key components of your clinical question would be created using the acronym PICO:-
Patient or problem: 4-month-old baby with viral bronchiolitis.
Intervention: corticosteroids.
Comparison: no corticosteroids.
Outcomes: clinical score, length of hospital stay.
In other words, *"In a 4 month old baby with viral bronchiolitis, does the administration of corticosteroids compared with not giving corticosteroids improve clinical score and reduce length of hospital stay?"*

Step 2: the next step is to find the best evidence that will help you answer the question. Traditional sources of information such as textbooks and journals may be out of date. Asking colleagues or "experts" will be quick and potentially requires little effort on your part. But again, the quality of information obtained from this source will be variable. The EBM approach involves searching the online electronic bibliographic databases such as Medline, which allows hundreds of thousands of articles to be searched in a relatively short period of time.

Studies looking at how well doctors could undertake such searches showed that they often conducted searches which resulted finding in too few or too many articles. Too few and they risked missing the best evidence; too many and there was too much information for the search to be useful. An early component of EBM was running basic training courses in database search skills so health care professionals could accurately find the best evidence.

Step 3: Having found some relevant and published research, the next step would be to appraise the evidence for its validity and clinical usefulness. The quality of each study may not be universally high. If the research has not been well designed, conducted and reported then putting unreliable evidence into practice could lead to harm being caused or limited resources being wasted.

Research evidence needs to be appraised regarding three main areas: validity, importance, and applicability to the patient or patients of interest. Critical appraisal provides a structured but simple method for assessing research evidence in all three areas. Developing critical appraisal skills involves learning how to ask a few key questions about the validity of the evidence and its relevance to a particular patient or group of patients. Health care professionals needed to be taught these new skills and they were key components of the new EBM courses, and critical appraisal even penetrated patchily into routine postgraduate training and examinations in some but not all specialties.

But the harsh reality is that the pace and effort required to survive clinical as a doctor means that few to none will have the time, energy and skills required to undertake steps 1, 2 and 3 of the traditional EBM model. And then there is Step 4:-

Step 4: Then, having decided that a piece of evidence is valid and important, the crucial step is how to decide whether that evidence can be applied to an individual patient.

Looking back with the benefit of almost 30 years of hindsight, this last step was given least attention in the development of evidence-based medicine. The original definition of EBM in the Sackett BMJ paper had considering the patient's own personal values and circumstances front and centre. But to this day, the evidence-based movement has concentrated on collecting evidence into systematic reviews and clinical guidelines, and then making recommendations which usually are expected to be applied to everyone with the condition. Only in the last few years is there some recognition that more work is required in the decision making for the individual patient. We are only now beginning to work on Sackett et al's original definition. Until recently no one was working out how best to use the best available evidence optimally in consultations alongside clinical expertise and the patient's values and preferences. Instead, evidence-based medicine has spent the best part of 30 years creating information overload.

There has been great progress in two areas where the effort has been expended. Methodological and statistical approaches to better undertake systematic review and meta-analysis are now well established. And how to best collect the best of the evidence together into clinical guidelines has well described, formal processes. There can be no doubt about the importance and value of having the best of the evidence available to inform decision making, at the level of the population, whether for diagnosis or for treatment. The evidence is absolutely necessary, but alone it is not sufficient for decision making with individuals. We will move onto cognitive psychology - how humans use information to make decisions shortly.

Discussing the efficacy and risks of treatment is easy to say, but how to do it optimally is a highly complex skill set. And with potentially thousands of systematic reviews and hundreds of clinical guidelines, how to get up to date and then stay up to date as a practicing clinician is another skill set requiring an optimal approach to be developed. We shall cover that issue too shortly since it also involves cognitive psychology.

It is easy to see why the areas of decision making with individual patients and optimising knowledge management have been relatively neglected until recently. When the best available evidence is scattered across individual scientific papers in

170

multiple medical journals it is only right to make the bringing together of that evidence with systematic reviews and guidelines the priority. In the early 1990s it was quite common for babies with viral bronchiolitis to be given corticosteroids. Thanks to evidence-based medicine very few babies will now receive that ineffective and potentially harmful treatment because, in the UK at least, the national guidelines are very clear that corticosteroids and several other treatments used for bronchiolitis in the past should no longer be given.

In addition to there being a need to bring the evidence together, the other early driver for EBM was to use it to address variation in clinical practice. This was not just about more people having their gall bladders or tonsils removed in one area than another. When in some areas, and in some health systems in most areas, many people with diabetes are not getting their necessary checks to keep them well and to potentially prevent the very serious potential complications of diabetes then there is a serious issue of the quality of care being provided for large numbers of people.

What interventions might usefully improve the quality of provided care was an important question for the future. At the time there was much angst about high quality evidence not being implemented for everybody and everywhere. According to a 2003 report from the US National Committee for Quality Assurance, 57,000 lives were lost annually because US physicians had not been using evidence-based medicine to guide their care. "*We're literally dying, waiting for the practice of medicine to catch up with medical knowledge,*" said Margaret O'Kane, president of NCQA. The report, *The State of Health Care Quality 2003*, said that the deaths "*should not be confused with those attributable to medical errors or lack of access to health care. This report shows that a thousand Americans die each week because the care they get is not consistent with the care that medical science tells us they should get.*"[cxix]

In the face of such serious issues, it seems entirely reasonable that the early priorities in EBM were gathering evidence about what really worked and what did not work for patients in one place so it was accessible. Focusing on technical developments which would enable evidence to be better collated was also entirely reasonable at the time. All this was helped by the fact the leaders of the evidence-based movement were intellectually strong in those technical, numbers-based aspects.

But the downside was little or no discussion about how to actually use the evidence in individual consultations. And there was little or no discussion about the truth at the core of EBM which was that the evidence could only indicate how the probabilities changed if the evidence was or was not used. There was no way of predicting whether an individual patient would or would not benefit. Such subtle but critical aspects were for the future. At the time, it was all about collecting the best evidence into accessible formats, and applying the evidence to everyone with the disease. This reduced variation but meant little or no thought about what was best for an individual patient.

Step 5 of EBM was evaluating performance. There was no getting around the inconvenient truth that data on clinical performance of doctors in the early and mid-1990s was largely absent. The work I did with prescribing data in North Yorkshire in the 1990s was novel and met some resistance. More was needed to explicitly demonstrate that the health system as a whole and individuals within it were providing competent care. Formal auditing of performance would be needed to show whether the EBM approach was being applied consistently, and whether it was improving patient care.

In the UK, clinical audit was rarely undertaken in the UK until 1989. But the concept was not new. As early as 1750BCE King Hammurabi (the sixth King of Babylon) instigated audit for clinicians by instructing them to measure their care against agreed standards. The detailed data analysis carried out by Florence Nightingale between 1853-55 during the Crimean War which improved sanitary conditions and resulted in decreasing the mortality rates from 40% to 2% was a form of clinical audit.

But it is twentieth century healthcare thinkers such as Ernest Codman and Avedis Donabedian who are generally regarded as the true forefathers of clinical audit. Codman, an orthopaedic surgeon at Harvard Medical School took the, at the time, unprecedented step in 1912 of monitoring surgical outcomes. Donabedian was an academic at the University of Michigan who in 1966 proposed his conceptual model that provided a framework for evaluating quality in healthcare. He collated the growing literature of health services research as it appeared through the 1950s and early 1960s and presented his findings in a lengthy paper with the title "Evaluating the Quality of Medical Care".[cxx]

This summation and analysis brought him immediate fame and is still widely cited and read. In it he sets out the necessity of examining the quality of health provision in the aspects of structure, process, and outcome. In 20 years of scholarship Donabedian strove to define every aspect of quality in health systems and proposed models for its measurement in over 100 papers and 11 books.

Yet despite a focus on measurement and health systems management in all his work, Donabedian recognised that there was a difference between providing and measuring the quality of health care for a group of people and providing health care and measuring its quality for an individual. He wrote that *"Systems awareness and systems design are important for health professionals, but are not enough. They are enabling mechanisms only. It is the ethical dimension of* **individuals** *that is essential to a system's success.* **Ultimately, the secret of quality is love.**"

Nightingale, Codman and Donabedian all played a central role in highlighting the importance of evaluating and measuring healthcare. Eventually their work became UK health policy when in 1989 the Conservative Government published the "Working for Patients" White Paper which formally introduced clinical audit to the NHS.

What started out in 1989 as a reflective opportunity for doctors to improve their care has evolved dramatically. National clinical audits are now mandatory and regularly published, most healthcare staff have audit written into their job contract, patients can increasingly access audit results and the healthcare regulator, the Care Quality Commission, routinely ask for clinical audit data whenever they carry out their inspections. But it is all based on what has happened to groups of people. It is much harder to measure the "love" involved in caring for another sick or worried individual.

Despite some dissenting voices, there was a general acceptance that evidence-based medicine was a better basis for modern medical practice than the alternatives - intuition, emulating unthinkingly what others or so-called "experts" do, unsystematic clinical experience, or using superficially rational, but often flawed basic scientific principles such as how the body worked at cellular and chemical levels in health and disease to guide treatment without measuring whether such approaches actually meant patients lived better or longer.

It is difficult to now contemplate that only thirty-five years ago, being able to readily access the best evidence was difficult if not impossible for almost all clinicians. There was no Internet, no smart phones and very few personal computers. Measurement of almost anything important in health care was a rare event, and there were only the first whisperings about the new science of health economics. And there were no clinical guidelines. All that was about to change.

CHAPTER THIRTEEN

NICE

Documents summarising how to diagnose and treat a specified condition have been in use throughout the history of medicine. Ancient medical textbooks were written for that purpose. However, modern textbooks are written by one or more authors and usually state considered opinions rather than being an up to date "state of the evidence'. The moment a textbook is published it is potentially out of date, as research continually progresses. Where there are references to published studies, it is often difficult to know how those references were identified. Did the authors undertake a comprehensive literature search before writing the content? Or did they write the content and then seek published research which confirmed their existing opinion?

Modern clinical guidelines should identify the most important questions related to an area of clinical practice, search for and critically appraise the evidence, and summarise the decision options. Well-constructed guidelines are based on a rigorous examination of all the valid and relevant current evidence, and it is very easy to produce a poor guideline. Even in 2021, when they were reviewed only a third of guidelines met acceptable standards for their development processes.[cxxi]

In the UK one of the earliest guidelines produced was for the diagnosis and management of asthma. It was produced by the British Thoracic Society in 1990, largely in response to the gap between the effectiveness of new corticosteroid inhalers which prevented asthma attacks, and their underuse in the real world. There were avoidable asthma deaths, and the guideline aimed to do something about that toll by collating the best available evidence and making a large number of recommendations that purported to represent best practice. This began the trend still seen in some countries for specialist medical organisations and sometimes pharmaceutical companies to be drivers of guideline development.

At one level, guidelines can be seen as an essential step towards improving the quality of care - compiling key knowledge and treatment options in a single document which if translated into clinical practice systematically would reduce unwarranted variation in care. At another level they can also be seen as a post-World War II reaction to standardise care as healthcare became part of the political arena, and because of that created an undermining of clinical autonomy. Representatives of specialist medical organisations might bring much technical knowledge to groups developing guidelines. But they might also potentially bring a resistance to recommending what the best evidence said should be usual practice. If the evidence pointed to a need to change, and those same representatives were currently using a now out of date treatment with their patients and had been doing so for many years, how easy would it be for them to follow the evidence? To repeat - for humans, learning stuff is hard and unlearning stuff is harder.

For many years, the effect of the evidence-based medicine movement was that there was little emphasis on where patient values and preferences sat in relation to all this activity. The focus was on critically appraising published research, differentiating important and well conducted research from the rest, and compiling summaries of evidence as guidelines or systematic reviews.

There were some discussions about how an individual clinician could be expected to get up to date, stay up to date, and if necessary, change the care they were providing to what now amounted to best practice. But aside from compiling the evidence, there was a rising concern about the cost of health care, pressure on health budgets, and in time what became cost-effectiveness.

Unsurprisingly, a new branch of economics was developing. According to the definition proposed by Lionel Robbins, *"Economics is the science which studies human behaviour as a relationship between ends and scarce means which have alternative uses.*[cxxii] I would emphasise three things that flow from that definition - economics is about human behaviour, it is about matching "ends" or "outcomes" to the available resources which are limited and, given that there are alternatives, there are decisions to be made.

The history of economics goes back to at least the Greeks, and their interest in the wealth of nations was continued by many including of course by Adam Smith in 1776.[cxxiii] The development of modern health economics is often credited to a 1963 paper by Kenneth Arrow, whose career spanned the RAND Corporation, Harvard, Stanford, and the Nobel Prize for economics in 1972.[cxxiv]

Arrow drew conceptual distinctions between health and other goods. Factors that distinguish health economics from other areas of economic study include extensive government intervention, intractable uncertainty including what would happen to individuals as opposed to the average benefit in a group, health care providers generally having more specialist knowledge about a condition and its treatment that do patients or those responsible for organising the health care system and paying for it, barriers to entry or to practice (for example, at the time only doctors could prescribe), the health or disease of one person may affect others, and in many health systems the presence of a third-party agent such as doctors themselves and insurance companies.

Arrow identified that in healthcare the third-party agent (the health care professional, usually a doctor) makes "purchasing" decisions (for example, whether to order a diagnostic test, prescribe a medicine, perform surgery) while being insulated from the price of the product or service. It should be noted that, typical of its time, the decision-making Arrow described was considered the sole responsibility the doctor and not the patient.

Despite the wider availability of technical knowledge about health and disease following the development of the Internet, there still usually exists a knowledge gap between a doctor and a patient - creating a situation of distinct advantage for the doctor, which is called asymmetric information. When the emotional context of being the ill person is added to the asymmetric information there is usually a significant power imbalance in consultations.[cxxv]

Externalities arise sometimes when considering decision making in health and healthcare, notably in the context of infectious disease. For example, taking antibiotics or getting a vaccination affects people other than that patient because of the risk of the development of antibiotic resistance or the transmission of infections which might then be a serious problem for the general population.

By 1977, Milton Weinstein and William Stason from the Harvard School of Public Health were publishing papers on the foundations for applying cost-effectiveness analysis to medical practice. They argued that the inevitable limits on health spending that applied even in the relatively wealthy United States – by far the world's biggest spender on health care – meant that *"we, as a nation, will have to think very carefully about how to allocate the resources we are willing to make available"*.[cxxvi]

Decisions had to be guided "by considerations of cost in relation to expected benefits." There were, however, ways of doing that, they argued, including using "Quality-Adjusted Life Years" a concept that became known for short as the QALY. Weistein and Stason were aware of work in the late 1960s and early 1970s by Alan Williams, a professor of health economics at the University of York, who had already started on the development of the QALY.[cxxvii] The QALY was a means of measuring the potential impacts of treatment by assessing not just the extra year or years of life an intervention might bring, but the quality of that life in terms of freedom from or reduction in pain, or the ability to perform basic activities of daily living such as feeding oneself or being mobile, or having a decent state of mental health. Crucially, it allowed a monetary value to be put on that quality of life in a way that provided a measure that could be used across all types of health intervention - whether from a new diagnostic test, a new drug, a new surgical procedure, or a new psychological treatment. This, at least theoretically, allowed the comparison of the value of one treatment against another.

To put this very simply, a cheap, easily administered, highly effective vaccine for polio, a sometimes-lethal disease that also

179

sometimes leaves profound disability in those who survive, has a very low cost per QALY even though millions of doses of it may be needed to protect all the individuals in the population. In terms of cost-effectiveness, it becomes obvious that a health system should fund it.

By contrast, a new medicine that costs many hundreds of thousands of pounds, dollars or euros for a course of treatment, but which extends life for only a few months in only a proportion of those treated, has a higher cost per QALY. That brings questions about whether health systems should fund such treatments over more cost-effective interventions even if the new treatment is more effective.

Those last eight words sound counter-intuitive; an example may help.

In a town, let us say that the available budget for treating condition X is £100,000. Treatment A is the standard treatment. It costs £10 a course and it cures 40% of people with Condition X. So, for the £100,000 we can treat 10,000 people and we cure 4,000.

Treatment B is a new treatment for Condition X. It costs £50 a course. It cures 50% of people, and so is clearly more effective. If you were a patient, you would want Treatment B, and if you were the doctor treating your patients with Condition X you would want to be using Treatment B too. However, for the available budget, if we use Treatment B we can only treat 2,000 people, and we would cure 1,000 people. Treatment A, despite being less effective, cures more people in the population if the budget is limited.

It is an uncomfortable truth that however rich a country is all budgets, including those for health, are ultimately limited. There are choices to be made over when that limit is reached, but there is a limit.

There might be some other factors to consider. The nature of Condition X would be one. What if Condition X was a fungal infection of a toenail? The downside of a treatment failure is the toenail still does not look very attractive. But largely that is the extent of failure. That might mean that many people would think it reasonable to have a policy of using Treatment A first. But what if the condition being treated was breast cancer? From the individual's perspective, most people would fight to get Treatment B – unless their general condition was so poor that they felt they were unlikely to benefit or they found the side effects intolerable. Health economics shines a light on the difference between "What is best for the population" versus "What is the best treatment for this individual"

QALYs are slightly more complicated. A person's state of health is expressed on a scale ranging from 0 to 1, in which 0 represents "death" and 1 "perfect health". The QALY assumes that a year of life lived in perfect health is worth 1 QALY (1 Year of Life × State of Health of 1 = 1 QALY). A year of life lived in a state of less than this perfect health is worth less than 1. QALYs are therefore expressed in terms of "years lived in perfect health": half a year lived in perfect health is equivalent to 0.5 QALYs (0.5 years × State of Health of 1). This would be the same as 1 year of life lived in a state of health of 0.5 (1 year × State of Health of 0.5).

So, we find from a study that when we treat Condition Y with standard Treatment C, the average length of survival is 2 years and the average state of health is 0.5. That gives us 1 QALY, and the cost of treatment per patient is £1000. But when we use Treatment D for the same condition, the average length of survival is 4 years, and the state of health is 0.9. That gives us a QALY of 3.6 (4 x 0.9). The cost per patient with Treatment D is £1500 per patient. So per patient we gain 2.6 QALYs at an extra cost of £500. The incremental cost is £500 / 2.6 which is £192.61 per QALY gained.

It would be wonderful to be able to give the best treatment for every single patient with every single condition but that does not reflect reality. Imagine Disease Z which until now is incurable. There is a new Treatment E, but it costs £1billion a week, and there are thousands of people a week needing treatment. A course of treatment costing £1billion a week for many weeks for thousands of patients with Disease Z would be unaffordable by any health system. Of course, if the patient was us or one of our family we would want the treatment, but no health system can afford it.

In 1984 Bryan Jennett, a neurosurgeon from Glasgow, followed in Archie Cochrane's footsteps with his Rock Carling lecture, subsequently published as a book. Entitled *High Technology Medicine: Benefits and Burdens* it questioned not just the value in terms of health outcomes from some of the most recent high technology interventions, but also their cost-effectiveness.[cxxviii] The previous year Sir Roy Griffiths in his management inquiry into the NHS evoked the third part agent when he declared that hospital doctors needed to take responsibility for their budgets because *"their decisions largely dictate the use of all resources, and they must accept the management responsibility which goes with clinical freedom"*. Implicit in that was the requirement to spend money to best effect. Griffiths noted, disapprovingly, that the economic evaluation of clinical practice was still "extremely rare".[cxxix]

Then in 1991 as evidence-based medicine was beginning to take off, Sir Michael Peckham became the first director of research and development for the NHS, based in the Department of Health. After establishing the UK Cochrane Centre in 1993 with Iain Chalmers as Director, the following year he set up a Centre for Reviews and Dissemination at York University. This was established to push Cochrane reviews and other findings out into the NHS through 'Effective Healthcare Bulletins'. Health Technology Assessment units were also established at several other universities to evaluate, unsurprisingly, new technologies being introduced - be they medicines, tests or operations. Sometimes the evidence review would be of existing treatments for which were no longer supported by modern science. The department also began talking to the drug industry about the issue, and in 1994, in conjunction with the Association of the British Pharmaceutical Industry, it issued the first joint guidance on the economic evaluation of pharmaceuticals.

Throughout the 1990s, economic arguments about the cost of health care, how efficient current health systems were, and whether all the new technical developments offered good value and were affordable circulated at an increasing volume. Margaret Thatcher's 1990 health reforms introduced a quasi-market into health with health authorities and GP Fundholders able to purchase for their patients to meet the health needs of their populations from whoever they wanted.

There were some early efficiency gains from GP Fundholders who were no longer passive third-party agents in the delivery of health care. Suddenly costs and cost-effectiveness mattered to these doctors. And the reforms introduced the role of medical adviser in each health authority with one of their major remits to take data describing variations in prescribing by all general practitioners into every practice. I took up one of those posts in 1993.

Evidence-based medicine had found a good fit in relation to prescribing. There was an increasing number of useful randomised controlled trials demonstrating the value or otherwise of established and new medicines. And there was plenty of variation which could be a legitimate subject of discussions. Clinical practice, however, did not automatically change in response to rational evidence. It was the first modern, concrete example that showed changing clinical practice was not as simple as providing rational information and expecting highly intelligent and very hard-working doctors to change their practice and follow the evidence. Once again, unlearning stuff is hard for humans.

The Thatcher health reforms and the debate about funding and affordability that surrounded them brought into sharper focus the historic issue that health services had never been evenly distributed across the country since the NHS was created in 1948. But now it was evident that patients, very occasionally quite literally on different sides of a street, might find they did or did not have access to certain treatments or procedures, depending on the decision of their GP Fundholder or health authority. This led to complaints about a "postcode lottery", and those complaints became increasingly fraught politically. That issue would lead to the creation of the National Institute for Clinical Excellence, soon to be known to many just by its acronym NICE.

I ended up working for NICE and worked alongside NICE colleagues whilst at the National Prescribing Centre during NICE's creation and its early years – all told about 14 years. It is now the National Institute for Health and Care Excellence but retains NICE as its acronym. Despite my personal experience, much of the following history relating to NICE's creation is closely based on an account set out in 2016 by Nicholas Timmins, the Health Correspondent of the Financial Times, John Appleby from the Kings Fund, and NICE's first Chair Professor Sir Michael Rawlins. It is a story worth retelling - all be it in abbreviated form.

A growing part of the debate - in health care generally and about new medicines especially[cxxx] involved cost-effectiveness. The underlying argument was what the economists define as "opportunity cost" - money spent from a limited budget on one thing, cannot be spent on another. Something else goes by the wayside. And, without careful health economic analysis, the value of new and, on the face of it, expensive treatments not provided might be greater than established practice that the money was currently spent on.

A Conservative government white paper in 1996 began with a lengthy defense of the NHS and of its tax funded nature, arguing that the model was sustainable not least because "*there continues to be scope for funding desirable improvements in part by offsetting savings elsewhere, such as reducing expenditure on those treatments which are now recognised to be less clinically and cost-effective*". [cxxxi] And in the grass roots NHS, the new purchasers in the NHS – the health authorities and GP fundholders – felt the need for advice on what to buy. As early as 1991, the then Wessex region of the NHS had established a "Development and Evaluation Committee" to provide just that, evaluating not just new technologies but some aspects of current practice.

By the end of 1994, the Wessex DEC had made recommendations from 'strong support' to 'not proven' or 'not recommended' on well over 50 topics, including pharmaceuticals, devices, procedures, and service design. For example, these included whether to introduce an "observation ward" into accident and emergency departments. When the DEC recommended something, the regional health authority would insist it went into contracts. When it judged something to be poor value for money, the purchasers could use its advice to resist funding. The Wessex DEC was followed by others - notably in the West Midlands and Trent regions - while most parts of the country developed at least some form of advice mechanism for purchasers on what was and was not worth buying. There was the Centre for Reviews and Dissemination in York. The North of England had a guidelines group while Oxford had a regular bulletin with the imaginative name of "Bandolier" which aimed to provide "bullets" of evidence for clinicians and commissioners on what was and wasn't worth doing.

Valuable though their work was, however, it had limited fire power. It remained well short of a national, authoritative voice recommending what the NHS should or should not adopt, and it did not prevent the controversy over the so-called "postcode lottery".

That national programme, which became NICE, emerged from events in which I played a peripheral role. The story here relies almost entirely on the Nicholas Timmins telling. In 1995 Gerry Malone, the minister of state for health, was asked to take a decision on whether the NHS should provide Beta-interferon, a new treatment for multiple sclerosis which was about to become available. There were three problems. First, Beta-interferon was expensive. Second, while it appeared to reduce the number, and possibly the severity of attacks in patients with the relapsing-remitting form of the disease, it was far from clear that the effect was dramatic, or indeed lasting. And third while there were some 70,000 MS sufferers in England, the proportion with the relapsing-remitting form could only be estimated at around 45 per cent. There were fears that the NHS could easily face a £100m a year bill and possibly even a £380m one – 10% of the then NHS drug budget - for a medicine whose long-term impact was uncertain.

Malone was married to a doctor. But his own background was that of a lawyer and journalist - he was a former editor of the Sunday Times in Scotland. He later said "*My reaction when I was told I needed to take a decision on whether the NHS would provide Beta-interferon was "how the hell am I meant make that decision?" The answer was "because you are the minister." But I pointed out that I was probably the least equipped person to make the judgement around its efficacy and its costs and benefits, even with the no doubt excellent advice of my civil servants.*"

Malone was acutely aware that if he restricted its use, the likelihood would be a storm of controversy. His response was to get together "*the great and the good among the neurologists and others who did know something about all this while bringing the MS Society into the frame… I basically said to this group 'I really don't want to ban this. But we are going to have to go fairly slowly to prove it, and to discover whether it is in fact effective'. Fortunately, everyone was very reasonable, and they all bought into that.*" The result was an instruction to the NHS in the form of an "executive letter" in late 1995 that permitted its use where NHS purchasers chose to adopt it but did so in somewhat discouraging tones and carefully defined circumstances that limited the cost, and with an inbuilt evaluation scheme stood some chance of providing better evidence of its efficacy.

When the dust settled, Malone got together some of the key people in the department and said "*Look, we have got away with this on this occasion. But I never want a minister to be put in this position again. Go away and devise some scheme where ministers do not have to take these decisions. This is not something that in my view should ever again land on a minister's desk.*" He knew that Beta-interferon would be the first of many.

In 1996 Graham Hart, the Department of Health's permanent secretary went on a 6-month sabbatical to Australia, Canada, New Zealand and the US. His remit was to study where the NHS was falling behind other health systems. He came back convinced that one of those areas was in cost-effectiveness evaluation of new medicines. The Australian Pharmaceutical Benefits System was already established and doing just that work - with Canada, New Zealand, and the relatively new Health Maintenance Organisations in the US not far behind. Early the following year Tony Culyer, another of the professors of health economics at York, was asked to chair a Department of Health Expert Workshop on Guidelines for Pharmaco-economic Studies – a high powered follow-up to the guidelines the department had first agreed with the drug companies in 1994.

In the campaign for the general election of May 1997, issues around the NHS, cost-effectiveness and evidence-based medicine were firmly in the public domain. In the February, Chris Smith, Labour's shadow health spokesman, made a speech on "Putting Quality at the Heart of Healthcare." His special adviser at the time was a young and fiercely bright health service manager by the name of Simon Stevens. Stevens would go on to be first Frank Dobson's special adviser, then Tony Blair's, and went on to be Chief Executive of the NHS from 2014 to 2021. He is now Baron Stevens and sits as an independent member of the House of Lords.

Stevens was also informally being advised by Alan Maynard, yet another health economics professor from York. Working at the health authority in York at this time, I can testify to the energy and intelligence of the health economics academics there. Chris Smith's speech included a passage on national standards for clinical effectiveness. He said there should be a system that provided guidance on "optimal quality care the NHS needs to ensure the speedy uptake of cost-effective innovations; the non-uptake of ineffective innovations; the regular assessment of current practice; and thorough testing of those not yet shown to be effective". He added that "evidence-based medicine, and active research programmes, can identify which treatments work; but you still have to persuade clinicians to use appropriate - and to avoid inappropriate - interventions." But there was no proposal in Smith's speech for a national body to undertake such work.

The UK electorate on the eve of polling were told that they had "*24 hours to save the NHS*", and Labour was elected in a landslide with Tony Blair as Prime Minister. But ironically any plans to save the NHS were sketchy to non-existent. There had been a string of short-lived appointments to the health brief when in opposition and as a result there was no coherent Labour policy alternative to the Thatcher reforms, save the abolition of GP Fundholding.

Blair's choice of Secretary of State for Health was inspired. It was, much to everyone's surprise, including apparently his own - Frank Dobson. A bluff and bearded Yorkshireman with a robust sense of humour and a passionate commitment to the NHS, he had last been the party's health spokesman in opposition in the mid-1980s. He was a far shrewder politician, and a much more effective manager, than his public persona sometimes portrayed. He proved to be a good delegator to an impressive bunch of ministers. They included Alan Milburn who was a dynamo of energy in creating the 1997 Health white paper. This was published in December 1997 when the government had only been elected in May when it had no clear strategy. Like Tessa Jowell, the public health minister, Milburn would go on to be a Cabinet minister.

And in the House of Lords there was Baroness Jay. Margaret Jay was the daughter of former Prime Minister James Callaghan. Educated at Oxford, Jay had been a journalist on the Panorama and This Week television programmes and had presented a BBC2 series on the Social History of Medicine. The health brief in the House of Lords is often a relatively lowly ministerial appointment but Blair gave her the rank of minister of state, and she brought to the task both a background in health and a brain to be reckoned with.

This formidable ministerial team were committed to improving quality and reducing geographical variation – as they put it "putting the National back into the NHS". After at least two dysfunctional discussions, it was Clive Smee - the Chief Economic Adviser to the Department - that was finally able to conceptualise on a few sheets of acetate and an overhead projector a policy that would capture the hearts and minds of the Labour health team. And in that proposal was an organisation, outside of the Department of Health that would produce both evaluations of new technology and clinical guidelines - using evidence of both clinical and cost-effectiveness, and would also devise the relevant audit tools.

Timmins tells us that Baroness Jay took the unusual step of asking to see Professor Mike Rawlins who was the current Chair of the Committee on Safety of Medicines - one of the three advisory committees of the UK's medicines regulator. Rawlins was a star - an academic clinical pharmacologist appointed a full professor at the age of 32, and a well-regarded honorary consultant physician in Newcastle. He had a reputation for getting things done, was regarded as an extremely wise source of advice, was utterly charming, and tough as old boots. He was also very well connected. He had experience as vice-chairman of the Northern Regional Health Authority, a position in which he had come to know Liam Donaldson who had been both its chief medical officer and general manager. Donaldson succeeded Sir Kenneth Calman as the government's Chief Medical Officer in 1998. I remember visiting Mike in his office in the Wolfson Unit in Newcastle in the summer of 1996. It was a small meeting, and from the wide-ranging conversation I was in no doubt he was clearly thinking about one last big job, but was not clear at the time what that was to be.

Jay told Rawlins the government was thinking of introducing an element of cost-effectiveness into whether the NHS should fund medicines, and she wanted to know whether Rawlins' Committee could do that job. Rawlins had no notice of the question but said he would not advise it.

He felt that the licensing body – the Medicines and Healthcare products Regulatory Agency - and its independent

189

advisory committee - the Committee on Safety of Medicines, had a difficult enough job in assessing the effectiveness, quality and safety of new medicines. Since the days of thalidomide the work of medicines regulation had become highly technical. Relatively small numbers of patients would have taken a medicine in the research studies necessary to get to a point where a drug company would be able to put a case together that their medicine could be licensed. There was a difficult balance to be struck by Rawlins, his colleagues, and the medicines regulators. Refusing or delaying a license based on insufficient evidence would potentially deprive some patients of benefit, perhaps with catastrophic consequences for those individuals. Approving a license for a medicine which subsequently was withdrawn from use because of a serious side effect also had potentially catastrophic consequences.

Rawlins immediately recognised that the cost-effectiveness decisions would be awkward and would at times be marginal. Adding in an additional fourth requirement for a new medicine - that of cost-effectiveness - Rawlins felt would contaminate the responsibility to assess and provide a license for a new medicine, and build in delays. Rawlins advised it was best to make decisions about cost-effectiveness through a different body to the one asked to judge quality, safety and efficacy.

In Frank Dobson there was a Sectary of State who saw the big picture, including all these difficulties. He knew about QALYs and Alan Williams' work from the 1980s when he was Labour's opposition health spokesperson. His parliamentary private secretary – an unpaid post that supplies an "eyes and ears" role for Cabinet ministers on the views of their back-bench MPs - was Hugh Bayley, the Member of Parliament for York MP and someone who had previously worked in the university's health economics department. Dobson himself had a cottage just outside York. Almost unbelievably, and as a result of great fortune and not design, cost-effectiveness was not a concept that required explaining from the ground up to the new secretary of state.

NICE as it was to become - became very much Dobson's baby. It offered a potential solution to a bunch of disparate and at times conflicting problems – the proliferation of guidelines, too little assessment of the cost-effectiveness of treatments, the so-called postcode lottery, and at least some answer to the "rationing" debate, allied to the fact that the NHS was demonstrably slow in international terms in adopting new drugs and treatments.

Pre-NICE *"the whole situation was totally unsatisfactory,"* Dobson said, *"and virtually everyone agreed it was unsatisfactory including the pharmaceutical industry. Trevor Jones, the director general of the Association of the British Pharmaceutical Industry, was endlessly pointing out that the companies would introduce a new drug that was clearly beneficial, and it would only be used in half a dozen places instead of across the NHS. There was a clear issue over take-up. And from the industry's point of view, while something like NICE might give the thumbs down to some things, it was likely that more things would get the thumbs up, and once that happened, it would be used across the board. So, there was something in it for the industry as well as for the NHS."*

It helped that whilst the discussions about establishing NICE were going on, Dobson had his own beta-interferon moment when he had to decide about whether to fund Viagra. As with Beta-interferon, without NICE all that was possible was an unsatisfactory fudge.

NICE was announced in Milburn's White Paper in December 1997, alongside an organisation to inspect NHS bodies and their development of clinical governance. Standardisation as the counterweight to variation, was gaining momentum and attracting lots of government funding. NICE did not initially get the nod to undertake technology assessment. There were doubts about the ability of one body to take it all on, but in the end it all went to NICE, and a recognisable remit was published in July 1998.

There was to be wide consultation before NICE decisions were made. And while purchasers and clinicians would be expected to follow NICE's guidelines and recommendations, no decisions in guidelines would be mandatory. This was a crucial distinction to what was happening in Health Maintenance Organisations in the United States where doctors were required to follow protocols - an approach that tied them into a system of formulaic medicine, even though it was normally underpinned by bureaucratic appeal mechanisms, and which the critics called "cook book medicine" - repeating the criticism hurled at evidence-based medicine from the start. In the NHS, by contrast, purchasers and doctors would be expected but not mandated to follow NICE's guidelines. That is still the case but, as we shall see later, other forces have incentivised "following the rules". From the start clinical audit would be in place to measure how far they did follow guidelines. In 1999 how that would play out was unknown. It was also unknown whether NICE would increase or reduce expenditure on health - but it should be more rational, making the best use of the money available would be explicit, and most importantly the difficult and unpopular decision making would be distanced from politicians.

Rawlins was appointed NICE's first Chair by Dobson. Dobson's first choice was unavailable, and he won Rawlins' long-term respect for telling him that before he heard it from anyone else. Rawlins recruited Andrew Dillon, who at the time was Chief Executive of a large London teaching hospital, as Chief Executive, and Tony Culyer from York as Vice-Chair. Rawlins would get the early morning train from Newcastle, Culyer would join him when the train stopped at York and the two of them would plan NICE on their journeys to London. The reaction from the pharmaceutical industry was not entirely negative, based on the promise of faster uptake of new medicines - a mantra that continues to this day. Rawlins and Dillon were responsible for much of NICE's success. Trevor Jones from the Association of the British Pharmaceutical Industry said "*I knew he [Rawlins] had huge integrity and intelligence. And I thought we would get a better judgement from him than from some lackey of the government who might simply have looked at the price and not the science*".

NICE's opening budget was tiny. While its initial work programme was small - it was only just getting going - its direct

192

turnover in its first financial year between 1999-2000 was a mere £600,000 and its full-time staff was just ten people.

Initially NICE outsourced much of its work - both guidelines production and technology appraisals - to the DEC's, the university-based HTA units, and for guidelines, the Medical Royal Colleges. Over time, the work moved in-house to NICE itself, but Rawlins and Dillon were masterful in establishing an initial work programme largely from existing resources. This also had the bonus of drawing in those collaborating bodies as real partners and in establishing NICE quickly as part of the "NHS family", rather than existing expertise becoming threatened, duplicated, eventually replaced and resentfully critical.

NICE became a legal entity on 1st April 1999 and was immediately plunged into its work. Glaxo Wellcome, then Britain's largest pharmaceutical company, had developed a new treatment for influenza called Relenza. NICE was still recruiting staff and was barely up and running. But the health department had known Relenza was coming and Dobson had asked NICE if it was willing to make an early rapid appraisal of the drug, ahead of the 1999/2000 flu season. "I put no pressure on them," Dobson said. "I only asked. I would have understood if they had said it was too early."

Rawlins and Dillon felt this was exactly the sort of problem NICE had been set up to sort out. Glaxo too agreed to a speedy process as it expected to get a positive recommendation ahead of the winter. An ad hoc "rapid appraisal process" was set up. NICE reached its judgement at speed and concluded that there was insufficient evidence that Relenza in fact reduced the severity of the illness in high-risk groups - the elderly, those with asthma, and other co-morbidities.

A mere 70 patients out of the 6,000 people in the clinical trial had been elderly. Relenza appeared to reduce the duration of symptoms from six to five days – but only if it was taken early enough when the initial symptoms differ little from a bad cold. There was no evidence that it reduced complications in the high-risk groups. Furthermore, it cost £24 for a five-day course of treatment. In an epidemic year, NICE calculated, the cost to the NHS might be close to £100million at a time when the drug budget for the NHS, outside hospitals, was under £4billion. Even in a non-epidemic year, the additional load on Britain's family doctors for what might or might not turn out to be 'flu' would be potentially overwhelming - displacing the rest of their work.

NICE then handled the appeal process, which Glaxo Wellcome took advantage of, in days. As it did so, it made clear that the guidance was only for the forthcoming flu season. It would review the advice if further evidence emerged. Indeed, a year on, as evidence started to suggest that Relenza did reduce hospitalisation among the most vulnerable, the Institute recommended limited use in high-risk patients in years with a significant flu outbreak. Many years later, when a global pandemic of swine flu threatened in 2009, the NHS was controversially to stockpile £136m worth of the drug.

NICE's initial decision about Relenza took many in the industry aback. There were predictions of a "gloves off fight". Glaxo Wellcome's Chief Executive, Sir Richard Sykes, stormed into 10 Downing Street to see Blair. Dobson had briefed Blair that he had to defend NICE's first decision, and he did so robustly. As tempers cooled neither the threatened judicial review of NICE's decision nor the threat of the company's withdrawal from the UK materialised.

Glaxo Wellcome did place advertisements in the medical press urging GPs to use the product. In the event, just 212 prescriptions for Relenza were dispensed between September 1999 and January 2000 compared to the many hundreds of thousands that might have been in the absence of NICE's national guidance.

Relenza illustrated another key feature of the NICE arrangement. It worked because ministers allowed it to. Like clinicians and health authorities, ministers were not bound by NICE's recommendations. But as well as standing up to Glaxo Wellcome's fury, they in effect stood back, allowing the organisation they had created to do the job which they had envisaged it doing.

NICE's first proper technology appraisal on the extraction of wisdom teeth was published in March 2000, their first clinical guideline on schizophrenia was published in December 2002, and the first interventional procedures guidance in July 2003. They now have responsibility for developing public health guidance and social care guidance and in January 2018 they published their 500th technology appraisal. By the end of 2023 NICE had produced nearly 400 clinical guidelines.

Whilst many doctors might criticise NICE's intrusion into their decision making, they are often pleased to have someone else make the difficult decisions about what should and should not be funded. And since it came into being there has never been a whiff of a suggestion from any politician from any political party that NICE should be abolished. They know too well that they would end up with the tricky decision making back on their own Ministerial desks. They both much prefer NICE to take the flak.

CHAPTER FOURTEEN

Information Mastery

"The art of medicine is to cure sometimes, to relieve often, and to comfort always."

This saying is often attributed to Hippocrates. Except the "Works of Hippocrates" would be better described as "the accumulated manuscripts of the library of the medical school at Kos named after a doctor called Hippocrates who may or may not have existed around about 300 BCE".[cxxxii]

Other sources attribute it to Ambroise Paré (1510-1590) who was physician to King François I of France, or to Edward Livingston Trudeau, founder of the tuberculosis sanitarium at Saranac Lake in New York's Adirondacks, or it might just have come from a 15th Century folk saying, and others think it was Sir William Osler (1849 – 1919).

Whoever it was, the words have been used as wise counsel to generations of doctors. But in the first few years of the 21st Century the bar was being set ever higher. An industrialised and globalised pharmaceutical industry was still developing new and expensive medicines. More and better options for treating patients ought to have been a good thing, but that was not always the case. Sometimes claims were made for medicines that did not stand up to critical appraisal. In the pursuit of potentially billions of dollars of sales worldwide, science would sometimes be distorted.[cxxxiii]

The drug companies themselves financed most of the clinical trials for their own medicines. Plenty of conflicts of interest there, but few people bothered much about it. The same companies funded much of doctors' continuing education, providing paid-for "expert" speakers that would be favourable to the sponsors products. Was the important postgraduate education of doctors in safe and unbiased hands? Clinical trials are often conducted on small groups of unrepresentative subjects, and negative data would sometimes remain unpublished – sometimes hidden deliberately. Apparently independent academic papers were actually planned and even ghost-written by pharmaceutical companies or their contractors, without disclosure.

I was medical director of the National Prescribing Centre for the NHS in England at the time, and it was frustrating. Some medicines were big game-changing advances – for individuals and for populations. Other new medicines most definitely were not, but despite the science being poor the pharmaceutical companies with lots of money and people would do their very best to maximise sales using every means at their disposal.

NICE guidelines and technology appraisals were starting to come through, and we had good in-house systems and were writing and disseminating short summaries of evidence for our core audience of the health authorities prescribing advisers. But it did feel adversarial at times with the drug companies, and we were very conscious that our critical appraisal of published research should be scrupulously fair and balanced. We were confident of our abilities and proud of our evidence summaries, but a serious lawsuit would occupy too much time and mean us using taxpayers' money on lawyers instead of evidence-based summaries.

The other frustration was the enduring nature of the gaps between evidence and practice. In addition to written bulletins we had a rolling programme of therapeutic topics which we covered in workshops for prescribing advisers. One year we would cover, say, diabetes, cardiovascular risk (high blood pressure and lipids), central nervous system topics, and common infections (antibiotics in the main). The next year it might be heart failure and treatment after a heart attack, gastrointestinal, pain (including non-steroidal anti-inflammatory drugs), and respiratory (largely asthma and chronic obstructive pulmonary disease).

When we prepared for every set of workshops we looked carefully at the national and local prescribing data. Everywhere we looked there was a gap between what the evidence suggested should be prescribed and what was, and of course we found variation between localities. Quite often one locality in one therapeutic area would be prescribing three times more or less

198

than localities with apparently very similar demographics and needs. And then on a different topic it would be other localities that were the outliers in the data. At the time our thinking was pretty much entirely transactional. If we could produce more and better summaries of evidence, if our therapeutic workshops were even better run and attended, then those gaps would narrow and so would the geographical variation. Or so we hoped.

I was appointed Medical Director at the NPC in January 2001. As we rolled through the first couple of years of writing bulletins and the cycles of workshop topics I began to look for alternative explanations to what looked like sub-optimal knowledge transfer. We now had good summaries of the evidence, and good dissemination networks, but practice did not always change in line with the summaries. It was a worry.

A 2001 study shed a little light on what sources doctors in hospitals and GPs used as sources of information about medicines.[cxxxiv] Information on the last new drug prescribed was derived from a broad range of sources: colleagues, 29%; pharmaceutical representatives 18%; hospital clinical meetings 15%; journal articles13%; and lectures,10%. GPs and hospital doctors differed significantly in their use of pharmaceutical representatives (42% vs 18%) and colleagues (7% vs 29%) as sources of prescribing information. As the authors concluded,

"The sources most frequently rated important in theory were not those most used in practice, especially among GPs. Both groups under-estimated the importance of pharmaceutical representatives. Most importantly, the sources of greatest practical importance were those involving the transfer of information through the medium of personal contact."

It did not make for comfortable reading.

A few years earlier a review of eleven individual descriptions of information sources used by family physicians found they used colleagues most often as information sources, followed by journals and books. Several factors influenced the use of information sources, and this included the convenience of the source.[cxxxv]

At the end of the 20th Century, evidence-based medicine was still being promoted as a route to keeping up to date with the published research with its now traditional approach of identifying the clinical question, finding the published research, critically appraising it, and so on.[cxxxvi] That approach did not seem to fit at all with how doctors actually went about finding and using information.

Even more questions were raised by a study of general practitioners in North America which found that two clinically important questions arose for every three patients seen.[cxxxvii] But those general practitioners pursued very few of those uncertainties, and when they did it was by talking to other colleagues or brief reading of a convenient source. There were 9 million new research papers being published every year. It was estimated that a generalist needed to read 19 papers every day to stay up to date. Evidence-based medicine was still pushing critical appraisal, but that did not seem feasible or to fit with what hard working, intelligent, conscientious doctors actually did. And no doctor would be reading 19 research papers a day – even if that was feasible and they had the skills to critically appraise those papers, they were already fully occupied looking after sick patients.

There was nothing wrong with our summaries of evidence or our therapeutic workshops for prescribing advisers. The content was accurate and fair, or at least no one ever sued us – and if we had not produced defendable summaries with a defendable process I am sure pharmaceutical companies would have. The workshops were well received, and prescribing advisers were using our materials in their discussions with prescribers. But if we were to reduce the gaps between evidence and practice and reduce variation between localities we needed to better understand what the prescribers were actually doing and why.

I discussed my thinking with my Chief Executive. If our current NPC programme was only partially addressing the issues prescribers faced, we needed to be doing something different. But it was not yet clear what. Then early in 2002 in own my reading of journals, I came across a course for doctors entitled "*How to Feel Comfortable with Not Knowing Everything*". It looked like it might explore the gap between the ivory tower of evidence based medicine and the real world - something I badly needed. The course was run by a couple of American academics – Dave Slawson and Allen Shaughnessy. I looked at a few of their academic papers.[cxxxviii cxxxix cxl] This was now very interesting. The only problem was that the course was in Charlottesville, Virginia – and I worked for the always cash-strapped NHS.

To his endless credit our Chief Executive, Clive Jackson, was immediately supportive and somehow found the cash. I was flying economy and staying in the equivalent of a poor-quality Travel Lodge but I was there. In Charlottesville on the first morning as we arrived at about 7am for a breakfast of coffee, fruit, muffins and "donuts" I was surprised but delighted to find one of "my" old North Yorkshire GPs on the course too. We reminisced cheerfully about my prescribing visits to his practice and settled down for the start. Dave Slawson was ill with influenza and only appeared in a weak and feeble state on the last of the three days.

Allen told the story of what they had for some years been calling "Information Mastery". They had both been enthused by people at McMaster and had been on courses there in the early days of evidence-based medicine. Bringing the traditional approach back to their own teaching, however, they had been disappointed. They had run courses on critical appraisal and the attenders had loved them. But when they went back six months later to find out how people were getting on with evidence-based medicine they found people were not able to use the skills they had acquired. Doctors were simply unable to find the time to go to the library in an evening or during the weekend to spend hours on a personal computer, find the relevant research, critically appraise it, and then use it in the treatment of their patients. The

201

patient had needed to be treated earlier in the week and their clinical state meant they could not wait for the evidence-based medicine process to unfold. And the pressure of clinical workload meant that the doctor could not abandon the rest of the day's patients and pursue the answer to the clinical question for just the one patient right there and then. The traditional EBM approach just did not fit with the reality of the way people acquired and used information.

Allen and Dave had created the "Usefulness Equation". This stated that the usefulness of information was first a product of how "relevant" the information was to the patient, then secondly whether the research was "valid". The conclusion was relevancy should be assessed first. If the study does not measure whether patients are living longer or better, then it has low relevance to clinical practice. If the research was, for example, on animals or measured some clinical marker of a condition then it was of low relevance. Only when a study passes the relevance test should validity be assessed. Well designed, well conducted and well reported randomised clinical trials will have high validity. Assessing validity was territory familiar to those of us with some critical appraisal training and experience.

The final part of the relevance equation was "convenience". Allen and Dave had taken on board the research showing clinicians prefer talking to other people or brief reading as information sources. The usefulness of information was inversely proportional to the convenience. Put more simply, high convenience means high usefulness. High convenience might have greater utility to a busy doctor than validity or relevance. Asking someone else who was a trusted colleague was quicker, easier, feasible, and actually more fun than EBM's five steps of finding the best evidence and critically appraising it. The usefulness equation fitted the evidence describing how people actually acquired and used information, and it was a big contrast with the traditional EBM exhortations to doctors to search for and then critically appraise the evidence themselves.

There were about a hundred people on the course, and we all held our hands up sheepishly when we were asked about whether we had a "guilt stack". We would be reading a piece of original research in one of the major medical journals. It looked either interesting, or important, or both. But we did not have the time right then to read it all, so we would rip the paper out of the journal and put it aside to read later. Except that we never got to read the paper, because there was always other stuff to do including other journals to read. Over time the stack of papers would get higher and higher, and the task of reading those papers became greater, to the point where we did know that we were never going to get round to reading all of those papers. But we could not bear to throw the stack away, because we felt guilty. Each of those papers looked so important and so interesting, and yet we just could not find time to read even the stuff we had identified. I had three guilt stacks – one in the office, one in the study at home, and one at my bedside.

Some of the skills of evidence-based medicine do have great utility, if only the numerophobic health care professionals could overcome their resistance to applying just a little arithmetic to their daily work. We heard about the relevance of the "sums" involved which enabled us to tease out better the actual probabilities for our patients when we were using screening and diagnostic tests – and communicate those probabilities in terms the patient could understand. I had already worked through that learning myself but was spellbound as we were taken through the story of "Baby Jeff" – a tale I still use today in teaching and which we will come to in a later chapter. The thorny issue of how to convey risks and benefits in a consultation got an airing too - another potential use of numbers.

Finally, we got to the nub of Information Mastery. Firstly, the volume of potentially useful information could be substantially reduced by only considering research with measured whether the patients lived longer or better. The outcomes of the research should be "patient-orientated".[cxli] No longer should we consider changing our practice based on "disease-orientated outcomes". The coroner is not going to be impressed if we base our practice on some biological marker which the research measured, yet when we come to look for whether people live longer or better, more people die despite the favourable improvement in the marker. This happens, and more than one would think. On the other hand, if people live longer or better, and we are not currently using that treatment, that is for sure worth looking at. In the Information Mastery bible, we pay attention to POOs, and we ignore DOOs.

Secondly, the start of looking for information to inform clinical decision making should be summaries of evidence and not original research. The volume of research was too great, the pressure of clinical work meant appraising primary research was unrealistic, and clinicians if they tried to do it were doing it so infrequently they were not confident that their skills were up to the task even if they had received substantial training in evidence-based medicine. There was a caveat though, about who produced the summary of evidence. The authors of the evidence summary should be a trusted, public-sector source. After all, pharmaceutical companies produced summaries of evidence, but they had proven that they could not be trusted to always write an unbiased summary. As a public sector producer of evidence summaries in the UK this was of course music to my ears, but it was Slawson and Shaughnessy in the United States who had come to this conclusion completely independently.

Even today I still talk with many young doctors training to be general practitioners who have given little thought to where they might go to get their clinical information. They cast around randomly it seems, with little consideration about whether what they are reading comes from a trustworthy source. If they use the British National Formulary for medicines and prescribing, Clinical Knowledge Summaries produced by NICE for summaries of guidelines, and the Oxford Handbook of General Practice to refresh their background knowledge covered in their undergraduate training across the vast range of potential conditions they may encounter, they seem to do quite a lot better in career-critical, applied knowledge examinations.

The same applies to patients of course. Every medicine box contains a leaflet, authoritatively provided by the UK licensing body. That leaflet tells them the truth, the whole truth and nothing but the truth about the medicine they are taking. But many a patient of mine would believe what someone else told them, or these days what someone with no expertise or even someone deliberately spreading mis-information for malign, state-based purposes was saying on social media. Almost nobody reads the patient information leaflet.

Coming back to Information Mastery, there was the question of how to use the trustworthy summaries of evidence to inform and potentially change practice. Three approaches are required – "hunting", "foraging" and "hot synching".

Foraging means having a reliable system to highlight new, important, relevant, valid information that requires a change in practice. The same trustworthy public sector orientated organisations that produce the summaries of evidence were, even then, producing short lists of potentially relevant and valid new research that might impact practice. A quick scan of those listings sent in an occasional e-mail means someone who is used to sifting evidence has done some of the work to identify the reliable and valid evidence, something that individual clinicians might never manage themselves.

"Hot synching" means purposefully checking and updating one's personal mental map of knowledge and skills once or twice a year for each of the 30 to 40 conditions seen frequently. This was the first time I had encountered the concept of a mental mind map influencing clinical decision making and it made perfect sense. Allen described young doctors in the United States working in two different hospitals both dealing with people who had scratched to front of the eye - a corneal abrasion. In one hospital the specialists wanted people with a corneal abrasion to have an eye pad placed on top of the closed eyelid. That would, they said, stop the eyelid rubbing across the front of the abraded cornea and so speed healing. At the other hospital the other specialists advised not to pad the eye for corneal abrasions. They had read the randomised controlled trial which said padding the eye surprisingly made no difference to healing rates and they had changed their practice in line with the evidence. Two different mind maps, and it was the mind maps that determined clinical decisions. And the trick was to quickly review what one did for a frequently encountered condition against a trustworthy summary of evidence. "Am I doing what the updated guideline says I should be doing for this condition? Yes I am, so all good and nothing to do differently. Great job." "Am I doing what the updated guideline now recommends? No I'm not. Maybe I need to have a good think about that and change my practice so that I am". It was something to think hard about on the plane home.

"Hunting" means having a reliable system to find relevant, valid information that answers specific questions quickly and efficiently. Even when using foraging and hot synching there will be times when a clinician needs to find information which is relevant and valid for an infrequent clinical situation. Traditional evidence-based medicine approaches would begin with searching one of the online electronic databases run by the National Library of Medicine in the United States – the successor to the library started after the US Civil War by George Billings. Simple searching of Medline or PubMed would usually retrieve many thousands of potentially relevant and valid research. How is a clinician supposed to handle that? Just pick the top one? Scroll down the first page and pick out the one paper that looks most likely to be useful based on the paper's title? How would one know that there wasn't a much better paper hidden as paper number 25,486 on the list of papers the wonders of personal computing linked to the Internet could now retrieve from the database (in less than a second)?

The Information Mastery approach was to turn things on their head and recommend that clinicians begin searching with pre-digested summaries of evidence from trustworthy sources. Only if they did not find an answer there did they need to drill down further into more extensive summaries such as the Cochrane Library, then the major journals perhaps, and as a final resort then perhaps Medline or PubMed was worth a try, despite the previous caveats.

It was a great course. There was an abundance of information, education, and entertainment. Lord Reith, the first Chairman of the BBC had those as the aims of the BBC in its early days and he would have been very happy with Dave and Allen's course. On the last evening there was a course dinner. The food was not at all memorable – traditional conference rubber chicken. But the setting was, at least for me, spectacular. I don't know how they had managed to arrange it, but we had dinner in a marquee actually in the grounds of Monticello – the home of Thomas Jefferson and familiar to many because it is the house pictured on the obverse of every US 10 cent piece.

I have always been a sucker for American history, and especially early history. Presidents George Washington, Thomas Jefferson, James Madison, and James Monroe were all born in Virginia. It was of course Jefferson who had drafted the Declaration of Independence, and it was a magical evening. We had the place to ourselves and wandered awestruck around the house and grounds, paying homage to Jefferson's grave, and saddened by the evidence that despite great deeds, Jefferson had kept slaves.

Back in the UK, I relayed my learning to my colleagues at the National Prescribing Centre. I tried to temper my enthusiasm, but to my colleagues' great credit my dissemination of Dave and Allen's generously donated teaching resources was met positively. We had known we needed to be more imaginative if our work was to have a greater impact, and challenging the orthodoxy of how evidence-based medicine should be practiced in those heady days was certainly imaginative. My colleague Jonathan Underhill went to Charlottesville the next year, and in 2004 Dave and Allen came over to the UK to run their workshops for our audiences in England and Wales.

Before Charlottesville we knew using evidence to change clinical practice was complex, the interventions that might be successful were unlikely to be straightforward to implement, and results were sometimes unexpected. After Charlottesville we had started to begin to understand some of the reasons why.

CHAPTER FIFTEEN

Pain

Pain is useful to humans. It tells us not to go too near to fire or mess about with very sharp things. It often alerts us to the possibility of disease. Pain of any degree is unpleasant, but when it becomes severe or lasts a long time or has a psychological element or has a cause other than a mostly physical one, it can be incredibly difficult to treat.

History documents that if humans have experienced pain, they try to give explanations for its existence and seek soothing agents to dull or cease the painful sensation. A Sumerian clay tablet from about 2100 BCE referred to the opium poppy. Some objects from the ancient Greek Minoan culture may also suggest the knowledge of the poppy and in 800 BCE, the Greek writer Homer wrote in his epic, The Odyssey, about Telemachus, a man who used opium to soothe his pain and forget his worries.[cxlii]

In the first century CE the opium poppy and opium was known by Dioscorides, Pliny and Celsus, and later by Galen. About 1000CE it was recommended by Avicenna especially in diarrhoea and diseases of the eye. The indigenous people of North America relied on the bark of the willow tree, the original source of our modern-day aspirin. Inca shamans chewed coca leaves, which contain a version of cocaine.

But the causes of pain were unknown. Even among the ancient Greeks, there were competing theories. Aristotle did not include a sense of pain when he enumerated the five senses. Like Plato before him, he saw pain and pleasure not as sensations but as emotions - "passions of the soul". Alternatively, Hippocrates believed that pain was caused by an imbalance in the vital fluids of a human. For many centuries it was not recognised that the brain had any role to play in pain processing, and instead theories implicated the heart as the central organ for the sensation of pain.[cxliii]

As late as the scientific Renaissance in Europe in the 15th and 16th centuries, pain was not well understood. Pain was often viewed as a punishment from God. Alternatively, pain was theorised to exist as a test or trial on a person to reaffirm their faith. As late as the 19th Century, there were echoes of this philosophy about pain being "a necessary part of life" in the debate about the use of anaesthetics based upon the notion that pain was necessary for healing.

In his 1664 Treatise of Man, René Descartes - who was French but actually spent a large part of his life working at the University of Leiden in the Dutch Republic - theorised that the body was more similar to a machine. He suggested that pain was a disturbance that passed down along nerve fibres until the disturbance reached the brain. Descartes proposed his theory by drawing a man's hand being struck by a hammer.[cxliv] In between the hand and the brain, Descartes described a hollow tube with a cord beginning at the hand and ending at a bell located in the brain. This would now be regarded as grossly simplistic, but it began the transformation of the perception of pain from a spiritual, mystical experience to a physical, mechanical sensation - leading the way to our current, highly complex theories about pain and its treatment.

Alongside opium, ancient pain relief could be obtained from numerous plant products such as marijuana, mandrake, belladonna and jimsonweed. These would sedate but, in the case of surgery, not truly anaesthetise. In the Middle Ages the soporific sponge included as - well as opium - mulberry juice, lettuce seeds, mandrake, ivy and a touch of hemlock.[cxlv] A fresh sea sponge was soaked in the liquid and allowed to dry in the sun; it could then be reconstituted by dipping it in water and squeezing the contents into the mouth or nostrils.

In 1805 a brilliant young chemist called Friedrich Serturner, when he was just 23 years old, successfully extracted morphine crystals from the raw poppy seed juice.[cxlvi] By trial and error, through self-administration and dosing three young volunteers, he noticed that one-fourth grain (30 milligrams) of the drug induced a happy, light-headed sensation, the second dose caused drowsiness and excessive fatigue, while the third caused participants to become confused and somnolent. He suggested

211

that 15 mg of the drug as the optimal dose and named the substance 'Morphium' after the Greek god of sleep and dreams.

Serturner's discovery enabled physicians to prescribe morphine in regulated dosages for easing pain and to a large extent eliminated the dangers of overdose associated with raw poppy juice, which varied unpredictably in its concentration of morphine from one batch to another. The identification of alkaloids was also a significant event in chemistry resulting in conceptual changes, leading to the French researchers Pierre Joseph Pelletier and Joseph Bienaimé Caventou, discovering strychnine in 1818 and quinine in 1820. Several other medically useful alkaloids were discovered around that time including atropine (1819), caffeine (1820), nicotine (1828), colchicine (1833), and cocaine (1860).[cxlvii]

In the 18th century, malaria was a prominent disease in many parts of Europe. The bark of the cinchona tree (containing quinine) was one of the earliest drugs discovered to be effective against fever. Since cinchona bark turned out to be effective, why shouldn't European barks be tested? First, willow bark was confirmed to be effective, and then the natural ester of salicylic acid was isolated as the willow's active ingredient. Later, salicylic acid itself was isolated, pure salicylic acid was synthesised and the first "scale up" of a synthetic process created the first drug factory in Dresden in 1874.[cxlviii]

In Strasbourg, two young physicians, Cahn and Hepp, tried to eradicate intestinal worms with naphthalene. They were amazed that the worms survived in one patient, but the patient's fever resolved. An analysis of this unusual result revealed that the pharmacy had incorrectly provided acetanilide rather than naphthalene for treatment. This led to the discovery of the pharmacologic activity of acetanilide, which was marketed soon by another small dye factory close to Frankfurt (Kalle) under the name Antifebrin. Bayer further investigated acetanilide and found that a derivative (a by-product of aniline dye production), namely, "acetophenitidine," was equally effective. They marketed it under the brand name Phenacetin.

As soon as salicylic acid and phenacetin became widely used, physicians and patients came to recognise the disadvantages of these painkillers that also lowered the patient's temperature. Each was of relatively low potency, and patients needed to take them in multiple-gram quantities daily. Ingesting up to 10 spoonfuls of sodium salicylate was extremely unpleasant and unpalatable. Taking several grams of phenacetin led to potentially dangerous methemoglobinemia. The expanding drug industry, especially Bayer in Wuppertal and Hoechst in Frankfurt, put their chemists to work to produce improved derivatives.

Felix Hoffmann, a young chemist at Bayer, was motivated to improve salicylic acid since his father had rheumatoid arthritis and he found taking salicylic acid increasingly unbearable. On the suggestion of A. von Eichengrün, who was at that time in charge of chemistry at Bayer, Hoffmann researched the literature thoroughly and learned that C. F. von Gerhardt in Strasbourg had produced acetylsalicylic acid a couple of years earlier. Hoffmann reproduced this synthesis and gave the acetylated product to his father, who preferred it. The company marketed it under the trade name, Aspirin.

To further improve the tolerability of phenacetin, Bayer, working together with the chemist Joseph von Mering, investigated a metabolite of phenacetin called acetaminophen (paracetamol). Sterling, a UK company, found that acetaminophen without impurities did not induce methemoglobinemia and marketed the product worldwide under the name Panadol.[cxlix]

The next phase developments in pain management occurred after World War II. Once again, an unplanned event paved the way. Hoping to reduce bone marrow damage attributed to another painkiller called phenazone, the company called Geigy in Basel synthesised a new agent, phenylbutazone. This turned out not just to reduce pain but to also have an anti-inflammatory effect in rheumatoid arthritis never seen before with salicylates or

213

phenazone. This was the first of what we now call nonsteroidal anti-inflammatory drugs (NSAIDs).[cl]

In the US, Charles Winter, initially at Merck, Sharp, and Dohme and later at Parke-Davis, identified another NSAID – indomethacin. In 1969 in the UK, Boots developed another - ibuprofen. In Europe, Geigy developed diclofenac (first marketed in 1974 in Japan), and Rhône-Poulenc, together with Bayer, contributed to the development with ketoprofen (marketed in 1973). By the 1990s there were approaching 20 different NSAIDs available. Treating pain was still difficult in many circumstances, but the explosion in drug development meant many more options for pain.

But of course all this came at a price. Widespread use of morphine in the 19th century meant many people became addicted. Recreational use of opium grew and by 1830 British dependence on the drug reached the point that warships were sent to the coast of China in 1839 in response to China's attempt to suppress the opium traffic, beginning the First Opium War.

Diamorphine was first synthesized in 1874 by C. R. Alder Wright, an English chemist working at St. Mary's Hospital in London who had been experimenting combining morphine with various acids. He sent the compound to F. M. Pierce of Owens College in Manchester for analysis, but his discovery was not taken up by a manufacturer. This only happened after it was independently re-synthesized 23 years later by Felix Hoffmann who was working for Bayer in Germany. His supervisor Heinrich Dreser suggested an approach to synthesise codeine from morphine. Codeine is a natural constituent of the opium poppy that is pharmacologically like morphine but less potent and less addictive. Instead, the experiment produced diamorphine - a form of morphine one and a half to two times more potent than morphine itself.

It seems astonishing now, but in 1895, Bayer marketed diacetylmorphine as an over-the-counter drug under the trademark name Heroin, and with advertising recommending

214

uses which included babies who were teething. For fifteen years Heroin was marketed as a non-addictive morphine substitute and cough suppressant. The effects – addiction and deaths due to respiratory depression - were entirely predictable, and provided ammunition for those introducing the first legal controls on medicines on both sides of the Atlantic.

The hope, or the marketing, that opiate-like painkillers could be developed that were not capable of creating dependence in their users continued throughout the 20th Century. Pharmaceutical companies created man-made substitutes for the natural chemicals isolated from the opium poppy. For example, Vicodin – a combination of hydrocodone and paracetamol – was launched in the US in 1984, but in 2009 was removed from the market. Percocet – a combination of oxycodone and paracetamol was launched in the US in 1976. In 2017 the US Opioid and Drug Abuse Commission reported:-

"Opioids are a prime contributor to our addiction and overdose crisis. In 2015, nearly two-thirds of drug overdoses were linked to opioids like Percocet, OxyContin, heroin, and fentanyl. [...] Americans consume more opioids than any other country in the world. In fact, in 2015, the amount of opioids prescribed in the U.S. was enough for every American to be medicated around the clock for three weeks.

"Since 1999, the number of opioid overdoses in America have quadrupled according to the CDC. Not coincidentally, in that same period, the amount of prescription opioids in America have quadrupled as well. This massive increase in prescribing has occurred despite the fact that there has not been an overall change in the amount of pain Americans have reported in that time period. We have an enormous problem that is often not beginning on street corners; it is starting in doctor's offices and hospitals in every state in our nation."

But the problems with treatments for pain did not just sit just with addiction to opiates. High doses of salicylates were good for pain relief in conditions such as rheumatoid arthritis, but their use was limited by toxicity. In addition, it was still unclear until the 1970s how aspirin, indomethacin and phenylbutazone actually managed to reduce pain and inflammation. It was a British pharmacologist John Vane who, with Priscilla Piper and others, discovered the relationship between pain and inflammation and key, natural occurring chemicals in the body called prostaglandins and cyclooxygenase.[cli] Vane described how NSAIDs reduced pain and inflammation by inhibiting cyclooxygenase (COX) – if the complex biological pathway leading to pain and inflammation was interrupted the pain was reduced. Vane won the Nobel Prize in 1982 and was knighted in 1984.

After that discovery, alliances between academic pharmacologists and the pharmaceutical industry were able to produce similar agents. A procession of new NSAIDs were developed, each one, of course, being heralded by the marketing arm of the pharmaceutical company as either more effective or less toxic than its competitors. As new NSAIDs appeared, the indications steadily broadened from inflammatory diseases to almost any painful condition. Each time a new drug was launched the market expanded, resulting in annual estimated sales for NSAIDs of more than $20 billion worldwide.

The first big problem with a new NSAID occurred in the 1980s with benoxaprofen, known by the brand name Opren. Developed by Eli Lilly, it was marketed on the basis of a unique mode of action. But it soon became clear that its use was also associated with novel adverse events, including skin sensitivity to sunlight and liver toxicity. The company went on actively marketing the drug until forced to withdraw it when several older people had died of liver failure after using it.

But the NSAIDs as a drug class had a characteristic range of serious side effects. They could increase blood pressure, worsen renal function, and they could worsen heart failure. But the real bugbear was their effect on the stomach. Apart from common but less serious problems such as dyspepsia, a minority of patients would develop serious problems with ulcers which would cause severe abdominal pain. This was bad enough, but some of the ulcers would bleed or perforate. Those were serious emergencies, which were sometimes life-threatening and occasionally fatal. In 2005, NSAIDs were estimated to cause the deaths of 16,000 Americans a year.[clii]

In 1991 Dan Simmons at Brigham Young University demonstrated that the COX enzyme had at least two forms. The main ones are COX-1 and COX-2; COX-1 is responsible for the synthesis of prostaglandin and thromboxane in many types of cells, including the gastro-intestinal tract and blood platelets. Through prostaglandin and thromboxane, COX-1 maintains the health of the lining of gastrointestinal tract and keeps platelets in the blood from becoming sticky and clumping together. An intact lining of the stomach means we do not develop stomach ulcers. Sticky platelets are a good thing when humans cut themselves and the blood needs to form a clot to stop the bleeding. But sticky platelets when they are not needed could, at least theoretically cause clots where they are a very bad thing – in the arteries supplying blood to the heart and brain resulting in heart attacks and strokes. COX-2 is the naturally occurring chemical that plays the major role in increasing prostaglandin synthesis in inflammatory cells and in the central nervous system. As Vane had already shown, prostaglandin is a key factor in the development of inflammation and pain.[cliii]

Theoretically, inhibit COX-1 and we get stomach ulcers and clumps of platelets circulating in the blood potentially leading to circulating blood clots which cause heart attacks and other cardiac events. But if we inhibit COX-2 then we get less pain and inflammation without those problems. Theoretically we want an NSAID to be a COX-2 inhibitor and not a COX-1 inhibitor. We should at this point remember the Information Mastery maxim of patient-orientated outcomes, not disease orientated outcomes, and one of the reasons for evidence-based medicine developing was the importance of no longer relying on mechanisms of action as a basis for treating patients. Fancy science and mechanisms of action are all well and good, but what matters is what happens to real patients, not in laboratory test tubes.

However, the challenge of developing a COX-2 inhibitor was accepted by teams working in pharmaceutical companies on modern, structure-based drug design. If successful the development of COX-2 selective NSAIDs would further validate the now widespread general belief that a detailed understanding of the chemicals involved in biological processes, especially those involved in causing diseases, would lead to better medicine.

Rofecoxib was one of the first such "designer" NSAIDs. It was developed by the US-based, multinational pharmaceutical giant Merck and reached the market in 1999. From the early days of rofecoxib's development, some scientists at Merck were concerned that the drug might adversely affect the cardiovascular system by altering the ratio of prostacyclin to thromboxane, and so increasing the risk of clots occurring within blood vessels and causing heart attacks and strokes. When describing the rofecoxib story I have relied on the published research in the public domain; that work is referenced.

Despite Merck's knowledge that rofecoxib might increase clot formation, none of the intervention studies that constituted its new drug application to the US Food and Drug Administration in 1998 were designed to evaluate cardiovascular risk. The nine studies generally had a small number of participants, had short treatment periods, enrolled patients at low risk of cardiovascular disease, and did not have a standardised procedure to collect and adjudicate cardiovascular outcomes.[cliv] If there was an increase in cardiac events, those studies were very unlikely to find it.

In January 1999, a few months before its launch onto the market, Merck began its largest randomised trial yet of rofecoxib. This randomised controlled trial, called VIGOR, compared robecoxib to naproxen. The aim was to demonstrate fewer gastrointestinal side effects than naproxen when rofecoxib was used for people with rheumatoid arthritis. This trial also did not have a standard operating procedure for collecting information on cardiovascular events and did not have a cardiologist on the data safety monitoring board. Data safety monitoring boards are independent committees whose purpose is to review the results of an ongoing trial to ensure the safety of trial participants. The study, involving 8000 volunteer patients, was designed to continue until a predetermined number of confirmed uncomplicated or complicated gastric perforations, ulcers, or bleeds had occurred.

In October the VIGOR study's data and safety monitoring board met for the first time. The study results up to that time showed that rofecoxib patients had fewer ulcers and less gastrointestinal bleeding than patients taking naproxen. It looked as if the study would be a success for Merck.

But at the second meeting in November the focus was on heart problems. As of 1st November 1999, 79 patients out of 4,000 taking Vioxx had serious heart problems or had died, compared with 41 patients out of 4,000 taking naproxen. The difference was statistically significant, but the actual number of events was small. The panel voted to continue the study and to meet again in a month.

At the December meeting, the number of cardiac events remained twice as high on rofecoxib. It is often difficult to decide to terminate a randomised controlled trial early. As in this case, the numbers of adverse events were small when compared to the total number of patients in the study. They might have been a chance finding. Continuing the study to collect more data might have given a clearer picture, though the interim statistics showed that a change in the existing trend was unlikely.

In this case there was the complication of a proposed explanation that naproxen could be acting like low-dose aspirin and protecting people from heart attacks; what if naproxen was protective against clots and falsely making rofecoxib look risky by comparison? The board voted to continue the study, but decided Merck needed to develop a plan to analyse the study's cardiovascular results before the study ended.

Discussions about the cardiac events did not go well. Merck were not keen on developing the analysis plan. The company wanted to wait and combine the cardiovascular results of VIGOR with results from other rofecoxib studies. Michael Weinblatt, the safety panel chair and a rheumatologist with Brigham & Women's Hospital in Boston, pushed for immediate analysis. After further discussions, Merck and Weinblatt agreed to analyse cardiac events reported by 10th February 2000 — at least a month before the study concluded. Events that were reported after 10th February would not be included in the analysis.

According to good practice for trials and in accordance with Merck policies, the data safety board is supposed to be independent, without financial or emotional stake in the trial being monitored. Yet, on 7th February 2000 Michael Weinblatt disclosed family ownership interest in Merck shares worth over $70 000, and on 15th February 2000 he was awarded a two-year consulting contract for 12 days of work over two years at a rate of $5,000 a day. Although it is not possible to tell whether this financial relationship made any difference, the conflict of interest was not a matter of public record at the time the study was conducted or published, and of itself calls into question the independence of the safety board.

In May 2000 the VIGOR paper was submitted to the New England Journal of Medicine for publication. Because of the agreed cut-off date, the data included only 17 of the 20 heart attacks that patients had who were taking rofecoxib. The authors of the paper made corrections, presumably in response to the usual peer review process for scientific papers, in June and November 2000 but there was no mention of the three "missing" heart attacks. However, on 13th October 2000 Merck did tell the US drugs regulator, the FDA, about heart attacks 18, 19, and 20.

The VIGOR study had enormous financial implications for Merck. If it showed rofecoxib to have better gastrointestinal safety than naproxen, it could be used to petition the FDA for a new indication - rheumatoid arthritis - and no doubt sales would boom for other conditions in advance of future license extensions. However, if the study raised concerns about cardiovascular

220

harm, the entirety of a billion-dollar revenue stream would be threatened.

The published study showed that rofecoxib was as effective as naproxen but not more effective in relieving symptoms of rheumatoid arthritis, but it did halve the risk of gastrointestinal events. However, there was a five-fold relative increase in the risk of myocardial infarction. Yet the published paper obscured the cardiovascular risk associated with rofecoxib in several ways.

Firstly, the agreement in February to have different termination dates for cardiovascular and gastrointestinal events was a highly irregular procedure. It was not described in the publication and had the effect of favouring the drug's effect on gastrointestinal events while understating the risk of cardiovascular events. Secondly, the published cardiovascular risk was not accurate because three additional myocardial infarctions occurred in the rofecoxib group in the month after the researchers stopped counting cardiovascular events when none had occurred in the naproxen group.

Thirdly, the potential harms were further minimised by a subgroup analysis decided on after the trial was designed and probably after the cardiovascular risks became apparent. This was based on the 4% of trial participants who met the criteria for taking a preventative low dose aspirin based on their previous medical history of ischaemic heart disease, but who were not actually taking low dose aspirin. The analysis found that 38% of the heart attacks occurred in the patients who had an "indication for aspirin prophylaxis but were not taking it". This analysis had the effect of shifting the reason for the increase in cardiac events onto the patients and away from rofecoxib. The reality was that had the authors included the three missing myocardial infarction cases, the subgroup analysis would have shown an increased cardiovascular risk in people who were and who were not in the subgroup with an "indication for aspirin prophylaxis but not taking it".

Fourthly, the paper concealed the cardiovascular risk even further by presenting the hazard of myocardial infarction as if naproxen was the intervention group, and without reporting the absolute number of cardiovascular events, even though all other results were presented appropriately with rofecoxib as the intervention group.

And finally, the authors proposed the "naproxen hypothesis" that had been raised at the second data monitoring board - suggesting that rofecoxib had not been harmful but that naproxen had been protective. This was despite there being no accepted evidence that naproxen had a strong cardioprotective effect.

Merck strongly promoted the VIGOR study, paying over $900,000 to the New England Journal for nearly 1 million reprints of the paper to circulate to doctors and other health professionals. In academic circles there was discussion and concern about the cardiac events, but without the full facts being known at the time it was impossible to form a judgement. There was, after all, a big reduction in the gastrointestinal complications and it was difficult to assess where the balance of risks lay.

In February 2001 the FDA held a committee meeting to review the VIGOR trial and the rest of the data it held on rofecoxib. Importantly, it published the complete VIGOR data on its website, including the additional heart attacks and data on other cardiovascular events. This allowed Debabrata Mukherjee, Steven Nissen and Eric Topol from the Cleveland Clinic to reanalyse the VIGOR data - with the extra three heart attacks included for the first time.

Their paper, published in the Journal of the American Medical Association in August 2001, cast serious doubt on the hypothesis that naproxen protects the heart.[clv] However, over the next couple of years other studies using a variety of cohort and case control designs, some of them having authors who were associated with Merck, were published with conflicting results. There were also numerous opinion papers published largely

222

written by Merck's consultants and employees which supported this notion.[clvi]

Merck also selectively targeted doctors who raised questions about rofecoxib, going so far as pressurising some of them through their department chairs[clvii]. So convinced were Merck by their own arguments that for several years they continued to investigate other indications for rofecoxib, and to do so they conducted additional trials. And it was one of those trials that finally provided the evidence needed, demonstrating conclusively that rofecoxib increased heart attacks.

The evidence came from a trial comparing rofecoxib with placebo. This meant that this time there could be no "naproxen is protective" theory. The APPROVe study involved 108 hospitals in 29 countries around the world. From them, 2586 patients with previous large bowel polyps were recruited. The aim was to see whether rofecoxib compared to placebo reduced the recurrence of the polyps, and therefore provide evidence to support an application for a new license for rofecoxib – for nothing less than the prevention of colon cancer. Fewer polyps equated to fewer precancerous colon growths in the future. The stakes were as high as they could be. There must have been keen anticipation within Merck of the scientific kudos, not to mention future sales, from a once-a-day pill to - as it would no doubt have been presented - "prevent a common cancer".

But there was more. Merck had tried to engineer a win-win with this trial. It was no accident that the trial involved 108 hospitals. Merck had carefully identified doctors who were "opinion leaders" - people who were well known within the profession and speaking often at educational meetings to their colleagues. The marketing division at Merck knew that even without the data from the colon research, if they could have 108 influential doctors speaking to other doctors about rofecoxib that would have a significant and positive effect on the numbers of patients taking their NSAID, as opposed to one of the competitors, for all sorts of indications. Some of these "opinion leading" doctors would no doubt enjoy speaking about their role as an investigator on a large and prestigious piece of research. So, this was in effect a "seeding trial", designed with at least one eye on the increase in sales, with the result of the research in potentially reducing colon polyps not the only objective. And of course those doctors would not have to do too much work for the study to gain the "prestige". The average number of patients recruited per hospital was just 24.

Patients entered the study between February 2000 and November 2001. The trial was stopped on 30th September 2004, two months ahead of the planned date of completion, on the instruction of the data and safety monitoring board. The average length of time in the study was 2.4 years in the rofecoxib group and 2.6 years in the placebo group. The safety board found that after 18 months treatment, 46 patients taking rofecoxib had had a myocardial infarction compared with 26 of those receiving placebo. The results were published in the New England Journal of Medicine in March 2005.[clviii] The statistics showed that no difference in the rates, given those results, would only occur 8 times in 1000. The approximate doubling of cardiac events on rofecoxib was highly statistically significant, and there were significant implications.

The blows to Merck were immense not only because of loss of revenue but also because of expected litigation, to say nothing about reputation. One key question was when during treatment did the risk became manifest? If short term use was not associated with increased cardiovascular risk, Merck's liability would potentially be drastically reduced. The APPROVe authors, five of whom were Merck employees and the remainder of whom received consulting fees from Merck, asserted that the increased risk became apparent only after 18 months of use. Once again, this analysis, reviewed and then published in the most prestigious medical journal in the world was fatally flawed in favour of the drug manufacturer and sponsor of the study. The "nothing within 18 months" conclusion was based on an analysis that was not prespecified, and used a flawed methodological approach. Merck subsequently admitted that it had incorrectly described the statistical approach, and the New England Journal of

Medicine issued a correction indicating that statements regarding an increase in risk after 18 months should be removed from the article. Again, mistakes that favoured the company, with colossal economic implications, made it through the journal peer review process to health care professionals and the public.

In September 2004 Merck received notice that a team of researchers including senior analysts at the FDA had submitted a paper to the Lancet confirming an excess cardiovascular events in a new cohort study using a large patient data base from the US health insurer and provider Kaiser Permananete. A few days later Merck finally voluntarily withdrew rofecoxib from the market worldwide.

Although the increase in cardiac events due to rofecoxib seemed small at around only 3 extra events per 1000 people per year, it was estimated that by the time the drug was withdrawn, 20 million people were taking it. As a result of such widespread use, it was estimated that as many as 140,000 cases of serious coronary disease and 60,000 deaths might have been caused in the US alone.[clix] This sobering number was more than the number of deaths of Americans in the Vietnam war.

In August 2005 a Texas state jury returned a verdict against Merck in the first rofecoxib liability case to go to trial. By that time, some 13,000 lawsuits had been filed against the company on behalf of 23,000 plaintiffs who alleged the drug caused heart attacks and strokes. In May 2006, external analysis of data sent to the FDA from the APPROVe study showed conclusively that the cardiovascular risks from rofecoxib began shortly after patients started taking the drug. The data also indicated that the risks from Vioxx remain long after patients stop taking the drug. Merck continued to disagree with the analysis and maintained that patients were not at risk unless they had taken the drug for more than 18 months.

Finally, in November 2007, Merck announced it would pay $4.85 billion to end thousands of lawsuits over rofecoxib. The amount, to be paid into a so-called settlement fund, is believed to be the largest drug settlement ever. In making the settlement, Merck emphasised that it was not admitting fault. The settlement allowed Merck to avoid the personal-injury lawsuits of some 47,000 plaintiffs, and about 265 potential class-action cases filed by people or family members who claimed the drug proved fatal or injured its users.

In the UK the impact of rofecoxib was attenuated by the work of prescribing advisers. In October 2002 we at the UK National Prescribing Centre summarised the current state of the evidence on COX-2 inhibitors:

> *"The gastrointestinal safety of rofecoxib …..has been assessed in large clinical outcome trials which, on first analysis, show benefits over non-selective NSAIDs in the incidence of serious upper gastrointestinal complications. However, …. cardiovascular adverse event data from the rofecoxib study (VIGOR) have questioned the risk–benefit profile of these new drugs and, until they are better understood, it seems sensible not to use them routinely in large numbers of individuals"*.[clx]

At the peak of its popularity in 2003, rofecoxib accounted for just 10% of all NSAID prescriptions in England.[clxi] Few people come out of the rofecoxib story well, and certainly not the medical journals.[clxii clxiii clxiv clxv clxvi] The New England Journal published the VIGOR and APPROVe studies, and despite serious methodological issues in both studies neither the internal editorial processes nor the external peer review picked these up. Once alerted to the errors and omissions, the journal was slow to clarify and issue corrections.

But other academic medical journals also played important parts. In 2001, the journal Circulation published a pooled analysis of 23 studies examining the association between rofecoxib and cardiovascular risk.[clxvii] The paper had no editorial commentary or critique; the study was coordinated internally at Merck, the results highly favoured the safety of rofecoxib, five of the seven authors were Merck employees, and the other two academic authors acknowledged being paid consultants to Merck.

The Annals of Internal Medicine published the assessment of differences between Vioxx and naproxen to ascertain gastrointestinal tolerability and effectiveness (ADVANTAGE) study.[clxviii] It later learnt that article was written by Merck but the paper as published appeared to have been written by academic authors. This was "ghost-writing" – where pharmaceutical company employees or their contractors write the scientific paper and academics allow their names to be used as though they had conducted the research and written the paper themselves. Yet again, the paper contained errors in the presentation of cardiovascular events with rofecoxib which once again minimised cardiovascular risk, and this study was conducted for marketing purposes, another so-called seeding trial. The Annals were quick to condemn ghost-writing and a full correction of the errors was published after Merck scientists provided an initial, but incorrect explanation. Many other journals published articles with results favourable to rofecoxib that subsequent court documents have shown to be ghost-written by scientific writing companies hired by Merck.

The rofecoxib story was the worst of news for modern, scientific medicine. There are the most serious ethical questions about the conduct of the mostly medically qualified researchers, those doctors who allowed their names to be placed on ghost-written papers, and those doctors who participated willingly and were paid for their part in seeding trials. Internal and external review at journals was clearly inadequate, the drugs regulator could have been more proactive in mandating a placebo trial but did not, and the seemingly cosy relationship between the drugs regulators and the pharmaceutical companies could be questioned and was by the US Senate Finance Committee.

Looking at the big picture, science and the scientific method had apparently triumphed only to then slump to disaster. Science always "stood on the shoulders of giants". No dye industry, no phenazone. No development of pharmaceutical companies, no NSAIDs. No COX discovery, no Nobel prize, but also no rofecoxib. Science had produced many very valuable medicines,

227

but in the pursuit of sales the brand of "evidence-based" was often usurped by the marketing department of the companies. Their primary and legal obligation was to make a profit for their shareholders.

Of course, it was skills honed by years of practicing evidence-based medicine that had enabled the deceptions to be uncovered by brave, academic whistle blowers. Yet the episode left a nasty taste. Thousands of people had been harmed, trust had been damaged and it was difficult to know who to believe. It was as if the pharmaceutical companies had two heads – a "good head" which did great science and helped lots of people live longer and better, and a "bad head" that would exaggerate scientific claims for sales and even distort science in the pursuit of profit. We never knew which one was talking to us, but I did personally experience being put under pressure to change National Prescribing Centre summaries of evidence from people closely associated with pharmaceutical companies with COX-2 inhibitors, and received offers to put my name to ghost-written articles. All such invitations were, of course, promptly and firmly rejected.

But the most serious questions were faced by Merck. Once one of America's most admired companies, with billions of dollars at stake Merck conducted the trials, stored, and analysed the data internally, paid academic researchers as consultants to the investigative teams and the safety monitoring boards, and maintained heavy involvement in the writing and presentation of findings. It hoodwinked the journals and peer reviewers and used its huge marketing budget to sell over 100 million prescriptions of its drug in the US alone, based on false promises and incomplete data to unsuspecting doctors and patients. Until the drug was withdrawn from the market, none of the people writing or picking up those prescriptions had had the opportunity to consider the true balance of its risks and benefits.

CHAPTER SIXTEEN

Diclofenac, a Canoe, and Everything Changes

Merck were not the only pharmaceutical company to synthesise a COX-selective inhibitor. Originally developed by team at Searle and patented in 1993, celecoxib was launched onto the market a few months before rofecoxib in 1999. A series of company takeovers meant that two companies – Pfizer and Pharmacia – were jointly marketing it at launch, although a further subsequent merger meant that eventually Pfizer emerged as the multinational pharmaceutical giant that included celecoxib in its large portfolio of medicines.

In September 2000, more than a year after celecoxib reached the market, what should have been the definitive celecoxib randomised trial was published in the Journal of the American Medical Association.[clxix] Known as CLASS, the trial concluded that a celecoxib was associated with a lower incidence of principally ulcer complications than traditional non-steroidal anti-inflammatory drugs. The trial received a large amount of publicity and was quickly cited many times by other researchers. What was much less widely publicised were criticisms that contradicted this conclusion.[clxx]

CLASS was reported as comparing celecoxib 800 mg/day with ibuprofen 2400 mg/day and diclofenac 150 mg/day in osteoarthritis or rheumatoid arthritis. Clinically relevant upper gastrointestinal ulcer complications (bleeding, perforation, or obstruction) and symptomatic ulcers during the first six months of treatment were described as the two main outcome measures. The trial was funded by Pharmacia.

The doses used in the trial seemed strange. Ibuprofen and diclofenac were right at the top end of the licensed dose range - levels that were certainly not routinely used in all patients taking these long-established NSAIDs. And the celecoxib dosage was twice the licensed daily dose. But that was the least of the problems with the CLASS trial.

An article in the Washington Post in August 2001 and two letters published in JAMA in November 2001 drew attention to the fact that complete information available to the United States

230

Food and Drug Administration contradicted the conclusions of the published research. The paper reporting CLASS comprised a combined analysis of the results of the first six months of two separate and longer trials. The protocols of these trials differed markedly from the published paper in design, outcomes, duration of follow up, and analysis. Fundamentally, this was terrible science.

Two comparisons were originally planned: celecoxib versus ibuprofen, and celecoxib versus diclofenac, and the maximum duration of follow up was not 6 months, but 15 and 12 months respectively. Reanalysis in 2002 of the whole of the data according to the original trial protocols actually showed similar numbers of ulcer related complications whichever NSAID people took. Almost all the ulcer complications that had occurred during the second half of the trials were in users of celecoxib. Because the JAMA paper only reported ulcer complications in the first 6 months, that analysis made celecoxib looked less toxic to the stomach. The truth was that, despite being a "designer, COX-2 selective NSAID", it appeared now from the CLASS data that as far as protecting the stomach was concerned, it was no better than traditional medicines. These data were available when the manuscript was submitted by its authors but were neither referred to in the article nor reported to JAMA.

By this point it was clear that science could develop potentially wonderful new medicines, and proper trials could determine whether they truly did what promised. But if the conduct of the trials was contaminated by poor design, or poor or alleged fraudulent analysis and reporting, then the evidence-based "quality mark" of the randomised controlled trial could be misappropriated and distorted by vested interests.

To impartial observers, between 2002 and 2004 the balance of risk and benefits on the stomach, the heart and on the kidneys for traditional NSAIDs and the "coxibs" remained unclear. That did not stop the increased use of the coxibs, fuelled as they were by intensive marketing by their manufacturers. In 2003 in the US alone, sales of celecoxib were $3.1billion. When rofecoxib was withdrawn from the market in September 2004, celecoxib had a brief surge in sales. But then in February 2005 a trial of celecoxib designed to show it too prevented precancerous colon adenomas was stopped early because of a more than doubling of the of cardiac events in the celecoxib group.[clxxi]

Regulators of medicines around the world sprang into action issuing new warnings to patients and prescribers and new studies were commissioned to try and untangle the mess, not least because some traditional NSAIDs had COX-selectivity similar to the "designer-NSAIDs", and there was some early evidence that they too could increase the rate of adverse cardiac events.

The most robust piece of evidence came from a meta-analysis of randomised controlled trials in June 2006.[clxxii] If someone in a trial gets struck by lightning it gets recorded as a serious adverse event. If someone in a trial gets admitted to hospital for planned surgery, it gets recorded as a serious adverse event. No one would ever think that the medicine being trialled was responsible for either of those serious adverse events, but the data collection in trials must be this detailed to pick up the adverse events that potentially are caused by the new medicine. Because every potential adverse event in trials is recorded, up to and including being struck by lightning, it was possible to undertake a meta-analysis of many randomised trials of many different NSAIDs – some new and many not so new.

It found that the selective COX-2 inhibitors did indeed increase in the risk of vascular events, but so also did high doses of ibuprofen, and standard doses of several other traditional NSAIDs including diclofenac. Standard doses of ibuprofen (1200mg per day) and all doses of naproxen were not associated with such adverse events. The UK Medicines and Healthcare products Regulatory Agency's (MHRA) Commission on Human Medicines (CHM) issued guidance asking prescribers to review their prescribing of NSAIDs in the light of the new evidence.[clxxiii]

This meant that in the UK the issue was no longer rofecoxib – it had been withdrawn by the company almost two years earlier. And thanks to judicious summaries of evidence from us at the National Prescribing Centre and others, and diligent work by prescribing advisers raising awareness practice by GP practice, sales of celecoxib too were now relatively small. If the increase in cardiac events was 3 per 1000 people taking celecoxib poor year, with the current volume of prescribing about 250 premature or avoidable heart attacks per year could be potentially associated with celecoxib. Each one was important of course, but there was another and much bigger problem in terms of harm to the population, and that was diclofenac. Diclofenac was no better or no worse in terms of cardiovascular harms than many other NSAIDS. But it accounted for about half of all NSAID prescriptions, and many of those prescriptions could have been ibuprofen or naproxen – avoiding the risk of heart attack or stroke. With the increase in cardiac events, based on reasonable assumptions I estimated that diclofenac prescribing was responsible for around 2000 avoidable or premature cardiac events per year.

Within a few months of the letter from the CHM, two things were apparent. Firstly, there was more and more consistent evidence that standard dose ibuprofen and naproxen were as good at relieving pain as other NSAIDs, and they did not carry the cardiac risk. And secondly, the established patterns of prescribing of NSAIDs were not changing despite the new meta-analysis being published in the British Medical Journal and an advisory letter being sent to all prescribers by the expert committee of the drugs regulator. I sat in the meeting room at the NPC looking at the data and knew we would have to begin discussions about better dissemination of the risks of not changing prescribing practice for NSAIDs in general and diclofenac in particular. It was not that diclofenac was worse than most other NSAIDs; the problem was, as with rofecocib in the US, that it was prescribed for many people. The risk to an individual was, in absolute terms, small. But a small absolute increase in risk amounted to a large number of adverse of events if many people were taking the medicine.

I consulted with the MHRA about the evidence and my estimates of the numbers of premature or avoidable cardiovascular events. They agreed with my estimates. I talked to colleagues in the Medicines, Prescribing and Industry branch in the Department of Health. They too agreed with the data, and that the issue was worthy of more action and a raising of the priority of the topic by us in our discussions with prescribing advisers. We produced an updated summary of the evidence as MeReC Extra 30[clxxiv] and I prepared myself for potential interest from the media. Everyone agreed that 2000 potentially avoidable cardiovascular events each year being caused by a commonly prescribed medicine might be very newsworthy. I had my answers to potential journalists' questions ready; I had had my hair cut, and I had a decent suit and two clean shirts pressed, ironed and neatly folded in the boot of my car.

But on the day we published MeReC Extra 30 the story that headlined was that of John Darwin – a man from Seaton Carew in the North East of England. Five and a half years earlier Darwin had been presumed drowned when he disappeared, and his wrecked canoe was found on a beach. He had faked his death, his wife had claimed the insurance money, and he had now been discovered in Panama. MeReC Extra 30 did not make the front pages of any lay newspaper.

But the complete lack of lay media publicity about MeReC Extra 30 allowed us to undertake a natural experiment. We began raising the issue as a priority in our educational programme for prescribing advisers, and began intensive monitoring of NSAID prescribing. We published initial data in 2011[clxxv]. We continued to track the changes over time and this natural experiment beautifully illustrated the difficulties of incorporating evidence into practice. (See Figure 16.1).

Figure 16.1.

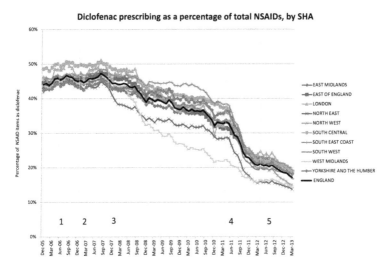

Line 1 is the date of the publication of the systematic review in the British Medical Journal.

Line 2 is the date of the advisory letter written to all prescribers from the Commission on Human Medicines.

Line 3 is the publication of the National Prescribing Centre's evidence summary and the start of its educational programmes for prescribing advisers.

Line 4 is the beginning of national payments to general practitioners for achieving locally-determined targets for prescribing. Most areas included NSAID prescribing as one of the targets.

Line 5 is the end of target payments for prescribing to GPs.

Simply making prescribers and prescribing advisers aware of the new evidence about cardiac risk and that the first choice NSAIDs for many people were now naproxen and low dose ibuprofen was clearly not enough to effect a quick and substantial change in prescribing. Change, even when it occurred was slow, even though it was related to patient safety. Evidence did not flow smoothly like water down a pipe to prescribers. Even when

235

patients were at risk, many prescribers found it difficult to change their established practice.

It was not a simple question of pressing "I" or 'N" on a computer keyboard instead of "D" to initiate safer prescribing. Prescribers had used diclofenac for their patients for many years. It appeared to help many of them. And they had not noticed lots of patients having cardiac problems with diclofenac. Even when it was pointed out that they would have been unlikely to notice that association because it had only just been described in the new research, the resistance to changing practice persisted for a long time in many parts of the country.

There were some discussions about the difference between the balance of risks for the population versus the balance of risks for an individual, and we included that issue in the MeReC Extra. The 2000 additional cardiac events data were not challenged, but prescribers, more implicitly than explicitly, recognised that the risk to an individual was of a different order. An increase in cardiac risk of 3 per 1000 people per year could be framed as 997 people out of 1000 not experiencing the adverse event. Weighing up the situation of someone with a painful condition that had significantly improved with diclofenac, both patient and prescriber might conclude that they, in that particular situation, would prefer to take the 3 in 1000 per year risk given the apparent benefits on pain that were already a big plus, rather than switching to a different treatment.

Yet, thousands of those decisions would cumulatively lead to the population excess of up to 2000 avoidable or premature cardiac events. That was the dilemma. How best to approach such decision making was not part of the our evidence summary at the time, but we were learning lots about decision making. We increasingly questioned our own awareness about how decisions were made we had those discussions; we were beginning to recognise we needed to think more about thinking.

Change in practice did begin to occur as conversations continued across weeks, months and into years. Gradually more naproxen and ibuprofen was prescribed, and less diclofenac. But this happened differentially, fastest in the North East and West Midlands, and slowest in the South Coast. It was counter-intuitive for evidence-based practice to be seen to widen variation in practice, at least in the short term. But the mean for the whole country was heading in the desirable direction, and the evidence indicated that at the level of the population change would be better for individual patients and for the population.

Progress was slow but steady because of education and summaries of evidence, and even the South Coast eventually began to change its pattern of prescribing. But when financial incentives accompanied by a local focus and local comparative data the pace of change accelerated (see lines 4 and 5 of Fig. 16.1). The educational "help it happen" approach was accelerated by the "make it happen" approach of finance and performance data. The variations in practice between regions rapidly narrowed. But when the incentives and focus ceased, the rate of change returned to its native path, all be it with preservation of the narrowed variation.

There was more work to be done in understanding how individual decisions were being reached by patients and prescribers in thousands of individual consultations, and more work to be done in understanding what approaches might work best at getting evidence incorporated into routine clinical practice. It was obvious that simply writing down or even telling people the evidence was not necessarily going to mean a large or rapid rate of change in clinical practice, even when high quality evidence was involved.

As all this was going on there were two very different pieces of academic work that helped us to a better understanding. The first was an incredible systematic review of the available literature on how to spread good practice in service organisations.[clxxvi] We spent a lot of time reading, discussing and debating the findings of this review both internally and with prescribing advisers. We invited the lead author, Trish Greenhalgh (who is now on her third professorship, this time at Oxford University) to come and

237

run workshops on her findings for us and many of our key audiences.

In short, there was great complexity, it was difficult to predict in advance what would work to change practice, but there were some things to consider. Among these were characteristics of the innovation (for example, was there a relative advantage, could it be tested out by the adopters, was the innovation complex or simple); what was the state of the health system into which the innovation was being introduced (for example, was there capacity within the system to accommodate the change); what was the implementation process (for example, was there a hands on approach by leaders and managers, was there feedback on progress); were end-users of the innovation involved in the design and was there attention paid to communication and project information; and what was the context for the innovation (for example, what was the socio-political context, were there incentives and mandates?).

Twenty years on, I still refer people to this review. It is still possible to broadly categorise implementation approaches as "let it happen" (publish information and let the system take it up, or not), help it happen (use education approaches to boost change, for example), or "make it happen" (regulatory or financial incentives / disincentives to boost change).

The other research approach could not have been more different in design. John Gabbay and André le May observed and interviewed in depth two general practices, one in the south of England and one in the north, over two years.[clxxvii] They found that instead of using guidelines,

"*Clinicians rarely accessed and used explicit evidence from research or other sources directly, but relied on "mindlines" - collectively reinforced, internalised, tacit guidelines. These were informed by brief reading but mainly by their own and their colleagues' experience, their interactions with each other and with opinion leaders, patients, and pharmaceutical representatives, and other sources of largely tacit knowledge. Mediated by organisational demands and constraints, mindlines were iteratively negotiated with a variety of key*

238

actors, often through a range of informal interactions in fluid "communities of practice," resulting in socially constructed "knowledge in practice."

This fitted well with the evidence we had explored with our Information Mastery colleagues – that brief reading and talking to other people were powerful influences on clinical decision making. But even when we focussed conversations between prescribing advisers and GP practices on NSAIDs in general and diclofenac in particular, the pace of change in the local NHS could be measured in years rather than weeks. And clinicians were generally overwhelmed with information. As the outputs from NICE increased in volume two hospital doctors compared the conditions the patients they had admitted as emergencies in one 24-hour period with guidelines issued in the previous three years advising how to treat those conditions. They found:-

"In a relatively quiet take, we saw 18 patients with a total of 44 diagnoses. The guidelines that the on-call physician should have read remembered and applied correctly for those conditions came to 3,679 pages. This number included only NICE, the Royal Colleges and major societies from the last 3 years. If it takes 2 minutes to read each page, the physician on call will have to spend 122 hours reading to keep abreast of the guidelines" (for one 24h on-call period).[clxxviii]

Medicine was changing. Rofecoxib and celecoxib were, sadly, only two examples where trust in science and medicine to always act in the best interests of both individuals and the population was shattered. There were too many others. At the Bristol Royal Infirmary in the 1990s, babies died at high rates after cardiac surgery. An inquiry found "staff shortages, a lack of leadership", "[a] ... unit ... simply not up to the task" ... "an old boy's culture" among doctors, "a lax approach to safety, secrecy about doctors' performance and a lack of monitoring by management". The scandal resulted in cardiac surgeons leading efforts to publish more data on the performance of doctors and hospitals.[clxxix]

Later scandals involving poor quality care included those at the Mid-Staffordshire NHS Trust, Gosport War Memorial Hospital, and maternity units at Morecambe, Barrow in Furness,

Shrewsbury and Telford. There were many others. And the Bristol scandal unearthed one at the children's hospital in Liverpool.

The issue was sparked by the death of 11-month-old Samantha Rickard, who died in 1992 while undergoing open-heart surgery at Bristol Royal Infirmary. Helen Rickard, Samantha's mother, demanded a copy of her infant daughter's medical records from the hospital. In the records she found a letter from the pathologist who performed the post-mortem written to the surgeon who had performed the operation, stating that he had retained Samantha's heart. Confronted with this evidence, the hospital promptly returned the heart in 1997. Rickard quit her job to find out exactly what had happened to her daughter. She set up a support group with other parents and ran a free phone helpline for the many other families affected. In September 1999 a medical witness to the Bristol Public Inquiry drew attention to many hearts that were in storage at the Alder Hey Children's Hospital in Liverpool.

The Alder Hey organs scandal involved the unauthorised removal, retention, and disposal of human tissue, including children's organs, during the period 1988 to 1995. During this period more than 2,000 body parts from around 850 infants were retained for unknown purposes without the knowledge or permission of the children's parents. There was a public inquiry into the organ retention scandal which led to the Human Tissue Act 2004, which overhauled legislation regarding the handling of human tissues in the UK and created the Human Tissue Authority.

There were other examples in addition to the coxibs where scrutiny by medical journal editors, their staff and their peer reviewers failed science, patients and the public. By far the worst was the claim in the early 1990s of a link between the Mumps, Measles and Rubella vaccine and autism. These have since been extensively investigated and found to be false.[clxxx] The link was first suggested in a research paper subsequently found to include fraudulent data authored by Andrew Wakefield and published by

The Lancet. It claimed to link the vaccine to colitis and autism spectrum disorders.

The paper was widely reported, leading to a sharp drop in vaccination rates in countries around the world. Promotion of the claimed link, which continues in anti-vaccination propaganda despite being widely and repeatedly refuted, led to an increase in the incidence of measles and mumps, resulting in deaths and serious permanent injuries affecting many thousands of children worldwide. Following the initial claims, reviews of the evidence by the US Centers for Disease Control and Prevention, the American Academy of Pediatrics, the Institute of Medicine of the US National Academy of Sciences, the UK National Health Service, and the Cochrane Library have all found no link between the MMR vaccine and autism.

The Lancet paper was retracted in 2010 but Fiona Godlee, editor of the BMJ, said in January 2011,

"The original paper has received so much media attention, with such potential to damage public health, that it is hard to find a parallel in the history of medical science. Many other medical frauds have been exposed but usually more quickly after publication and on less important health issues."[clxxxi]

And of course, there were shocking cases involving individual health care professionals. Harold Frederick Shipman was convicted on 31st January 2000 of the murder of 15 patients under his care. He is the only British doctor known to be guilty of murdering his patients. The public inquiry identified 215 victims of Shipman and estimated his total victim count at 250, about 80% of whom were elderly women.

And in Grantham, in 1991 Nurse Beverley Allitt attacked thirteen children, four fatally, over a 59-day period before she was brought up on charges for her crimes. It was found that Allitt was the only nurse on duty for all the attacks on the children and she also had access to the drugs. She was charged with four counts of murder, eleven counts of attempted murder and eleven counts of causing grievous bodily harm. On 28th May 1993, she was found guilty on each charge and sentenced to thirteen concurrent terms of life imprisonment, which she is serving at Rampton Secure Hospital in Nottinghamshire.

A hard lesson to be learned was that a centuries-long, implicit trust in the scientific method and healthcare professionals delivering safe and effective care was no longer possible. Checks and regulation of pharmaceutical companies in relation to new medicines and pricing of medicines, of device manufacturers, of health service organisations, and of health care professionals were all tightened. These changes would include greater availability and transparency of data, a requirement for the explicit demonstration of clinical competence and the incorporation of high-quality evidence routinely into practice. All this would need to be demonstrated, rather than this being assumed. Comparative performance and league tables were about to go mainstream. The impact of these changes on the practice of medicine would be profound, and the consequences would difficult to measure and sometimes unintended.

As Richard Smith, the editor of the British Medical Journal, wrote the week after the verdicts in the Bristol heart case, medicine was "All changed, changed utterly".

CHAPTER SEVENTEEN

Industrialised Medicine

From the start of the NHS until 2004, general practitioners were self-employed and contracted with the NHS as individuals to provide 24-hour care, 7 days a week, 52 weeks a year for their registered patients. They received a basic practice allowance and then most of their practice income came from for the number of patients they had registered on their list (capitation), with a number of additional payments – for example, for childhood immunisations, contraception, maternity care, and patients temporarily registered with them as holiday makers or students home from university and so on. These payments were governed by a complex set of rules called "The Red Book". Over time, most GPs formed small partnerships offering crossover for each other on a day-to-day basis. The Red Book also made provision for GPs to be reimbursed 70% of their staff costs and 100% of the cost of their premises, subject to specific criteria being met.

Out of hours care during evenings, nights and weekends in cities was often sub-contracted out to a "deputising service". In the 1990s, some smaller towns had created their own Out of Hours Cooperative in order to ease the increasing burden of an increased demand for 25-hour, round the clock care on individual GPs. I was instrumental in establishing one for our town. Rural practices still often covered their own out of hours calls but even then it was only those GPs in truly remote practices who were continuously available to their patients.

In the 1980s, the Conservative government under Margaret Thatcher increasingly looked for ways of linking GP's remuneration to performance. Constantly battling the growth in the costs of the NHS, in the 1990 GP Contract - given the government's enthusiasm for competition and unequivocal evidence of variations in practice - there was increased weighting given to the pay of GPs being derived on a per patient basis, a reduction in the basic practice allowance which everyone received whether they had 1 patient or 3000, and targets were set for cervical smears and immunisations. GPs were required to give health checks to new patients, patients over 75 and those who had not seen a GP for 3 years. The GP Fundholding scheme gave those practices who opted in the opportunity to manage a budget for purchasing hospital care for their patients. This certainly stimulated competition, with some Fundholding practices adopting an assertive approach to contract negotiations with their local hospitals. As a consequence, the culture of health care in those practices changed substantially, with a much greater awareness of and emphasis on the costs of care being provided.

However, costs of care continued to increase, as did waiting lists for planned surgery. So many people were waiting months for their hospital treatment that the Labour Party came to power in 1997 promising to "save the NHS". A year post-election and the health strategy emerged. It provided unprecedented increases in funding for the health service, but Prime Minister Tony Blair emphasised that the extra money must be linked to a 'step-change' in reform. It took four main forms: clear targets and standards set nationally; regulatory inspection and assessment; central support of professionally led collaboratives; and having earlier abolished GP Fundholding because of concerns about a two-tier GP service developing, it later introduced its own market-style incentives including a private finance initiative to fund the building of new hospitals to replace long-outdated NHS infrastructure.

Alongside guidelines from NICE, there was a blitz of National Service Frameworks to stimulate greater efficiency in the delivery of care of cancer, heart disease and mental health. Every year seemed to bring another bout of structural reorganisation. Despite increased health funding and a welcome reduction in patients waiting a long time for elective surgery, as the millennium turned general practice was on its knees.

Demand for care had continued to increase. The days got busier and busier. In general practice, recruitment was increasingly difficult. In the 1980s an advertisement for a partner might bring in as many as 120 applicants, which was equally worrying as a demonstration of workforce planning that was non-existent or wrong. By 2000 there were rarely more than a handful of applicants to replace a retiring GP and some practices got none at all leaving the existing partners to cope with an ever-increasing workload.

In a national ballot in 2002 GPs called overwhelmingly for a new contract. At the same time, under the influence of Downing Street advisors, the government had its own agenda including opening primary care to a wider variety of providers and introducing a form of performance related pay.

Regarding the Out of Hours part of the contract, the doctors were clear that the current model of individual GPs still having total responsibility both for organising and providing round the clock cover was unsustainable. In reality in all but the remotest practice, care was provided by other organisations. The Department of Health was attracted to the idea of an integration of out of hours care. They thought this was an excellent opportunity to redesign out-of-hours provision for the better, putting services around patients' needs and developing a new model of out-of-hours care that dovetailed with the wider economy of unscheduled care provision including A&E departments, ambulance services, GP emergency clinics, Walk-In Centres, NHS Direct, and local authority social services provision.

So, in the new GP contract in 2004 there was a clause in the new contract which allowed GPs to opt out of their 24/7/365 responsibility. This suited both GPs and the Health Departments. In England the responsibility for organising out of hours care passed to Primary Care Trusts (which had replaced health authorities), and they had transferred to them exactly that part of GPs' pre 2004 income which was earmarked for out of hours work. GPs gave up £6000 per year each to absolve themselves from out of hours care.

Almost all were very relieved to do so because there were many other changes afoot as a result of the 2004 contract, not least pay for performance. The "Red Book" was abolished, with each GP practice receiving a share of the money allocated to primary care (the "Global Sum") according to a new formula which used list size (weighted for age and sex), rurality, for the

246

differential cost of employing staff in some areas compared with others, the rate of turnover in the patient list, and for morbidity as measured by the Health Survey for England. For some practices this meant a substantial reduction in their income and a Minimum Practice Guarantee had to be introduced as a "safety net".

But then the Global Sum was reduced, with money reallocated to the largest pay for performance scheme in the world − the Quality and Outcomes Framework. Rapidly called the QOF by everyone, it was designed to give GPs the incentive to do more work and fulfil centrally set requirements.

At its heart was a frustration with the obvious variation in care provided for people with chronic conditions. People with chronic disease are more likely to be users of the health system, accounting for some 80% of all GP consultations.[clxxxii] And yet obvious, evidence-based approaches to managing those chronic conditions somehow did not always happen. People with diabetes did not always get their blood pressure and cholesterol checked. People with asthma were not necessarily regularly reviewed to check their inhaler technique or their understanding of the importance of regularly taking their "preventer" inhaler even if they remained well and without symptoms. And so on. There was little to no general discussion about why clinical management of chronic conditions quite often did not follow the evidence-base. This was going to be very much a "make it happen" approach.

The QOF did not lack ambition. It linked up to 25% of UK general practitioner income to performance on no less than 146 indicators. This huge number was deliberate. There were concerns that a much smaller number of indictors targeted on a narrower group of diseases where variation was widest or furthest from the desirable level of evidence-based care would mean clinical care being focussed on those to the detriment of other, "non-QOF'd" conditions. Whilst this was laudable, the sheer number of indicators resulted in a monumental effort being required to get the recorded data accurate and complete − which itself was distracting from clinical care.

About half of the indicators related to clinical quality indicators. Of those, ten related to maintaining disease registers, 56 to processes of care (such as measuring disease parameters and giving treatments), and 10 to intermediate outcomes (such as controlling blood pressure). It should be noted that controlling blood pressure is a disease-orientated outcome, not a patient orientated outcome. It was unclear from the start whether the QOF would mean people living longer or better.

The financial incentives built into the QOF created perverse incentives for the registering of disease. No one wanted a patient with diabetes on their list whose condition was not yet controlled, because the level of achievement for potentially several indicators might become compromised. If a patient presented with a QOF-related disease at the tail end of a financial year, thereby leaving little time for them to be treated, there was a real incentive to delay putting them on the disease register until the next financial year. There would be no detriment to their care, but they would appear on the disease register and be counted in the QOF data at the start of the next financial year.

Of greater concern was exception reporting. Practices were permitted to use their clinical judgment to exclude inappropriate patients from achievement calculations ("exception report"). This sounds like an opportunity for "gaming" the QOF but there are many good reasons for exception reporting. There are many circumstances in which treating a patient in line with evidence-based, QOF guidelines would be inappropriate - great age, a previous individualised lack of response to the evidence-based treatment, an unwillingness of the patient to be treated, and a contra-indication to the guideline-recommended approach. At the heart of this is the ability to treat people as individuals and to respect their individual wants and needs, rather than taking a broad brush, treating everyone in line with the evidence, and improving technical aspects of care and health.

If children who, for example, had parents who declined to have their children vaccinated were included in the QOF, it

248

could unfairly penalise practice income, produce perverse incentives for inappropriate treatment, or encourage practices to remove such patients from their lists to maximise payment. There has never been any evidence of practices gaming the system, but seven years on in 2011 the Audit Commission was criticising Primary Care Trusts for not monitoring exception reporting by practices more intensively.[clxxxiii] There was little recognition that good medical practice prioritised finding out whether patients were in agreement with proposed treatment, when explicit consent to treatment was remained an absolute imperative for clinical practice according to the General Medical Council..

To treat without consent constituted assault, or perhaps more often amounted to a bathroom medicines cabinet bulging with prescribed medicines which the patient did not take because they had never wanted them in the first place. But the more a practice found out what mattered to individual patients and tailored the care accordingly, the less it was following guidelines, and the more patients it needed to "exception report" for the QOF. A high level of "exception reporting" could be a marker of excellent, individualised care. But instead, there was the threat of GPs having to defend the care they had provided to NHS managers, many of whom did not have a clinical background and therefore struggled to understand why the Audit Commission, for once, had got it wrong. The effort involved for everyone was substantial, but "achieving maximum QOF points" seemed to have developed a momentum entirely of its own. Very quickly practices featured their "high QOF achiever" status in job advertisements.

Indicators were periodically reviewed with a whole team of people at NICE to ensure they were evidence-based and in line with NICE guidelines. Indicators were periodically adjusted or dropped from the scheme altogether, and new indicators introduced. A huge industry developed involving NICE, NHS England, and the British Medical Association representing the GPs. Participation in the QOF was voluntary but finances made it so imperative that almost everyone did. And since the standards changed each year, all practices participating had to do more work each year for the same income.

The effect on practice income could be substantial. Practices were awarded points based on the proportion of patients for whom targets are achieved, between a lower achievement threshold of 40% for most indicators (that is, practices must achieve the targets for over 40% of patients to receive any points) and an upper threshold that varies according to the indicator. In 2007 each point earned the practice £125, adjusted for patient population size and disease prevalence. A maximum of 1000 points was available, equating to £31,000 per GP.

Unsurprisingly, net effect of the QOF was a substantial, if temporary, increase in practice income. The Department of Health estimated that GPs would achieve 75% of QOF points, but in each of the first three years it was around 95%. Increased practice income did not last long; with the worldwide financial crisis of 2008 and subsequent public sector financial austerity imposed by the Conservative - Liberal Democrat coalition government, income in subsequent years did not keep pace with rising practice expenditure. And of course, this expenditure was required in part to maintain staff and systems to data collect for the reduced-value QOF points.

With all this effort, surely the increased focus on delivering evidence-based care made a real difference to patients? Given the spend on the QOF was more than £1billion a year it is unsurprising that a considerable amount of research has been undertaken to produce that evidence.[clxxxiv][clxxxv][clxxxvi][clxxxvii][clxxxviii][clxxxix] Unfortunately, the evidence that pay for performance improves health outcomes is lacking, and even worse there were unintended outcomes which may have worsened care considerably.

This is typical of the research findings:-

"Between 2003 and 2005, the rate of improvement in the quality of care increased for asthma and diabetes but not for heart disease. By 2007, the rate

of improvement had slowed for all three conditions and the quality of those aspects of care that were not associated with an incentive had declined for patients with asthma or heart disease. As compared with the period before the pay-for-performance scheme was introduced, the improvement rate after 2005 was unchanged for asthma or diabetes and was reduced for heart disease......... The level of the continuity of care, which had been constant, showed a reduction immediately after the introduction of the pay-for-performance scheme and then continued at that reduced level."

In other words, the quality of primary care was generally improving in England in the early 2000s and before QOF. Despite the constant barrage of policy initiatives from the Labour government, those initiatives alone seemed to the having a galvanising effect. The introduction of clinical audit, wider adoption of information technology, and the creation of quality oriented statutory bodies were having an effect in improving quality of care. This, of course, fits with implementation science and information mastery. Human beings respond well to talking to other people, educationally focussed input especially if led by credible peers, and brief reading.

The introduction of the QOF seemed to temporarily accelerate this trend for the QOF-incentivised activities, but a plateau was quickly reached. Incentives had little apparent impact on non-incentivised activities in the short term but seem to have some detrimental effects in the longer term, possibly because of practices focusing on patients for whom rewards applied. And of course, the QOF measured care processes; these are disease-orientated and not patient-orientated outcomes.

The adverse effect of this industrialised approach to delivering health care which may be of greatest concern is the loss of continuity of care. Patients were asked to attend for a review appointment with one of the practice nurses for their diabetes one week, their cervical smear with someone else the following week, and then someone else would be dressing their ulcerated leg. When actually the most important thing in her life that she wanted help with was that her son had been arrested for possession of a Class A drug and she was beside herself with worry. If only she could see a GP who knew her and her family?

For chronic conditions there is evidence of a strong association between higher continuity of care and reduced premature mortality rate, complication risks and health service utilisation but little to no improvement in various health indicators.[cxc] In other words, the markers of chronic disease do not seem to be any better when there is continuity of care, but people live longer or better. All-cause mortality is substantially reduced by continuity of care[cxci] – and yet the QOF reduces continuity of care. Premature mortality is the most important patient-orientated outcome for many people, and yet the QOF works against continuity of care which reduces premature mortality.

The reasons for this reduction in mortality are not simple, but from my twenty years of being a GP it seemed easier for patients to disclose embarrassing or worrying symptoms to someone they knew well rather than to a stranger. If those symptoms are rectal bleeding, or vaginal bleeding after intercourse, or "a silly cough I've had for a few weeks and then yesterday I coughed a bit of blood" that might be quite important. Continuity of care means fewer referrals to hospital, fewer tests, and less treatment "just in case". It seems as if avoiding some aspects of especially specialist care might confer health advantages. Less care can sometimes mean avoiding tests and treatments that benefit some people but harm others. Despite substantial, successive, scientific and technical advances in medicine, interpersonal factors remain important.

But instead, technical aspects of care came to dominate what mattered most to some patients. Whatever the patient had come for, if blood pressures were not recorded or patients asked about how much alcohol they drink every year or so, clinical care was judged to be substandard, and the practice lost income.

QOF and the associated NICE guidelines created a practice environment damaging to individualised care which has continued over the next twenty years to the present day. If I ask doctors about the standards for the good control of Type 2 diabetes, they will give me a number representing the level of glycosylated haemoglobin (HbA1c) in the blood. NICE guidelines rightly say that the target level of HbA1c should be individualised. A 90-year-old in a nursing home with advanced Parkinson's disease, glaucoma, and three other chronic conditions who also has a thirty year history of diabetes but no signs of complications and who takes no medicines for her diabetes could and should have a less rigid target for her diabetes control than a 50 year old man who smokes, has angina and also has diabetes. That sensible, flexible, individualised and kind care of the 90-year-old is sometimes driven out of mind by the presence of a QOF target, especially when it is accompanied by an erroneous mindline of what is thought the NICE guideline wants clinical care be. I still have the privilege to teach lots of doctors about evidence-based medicine. Such misunderstandings are not some rare occurrence. They are the norm.

We seem to have fallen into a situation known as the McNamara Fallacy.[cxcii] It goes something like this:-

1.   The first step is to measure whatever can be easily measured. This is OK as far as it goes.
2.   The second step is to disregard that which can't be easily measured or to give it an arbitrary quantitative value. This is artificial and misleading.
3.   The third step is to presume that what can't be measured easily really isn't important. This is blindness.
4.   The fourth step is to say that what can't be easily measured really doesn't exist. This is suicide.

It was the sociologist Daniel Yankelovich who coined the phrase "The McNamara Fallacy" in 1972. Robert McNamara was US Secretary of Defense from 1961 to1968, serving Presidents Kennedy and Johnson. His career was stellar. It started with a degree in economics from Berkeley, an MBA at the Harvard Business School, and staying on at Harvard to became its youngest assistant professor at the age of 24. During the

Second World War, McNamara served in the US Army's Department of Statistical Control. He applied rigorous statistical methodology to the planning and execution of aerial bombing missions, achieving a dramatic improvement in efficiency.

After the War, he joined the Ford Motor Corporation. Ford was in disarray and losing money. McNamara applied his skills of rational statistical analysis to the problems of the ailing giant and returned Ford to profit. He had a highly developed sense of the greater good and was a pioneer of passenger safety in car manufacture. In 1960, aged 44, he was appointed President of the Ford Corporation. After less than two months in this post, he was offered a cabinet position by President-Elect John F. Kennedy, which he accepted.

McNamara applied the same rigorous numbers-based analysis to the Pentagon that had worked at Ford. As the conflict in Vietnam escalated, he believed that if Viet Cong casualties exceeded the numbers of US dead, the war would eventually be won. The data, however, were flawed. The US-backed South Vietnamese army reported false and over-optimistic data on casualties that they thought the Pentagon wanted to hear. The US did not question the numbers. The Pentagon also failed to recognise the limitations of modern military equipment when facing highly unconventional, highly motivated people's movements.

Some problems do not submit to numerical analysis. In health care how do you measure kindness, compassion, continuity, and caring? Are these not important? It seems that because they are difficult to measure, they have become to be regarded as unimportant.

For those who believe in evidence-based medicine and patients living longer or better, what data there is shows the QOF was not associated with significant changes in mortality when the UK trends were compared internationally with other countries who did not have a comparable pay for performance system. The lack of evidence of benefits associated with the schemes, the loss

254

of focus on conditions not included in the schemes, that the schemes were not necessarily relevant to local health priorities, the evidence of mechanistic approaches to individual care as clinicians "followed the rules" irrespective of whether the intervention is appropriate for that patient (including their values and preferences), and the sheer burden of administration and management on the workforce means it is surprising that the QOF still exists. In Wales, Scotland and Northern Ireland the QOF approach to quality improvement has been quietly shelved But in England it continues, all be it in a reduced form. At the time of writing, it was suspended whilst the NHS attempted to cope with and then recover from the coronavirus pandemic, and there is a consultation on the value of such schemes. But it has not, at least yet, been quietly set aside.

And in the meantime it contributes greatly to over treatment, encourages the unthinking following of guidelines instead of individualising care, perpetuates the fragmentation of care, and works against continuity of care.

Whatever is the NHS in England doing, allowing this to continue?

CHAPTER EIGHTEEN

Uncertainty, Probability and Making Decisions

Most people have not studied how they and their fellow human beings make decisions. Yet we all make decisions – how much milk shall I put in the morning tea, which pair of shoes should I put on today, what television programme shall we watch tonight, shall I tell my bosses what I really think of them, should I propose marriage – and so on. Lots of decisions every day, and they just fly by, most without too much time or thought being given to the decision. Some decisions are, of course, more important than others, and we might give considerable thought, for example, about whether and who we should marry, and spend rather less time on the "which pair of socks" kind of decisions. But how human beings make such decisions is not prime time on many people's curriculum. We might give some decisions lots of thought, but have we been taught how we can make decisions better? Probably not. It seems we still just expect people to pick up by osmosis how to make decisions, never mind how to make them better.

When we are ill and we consult a health care professional the product of that consultation is a decision, or more usually several decisions. There will often be a decision called a diagnosis, and often a decision will be taken about treatment. There might be decisions about when to review the condition, or when to return for a further consultation. There might be a decision made about when to come back sooner if certain things get worse. And so on. It might be expected that at least one of the participants in the consultation, the health care professional, has had some education, training and skills in how human beings make such decisions, and it would be good if everyone knew a little more about making decisions better. But no. There is some work underway teaching "Clinical Reasoning" to medical students, but otherwise undergraduate and postgraduate training programmes concentrate almost entirely on technical aspects, and very little happens for the public – for example, in schools.

For health care professionals, when to begin learning about how to make decisions is not straightforward. Human beings first need to understand the basics which underpin the technical aspects of their tasks and roles.[cxciii] It is very difficult for someone to become an expert chess player without first learning how each of the chess pieces move as individual pieces. Their next stage is learning to put certain moves together in sequence to, say, create a strong opening set of moves to a chess game. That might need to be adapted according to how the opponent responds, so there are variants to be learned. Eventually, after much learning, repetition, and feedback from both winning and losing, the expert chess player can see a potential larger set of moves than a beginner can, and there is an automatic element to the making of the next move because the situation has been experienced many times before. Experts also see further ahead - they can envisage a wider range of opponent moves than a beginner can.

In healthcare, the equivalent of the chess piece moves that must be learned first is the basic sciences. The doctor, nurse, pharmacist or whoever will find it very difficult to manage the complex medicines needed for a patient with heart failure if they have not learned the basic anatomy of the heart, understand how the heart functions in its non-diseased state, and realise that how it functions is controlled by a complex system of automatic nervous systems and circulating hormones to make it beat faster or slower or push the blood around the body with more or less force.

The medicines for heart failure work on the nervous system controls of the heart and the hormones. How to use them judiciously in a patient with heart failure simply does not make sense to someone who does not have the basic scientific knowledge. Interestingly, lots of the details of that basic science cannot be recalled in detail even a few years out from medical school if it is not used explicitly in the day-to-day work. I once passed an examination in which I needed to recreate from memory a complex cascade of biochemical interactions called the Krebs cycle. I have never needed that knowledge since I passed the examination. But quite a lot of the basic scientific underpinning is important to the initial understanding and learning, and is necessary to create a solidly constructed pyramid of knowledge which enables how to later in the course begin to make accurate diagnoses and recommend safe and effective treatments. And then once those "disease scripts" have been learned, then they are readily recalled when needed.

There is lots and lots of basic science to be learned. Any health care professional has had to learn and recall in crucial examinations huge amounts of facts, and then learn the diagnosis and treatment "scripts", and then apply that knowledge accurately and appropriately in later clinical examinations in order to graduate and be able to have consultations with people who are ill.

The problem is, it is all technical and theoretical knowledge. As Joan in Chapter One dramatically demonstrated, whilst the technical knowledge is very, very important, it is not the whole story. Yes, woe betide you if you are a health care professional and you get important diagnoses and treatments wrong. Quite rightly, it is expected that health care professionals have great technical knowledge. But for great decision making there is a need for health care professionals to understand how they arrive at decisions, and how other people arrive at decisions, and then why those decisions might legitimately be very different. Only then can appropriate decisions be made for individual patients – decisions that are appropriate for them.

At the National Prescribing Centre around 2007 were already exploring how to make decisions better. We were reading and discussing with colleagues what we were uncovering, and how much it helped us to understand what we were seeing with individual patients and in the implementation of evidence in localities and in large populations. Trish Greenhalgh's systematic review on the influences of decision making when attempting to spread better practice, Gabby and Le May's mindlines paper and the real world use of information as described in the Information Mastery work were already at the front of our thinking. Joan was a stimulus and a vivid example, but not the beginning.

****

259

Putting the first pieces in place to begin constructing the jigsaw of decision-making theories, it seems best to start with Daniel Bernoulli who was born in Basel in 1700. Daniel came from a family with eventually eight gifted mathematicians, who were of course all called Bernoulli, and even their given names add confusion because in the eight there were two Jacob's, two Nicholaus's, and no less than three Johann's.

Daniel was a genius. He set out the basis for the kinetic theory of gases, made important mathematical developments in fluid dynamics and discovered how to measure blood pressure by sticking a needle directly into an artery and seeing how high up a glass column the blood flowed. His method lasted 170 years until Scipione Riva Rocci in 1896 discovered a less painful and less dramatic approach to measure blood pressure, which is still used today.

But it is his work on decision making which is of greatest interest here. Daniel noticed that when making decisions that involved some uncertainty, people did not always try to maximize their possible monetary gain, but rather tried to maximize "utility", an economic term encompassing their personal satisfaction and benefit. Bernoulli realised that for humans, there is a direct relationship between money gained and utility, but that it diminishes as the total money held increases. For example, to a person whose income is £15,000 per year, an additional £1,000 in income will provide more utility than £1,000 would to a person whose income is already £500,000 per year.

There were more insights as he addressed another thought experiment, the St Petersberg Paradox which had been created by his older brother Nicholaus I Bernoulli. The experiment involves a game of chance for a single player in which a fair coin is tossed at each stage. The initial stake begins at £2 and is doubled every time heads appears. The first time tails appears, the game ends and the player wins whatever is the current stake. Thus the player wins £2 if tails appears on the first toss, £4 if heads appears on the first toss and tails on the second, £8 if heads appears on the first two tosses and tails on the third, and so on. If a casino is running the game, what would be a fair price to pay the casino for entering the game?

The paradox is that there is the potential for a participant to win a great amount of money, and therefore theoretically a player could decide to pay a very high price for being able to enter the game. But when people are asked how much they would pay for a ticket to play the game, even a millionaire will be reluctant will risk £20. Other people with less capital are prepared to risk even less to play.

This approach of discrete choice experiments - setting out a scenario and asking people what decision they would make - has greatly informed those studying decision making in the last forty years. It has become a mainstay of those studying cognitive psychology and behavioural economics – both address the domain of human decision making. Much progress has been made, and a number of Nobel prizes awarded for the work.

Here are some modern examples of expected utility games:-
cxciv

Scenario 1:

You have no savings but if you are careful, you can live week to week and month to month within your means.

You acquire a lottery ticket which gives you a 50% chance of winning £200,000.

Would you prefer to

A.   Take a chance with the lottery.

B.   Accept a certain £90,000 instead of playing the lottery.

Please take a moment to think about your decision and then make your choice, A or B.

261

Most people, but not everyone, selects option B. Humans generally prefer certainty to uncertainty. And humans fear losses more than they value potential gains. This forms the basis for modern expected utility theory in economics – much of economics is about how people make choices, and often those choices can be measured in terms of how they spend their money. Of course, in the same way that setting a ceiling on what one would pay to play the St Petersberg game, this also shows that human decision making is not truly rational – selecting option B means that on an individual basis that every time that choice is made it involves giving away £10,000 against the mathematical expected value. It is important to note that people are different one from another – despite the preference at the level of the population for certainty which is represented by more people picking B than A, everyone does not select B.

Now try this second experiment.

Scenario 2.

You must choose between having
A: £5million for sure
or
B: This gamble………
An 89% chance of winning £5million, a 10% chance of winning £25million, a 1% chance of winning zero.

Again, spend a little time and make your decision.

Most people will go with Option A, but not everyone. Note again that people make different choices one from another. But again, certainty is preferred by most humans over uncertainty, and £5million is definitely a whole heap of utility and enough for most people.

Our next scenario was developed by a Frenchman, Maurice Allias. He first worked on fundamental physics but from the 1930s, following the great depression, he switched to economics.

It was a good choice – he won the Nobel Prize for economics in 1988.

Scenario 3.

You must choose between having:-

A: An 11% chance of winning £5million with an 80% chance of winning zero.

B: A 10% chance of winning £25million and a 90% chance of winning zero.

Again, spend a little time and make your decision.

Here, most people select the more uncertain option, option B. They usually reason that there is no great difference between the probabilities of winning (11% versus 10%), but the sum gained from the slightly lower probability of winning is much larger. Again, not everybody chooses the same option.

The Allias Paradox illustrates that in its pure form Expected Utility Theory describes too narrow a range of decision making behaviours. If the circumstances are right, some people, perhaps quite a lot of people, would go for a riskier option because it is not very much riskier, and the gains are so substantial.

In an earlier chapter we briefly considered decision making in the context of getting on a plane, driving a car and so on. The analogy in health care might be the person with cancer. Let's work on the scenario that their treatment has been evidence - based, the best they could get, and it has all been done in a timely way and with great skill, compassion and kindness. But it is not going well. They have had two significant operations, followed by radiotherapy and two different chemotherapy combinations – and yet follow up scans show their cancer is rapidly progressing. So far, the treatment has been gruelling. There are two options:

A: No further attempts at curative treatment. Management now is directed towards control of symptoms. Treatment so far has been unpleasant and unsuccessful, and the aim now is quality of life rather than extending life.

B: At least one further attempt at curative treatment. Evidence suggests there is a 1% absolute chance of a cure – in other words the probability of survival a year from now improves from 0% to 1% with treatment. The new treatment has several unpleasant side effects and will require spells of several days at a time in hospital to administer treatment and manage side effects.

Just about as difficult a decision as anyone could possibly face. Now we have done a few exercises in decision making we can readily understand why people make different decisions when faced with this dreadful situation. Some people will opt for the last resort treatment even though only one person in 100 will get a cure. Other people will abandon further attempts at a cure and opt for symptom control now.

Even though these are brief and relatively simple thought experiments, they have profound implications. Currently almost all clinical guidelines make recommendations for treatment for everybody with the condition, or at least that is the impression they have created – especially in the UK when the guidelines are reinforced with serious money in the form of QOF. Is it reasonable for guidelines to make recommendations for everybody when the evidence on decision making shows that people will make different decisions?

But we are getting ahead of ourselves. When we are making decisions, we are often attempting to predict the future. "I will accept this job offer, I will enjoy working here", or "I will watch this TV programme, it will be entertaining", or "I will buy this car, it will be perfect for what I need", or "I will marry this person and we will have a wonderful life together". And so on. So let us consider one last scenario:-

Scenario 4:

A 90 year old aunt offers to leave you her beautiful house on the seafront in Cannes worth £900,000 – but only if you provide her with £2,500 a month (£30,000 a year) to live on. She will bear the cost of drawing up watertight legal documents. Average female life expectancy is 82 years, and as it happens you are currently able to save regularly £2,500 a month (which earns only a very small amount of interest).

Please choose one of these options:-
A: Accept the offer

or

B: Not accept the offer.

Spend a little time and then make your decision.

Most, but certainly not all, people pick Option A. The probability is your aunt will sadly not live many more years and you will then have the nearly £1million capital value of her wonderful-sounding house having given her £30,000 a year for very few years. Rationally this looks like a superb investment, especially given your ability to fund her monthly allowance comfortably.

However, some people do pick Option B, on the grounds of preferring certainty to uncertainty, and perhaps because they have now seen a few of these scenarios and are beginning to understand just a little of what underpins their own personal and usual approach to making decisions.

This scenario is based on French woman Jeanne Calment, who made such an agreement with her lawyer Andre-Francois Raffray in 1965 when she was 90 and he was 47 years old. She survived for 32 years after the deal was signed, dying aged 122 years and 164 days. She outlived Raffray who died aged 77. By then he had paid twice the market value for her house which he never lived in. Raffray's family had to keep up the payments until she died.[cxcv] Even when it is relatively straightforward to work out the probabilities, sometimes the remotely unlikely does happen. Uncertainty is everywhere, it is the water in which we swim.

Turning to probabilities in medicine, let us use a very common clinical scenario to start with – one with which many people will be familiar. A 23-year-old woman develops pain when urinating for the last 24 hours, is urinating more frequently, and she thinks she might have seen a little blood in her urine on one occasion. She is on day 7 of her menstrual cycle, in a stable relationship, and takes a combined oral contraceptive. There are alternative diagnoses, but the probability is high that she has a simple urinary tract infection (cystitis, or UTI).

Treatment of a UTI is almost always with an antibiotic, and the UK guidelines recommend an antibiotic called nitrofurantoin. Most doctors dealing with people with UTIs quickly learn the treatment, what the dose is, how frequently it should be taken, and what advice and warnings to give the patient. What they do not give much thought to, until we have a conversation about it, is how many of their patients get better because of the antibiotics?

If we look at one of the biggest randomised controlled trials of nitrofurantoin versus placebo for uncomplicated urinary tract infections,[cxcvi] of the people given nitrofurantoin 88% of them are cured by seven days of treatment, but so are 52% of the people given placebo. What does our patient - who has symptoms of a UTI, gets treatment with nitrofurantoin - and gets better think?

Of course, she thinks that the antibiotics were the magical thing that got her better from those horrible symptoms. But the true probabilities are that of the 88 people out of 100 who get better, 52 of them would have got better anyway. For sure, the antibiotic meant an extra 36 were better. But no one could tell in advance - or indeed afterwards - which individual would recover without the antibiotics and who truly did get cured by the

266

wonders of modern medicine. Of course, the prescribing doctors largely also think that when lots of people get better with the nitrofurantoin that they did a good job. Well, they did do a good job, but just over half of their patients would actually have got better without an antibiotic. In advance of making a decision about treatment, nobody can predict who will get better without an antibiotic. Decisions have to be taken in the face of that irresolvable uncertainty.

Then there are the 14 people out of the 100 with a UTI who did get the nitrofurantoin who were not cured. What will they and their doctors be thinking? Obviously, they will both be looking for the reasons why. Was this a urine infection in the first place? Could it be something else? Is there an obvious reason the nitrofurantoin did not work in this patient - for example, is the patient taking another medicine that interacted with it? Did the patient understand when to take the tablets, and manage to do that without missing doses – or at least not very many doses? All those are reasonable questions. But the numbers game tells us that the antibiotics not having the desired effect is not unusual. If there are 100 people with a UTI and they all get exemplary management, even in the best of circumstances in 14 people of 100 the evidence-based treatment will not work. And of course, no one can tell in advance who those individuals are going to be. And when humans automatically prefer certainty to uncertainty, and in such decision making there is almost always residual uncertainty just like this, it means the best modern medicine can usually offer is an improvement in the probability of a good outcome, but not a promise. There is no absolute guarantee of a good outcome even with timely, modern scientific, evidence-based medicine. That comes as a surprise to plenty of doctors and patients.

Why does this matter? Well, in the UTI scenario both patients and doctor might look differently at treatment success and failure if they were better aware of the true probabilities. Some of the mystery of cure and failure is dispelled. And when we come to preventative actions – treatments or screening tests which might be offered to lots of well people who might never develop the condition that attempts are being made to prevent – the probability numbers start to assume much greater importance.

I have previously mentioned President Roosevelt, his stroke and the establishment of the Framingham cohort - the aim of the research being to uncover the causes of the cardiovascular epidemic. Within a few years the Framingham cohort and other similar studies around the world showed that several factors increased the risk of a heart attack or stroke. Age, male sex, and diabetes were some of the biggest – but it was difficult for modern medicine to make those risks go away. Reducing the number of birthdays someone had had would be a very popular medicine if it were possible, but unfortunately it is currently an unrealistic expectation. But smoking, high blood pressure, high cholesterol, diet, and a lack of exercise could be modified, and the pharmaceutical industry set to work – especially on potential treatments for "high cholesterol".

Cholesterol is an essential component of cell membranes, the structure that borders every cell in the human body. Cholesterol is also needed for the manufacture of steroid-based hormones, particularly the sex hormones testosterone and progesterone. Other hormones, produced mainly by the adrenal gland, also require cholesterol for production. Aldosterone (the hormone that makes the kidneys retain water) and cortisol (the hormone that is important in suppressing inflammation in the body) are two such examples. Cholesterol must also be present for the skin to manufacture vitamin D, which plays a role in how the body handles calcium and assists in maintaining bone density. Cholesterol also enables the body to form bile acids, which are needed to help breakdown fats in the digestive tract so that they can be absorbed into the body.

Thirteen Nobel Prizes have been awarded to scientists who devoted major parts of their careers to cholesterol research. Over the course of a century, science has uncovered several lines of evidence that have established the causal connection between blood cholesterol, atherosclerosis, and coronary heart disease. Building on that knowledge, scientists and the pharmaceutical industry have successfully developed a remarkably effective class of drugs - the statins - that lower cholesterol levels in blood and reduce the frequency of heart attacks.

The first hint that cholesterol was related to atherosclerosis was in 1910, when it was discovered that atherosclerotic plaques from aortas of human subjects contained over 20-fold higher concentrations of cholesterol than did normal aortas. But serious research on the role of cholesterol in human atherosclerosis did not really get underway until the 1940s, due to a prevailing view that hardening of the arteries (atherosclerosis) was a simple consequence of aging and could not be prevented.

The genetic connection between cholesterol and heart attacks was first made in 1939 by Norwegian clinician Carl Müller, who described several large families in which high blood-cholesterol levels and premature heart attacks together were an inherited trait. In the mid-1960s the genetic understanding of this syndrome, which came to be known as familial hypercholesterolemia (FH), became clearer. Two clinically different types were identified - the homozygous form, in which affected individuals have severe hypercholesterolemia at birth and heart attacks occur as early as 5 years of age, and the heterozygous form, characterized by premature heart attacks that occur typically between 35 and 60 years of age.

Then in the early 1950s, John Gofman at Berkeley found - in the general population without FH - not only that heart attacks correlated with elevated levels of blood cholesterol but also that the cholesterol was contained in the blood in low density lipoprotein (LDL). He also observed that heart attacks were less frequent when the blood contained elevated levels of high density lipoprotein (HDL).

Intense efforts were made in the 1950s to determine the pathway by which cholesterol was synthesised in the body. Most of the crucial steps in this complex pathway, involving 30 chemical reactions, were worked out by four biochemists - Konrad E. Bloch, Feodor Lynen, John Cornforth, and George

269

Popják. Bloch and Lynen were awarded the Nobel Prize in 1964. The hunt was already underway for medicines that would block part of the cholesterol-synthesis pathway.

Cholesterol has two sources – it comes from what we eat and from what is synthesised within the liver. In humans, cholesterol produced in the liver far exceeds what is absorbed from the diet, even when large quantities of cholesterol are eaten. Again, this comes a surprise to many – there are still plenty of health care professionals and part of the food industry advocating low cholesterol diets and foods which are low in cholesterol . It was realised that inhibiting a step in the chemical pathway that synthesised cholesterol in liver cells would reduce the circulating cholesterol. Inhibiting HMG-CoA reductase (3-hydroxy-3-methyl-glutaryl-coenzyme A reductase was the targeted, rate-controlling enzyme.

Other approaches had been tried. The cholesterol-lowering properties of nicotinic acid were discovered in 1955. Clofibrate was synthesized at Imperial Chemical Industries (ICI) in England and marketed in 1958. In the 1960s, many other fibrates, that were more potent and safer than clofibrate were developed. In most patients, the cholesterol-lowering effect of fibrates was minimal to moderate, and there was no evidence that heart attacks and strokes were reduced by their use. Cholestyramine interferes with the reabsorption of bile salts, enhancing their faecal excretion, which means it is not well tolerated by all patients. And there was still no evidence of people living longer or better with fibrates or cholestyramine, which in this instance would mean demonstrating that people taking them had fewer cardiovascular events than people who were not taking them.

In 1957, Akira Endo graduated from Tohoku University's College of Agriculture in Sendai.[cxcvii] Inspired by the work of Fleming, Flory, Chain and Abraham on penicillin and Waksman on streptomycin, he joined the pharmaceutical company Sankyo in Tokyo, where he was assigned to one of the applied microbiology groups. After eleven years working on other projects, he had an opportunity to work on a project of his own.

Antibiotics had been shown to work in part by inhibiting many kinds of important chemicals within cells, not only in bacterial cells but also in mammalian cells. Although no metabolites that inhibited any enzymes involved in cholesterol synthesis had been isolated previously, Akira speculated that fungi such as moulds and mushrooms would produce antibiotics that inhibited HMG-CoA reductase. He postulated that antibiotics would cause the cell walls to collapse because of the lack of cholesterol. If you could create a chemical that would inhibit HMG-CoA reductase and kill microbes, could the same chemical lower cholesterol and prevent heart attacks and strokes?

It was a long, hard slog, quite different from Al Schatz and the isolation of what turned out to be streptomycin. After a year of testing 3,800 strains of fungi, his team found a culture broth of mould that showed potent inhibitory activity. A few months later they found a second active culture broth of blue-green mould, which was isolated from a rice sample collected at a grain shop in Kyoto. Eventually isolating the active ingredient, which was called compactin, there was still a long way to go. Collaborative work with Michael Brown and Joseph Goldstein at the University of Texas had successes and failures. Results in animals gave initially unpromising results, which were eventually explained and overcome. Akira had now been working at the issue for ten years.

Eventually, in February 1978, Akira Yamamoto, a physician at the Osaka University Hospital in Osaka, started treating an 18-year old woman with severe familial hypercholesterolemia with compactin. Akira Endo was not a doctor so needed Yamamoto's help. The patient's serum cholesterol dropped by about 30% during treatment with compactin, but after treatment for two weeks, her liver enzymes became elevated which indicated possible early signs of liver damage, and the patient had muscle pains. Both adverse effects were reversed on discontinuation of treatment. Cholesterol deposits in her skin and in association with tendons were markedly reduced after treatment at a lower dose of compactin for five months. In the following 6 months, Yamamoto treated five heterozygous FH patients and three patients with combined hyperlipidemia with compactin, and their cholesterol declined by roughly 30% on average; no severe side effects were noted.

Larger clinical trials were started but were then abandoned when researchers performing safety studies elsewhere found huge doses of compactin caused lymphoma in dogs. Meantime other pharmaceutical companies were very busy looking for potential cholesterol lowering medicines, and in 1979 Alfred Alberts at Merck - after an agreement to share research findings between Merck and Samkyo - isolated a molecule very similar to compactin from the fungus *Aspergillus terreus*. The new molecule was called lovostatin, and now the pace increased again. In 1981 Brown and Goldstein and Hiroshi Mabuchi's group at Kanazawa University reported the impressive lowering of cholesterol with compactin treatment of severe heterozygous patients with familial hypercholesterolemia.

In July 1982, several clinicians - stimulated by Mabuchi's report - including Roger Illingworth of Oregon Health Sciences University and Scott Grundy and David Bilheimer of the University of Texas, treated patients with severe FH unresponsive to available agents with lovastatin. The drug showed dramatic activity in lowering LDL cholesterol, with very few side effects. This led Merck to begin large scale clinical trials of lovastatin in patients at high risk, and long-term toxicity studies in dogs in 1984. The drug dramatically reduced cholesterol levels was well tolerated and no tumours were detected. In November 1986, Merck sent the New Drug Application to the U.S. drug regulators and lovastatin was given approval to become the first commercial statin in September 1987. Two years earlier, in 1985, Brown and Goldstein were awarded the Nobel Prize in Physiology or Medicine for their discoveries concerning the regulation of cholesterol metabolism.

Progress was now rapid. Multiple other statins were developed, including simvastatin, pravastatin, atorvastatin, fluvastatin, cerivastatin, and rosuvastatin. Of these, only cerivastatin was found to have an unacceptable adverse event profile and was removed from global markets due to excess risk of muscle problems.

Whilst statins had definitively answered the disease-orientated outcome of lowered cholesterol especially in people with familial hyperlipidaemia, the remaining research question was did they also lower the patient-orientated outcome of heart attacks and strokes in people without FH?

The Scandinavian Simvastatin Survival Study (4S) was the first randomised clinical trial with a statin with patient-orientated outcomes, and the results were remarkable. All patients enrolled in 4S had established coronary artery disease. After 5.4 years of follow-up and a 25% decrease in total cholesterol and 35% decrease in LDL-cholesterol, all-cause mortality was reduced by 30%, risk of a major coronary event by 34%, cardiovascular death by 35%, stroke by 30%, and coronary interventions by 37%.[cxcviii]

Studies in people with established heart disease with pravastatin were also positive, if with less impressive relative reductions.[cxcix][cc] Prevention trials in people without established heart disease with pravastatin and lovastatin showed a substantial reduction in risk for first-time CV events.[cci][ccii][cciii]

Atorvastatin therapy was associated with significant reductions in risk for CV events in patients with diabetes mellitus or hypertension.[cciv][ccv] The Heart Protection Study demonstrated benefit irrespective of baseline LDL-cholesterol.[ccvi]

The Pravastatin or Atorvastatin Evaluation and Infection Therapy–Thrombolysis in Myocardial Infarction (PROVE-IT) and Treating to New Targets (TNT) studies both suggested that when it comes to LDL-cholesterol levels, lower is better.[ccvii][ccviii]

And so on and so on. Statins have become one of the most researched medicines in the history of medicine. There is no question that they can reduce subsequent heart attacks and strokes, by up to 40% in relative terms. Their widespread use in people with established cardiovascular disease in the form of a previous heart attack and stroke seems unquestionable. They were not available when Herbert had his heart attack, but Joan took them for years and the probability is that they, along with a cocktail of other medicines, were at least in part responsible for her long survival after a heart attack and with established cardiovascular disease.

However, there is a genuine debate over the use of statins in people who do not have cardiovascular disease to prevent such disease occurring. The discussion is polarising, and to understand why we need to consider probability a little more, and understand more about how humans make decisions.

Several cohort studies, including Framingham, have been used to develop online risk calculators which can estimate the probability of a currently well individual having a heart attack or stroke in the next 10 years. In the UK, NICE has consistently recommended the use of the latest Q-Risk calculator.[ccix] A 60 year-old, non-smoking man living in the North West of England without diabetes or hypertension, with average cholesterol and not over weight has a ten year CV risk of 9.9%. All these risk calculators have a margin of error so it is reasonable to say his 10 year risk is 10% and keep in mind (a) that really means his risk is somewhere between, say, 8% and 12% and (b) the incidence of heart attacks has been falling every year since the peak year of 1979 so if that continues over time 10%-ish might be a small over estimate.

On the other hand, in 10 years' time, if nothing else changes, his 10 year risk goes up to 20% just because he is 10 years older. Also, there are a few things that might be important but are not included in the Q-Risk calculations, at least not at the moment. He might take regular exercise and eat a healthy Mediterranean-type diet, both of which ought to reduce his calculated risk. But since, like alcohol consumption, they are not included in the calculator we cannot know how big and what effect they would have on those numbers. Let us have a look visually at what that means to the probabilities using a website "GP Evidence" created for just this purpose by Julian Treadwell at Oxford University and funded by the National Institute for Health Research.[ccx] (See Figure 18.1).

Figure 18.1.

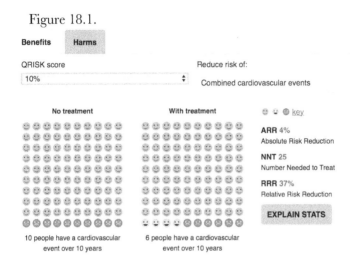

If 100 people with a baseline 10-year risk of cardiovascular disease of 10% take a statin, 4 will avoid a cardiovascular event compared with if they hadn't taken a statin

Look first at the left hand set of one hundred people - before statin treatment is considered. Whilst the Q-Risk calculation says there is a 10% risk of a heart attack or stroke in the next 10 years (and these are represented by the red faces), it could also say there is a 90% chance of NOT having a heart attack of stroke in the next 10 years (represented by the green faces). This "positive news" or "negative news" is called "framing" and can make a big difference to how human beings view risk.

Imagine someone going to see someone for a preventative consultation and being told "Good news, you have a 90% chance of NOT having a heart attack or stroke in the next 10 years". Then imagine someone else with the same risk factors and the same risk calculation being told "Bad news, you have a 10% chance of having a heart attack or stroke in the next 10 years". Are they likely to view their decision differently? Almost certainly yes. Were they given untruthful information? Definitely not. The words used matter a lot, and we will come to that in a later chapter.

Now look at the right hand set of one hundred people. All one hundred take a statin every day for the next 10 years. The statin is very effective at reducing heart attacks and strokes. It reduces them in relative terms by 40%. Who wouldn't want 40% fewer heart attacks and strokes?

But of course, 90 people out of the 100 were never going to have a heart attack or stroke anyway (the green faces). A policy of giving everyone with a 10-year CV risk of 10% a statin means will only prevent a heart attack in four people out of the hundred (the yellow faces). And there are still six people who have a heart attack or stroke (the remaining red faces) despite all 100 people having to undertake the effort and risk the side effects of taking a statin every day for the next ten years.

I have used this as an example in workshops on decision making for many health care professionals over many years. Remarkably, for prevention with statins in people without heart disease, very few health care professionals have an accurate understanding of the probabilities and the uncertainties, despite all of them having prescribed statins many times in such circumstances. And in general, for any medicine, healthcare professionals overestimate the benefits and underestimate the risks.

The optimum approach to risk communication is to use natural frequencies – "if there 100 people like you…..". Not every patient wants to know the probabilities of course – many of them will decide based on a different mental framework, often involving past experiences of illness in themselves or others, or simply an emotional response based on their life circumstances. But very few health care professionals use that approach. There is lots of "telling people", because that is what they think the guidelines say, and the QOF reinforces that approach. Given that statins and the better approaches to risk communication have been around for decades, most people find it difficult to accept that many consultations about statins are so often so far away from best practice. But I can assure you they are.

Even if risk communication was optimised, how someone views this decision depends on more than the numbers. Remember the expected utility choices where some people choose A and others faced with the same decision choose B? If you are a hospital specialist seeing lots of people who are seriously ill with heart attacks or strokes, then no doubt you would most likely be in favour of everybody taking a statin. If you are a GP working in an under-doctored and under-staffed practice still recovering from the coronavirus pandemic workload, then the extra work of counselling patients about these benefits and risks, advising them on how to take their medicines, making sure they know what to lookout for and how to report it if it happens, taking their periodic blood tests, issuing repeat prescriptions and occasionally but regularly reviewing how the patient is getting on............well, you might have a different view.

And, even more importantly, what if you are a patient? As we now know from our lottery scenarios, it will be no surprise to find that patients vary in how they view this uncertainty. Some people are not keen on taking tablets and say "Only four people? I'll take my chances". Others might say "I remarried a few years ago. Our children are still young. I know it's only four people out of a hundred, but I want to do everything I can to see the kids grow up". And then there is a third response. "Knowing my luck, I'll be one of the 6 who have the heart attack despite taking tablets for years. No thanks. I'll take my chances". It is not possible to predict in advance of such consultations what the preferences of individual patients are.

And meantime, other patients of the practice fall sick but find it difficult to see a health care professional because they are all busy attempting to prevent future illness in well people, or preventing future complication in people who have already developed one or more chronic conditions. All very laudable and valuable preventative work and what the QOF was designed to

277

ensure was done well – until there are no appointments today for the people who need an urgent appointment because they have a potentially serious set of new symptoms today. Prevention is a good thing. Until medicine becomes unbalanced by the volume of capacity within the health system that prevention consumes. Health care is indeed complex, many problems are without easy simple solutions, and unintended consequences are surprisingly frequent.

And what do those people who do start the statin think in ten years when they have not had a heart attack or stroke. Remember they are 94 out of every 100 people. They will all think the statin prevented the heart attack or stroke, as will most of their doctors. But we now know that 90 out of the 94 would never have the heart attack or stroke. We now know that they have only helped 4 out of the 100. We just do not know which 4.

Since it is not possible to predict in advance which response the patient will provide to an explanation of risks and benefits, it is important to set out the probabilities and see what each individual thinks would be the best decision for them. Even then there is even more complexity. Not everybody wants such probabilities explained using the best numbers we can find, nor are numbers necessarily the biggest factor in their decision making.

And in order to understand why that is, there is a bit more to explore about how humans make decisions.

CHAPTER NINETEEN

Choosing

Rationally, we are twenty six times more likely to be killed in a car crash than in a plane crash. But on average, people get more anxious getting on a plane than getting into a car.

One of my daughters loves mushrooms. If we go to a restaurant, she'll always pick a dish with mushrooms – it is a family joke. She never thinks that those mushrooms might be one of the many kinds that are poisonous to humans. But like most mushroom eaters, she doesn't go into the countryside at weekends, pick wild mushrooms, bring them back home and eat them. She knows that some mushrooms are poisonous. She can avoid that risk by buying mushrooms from a shop. Or can she? How sure are we that shop-bought wild mushrooms are not poisonous ones? Why do we trust the pickers, or the shops, or both, but not ourselves? What if the usual wild mushroom picker in some remote part of Tuscany was sick, and his untrained friend was deputising? Until recently, I have never given it any thought. Now I'm aware of it, I am thinking again about whether dried wild mushrooms from faraway places are such a good idea. The point is, often we are not at all rational in our decision making.

When it comes to choosing, let's start with another thought experiment. We all must do some shopping from time to time, whether we enjoy it or not. Let us imagine that today we need a new shirt - there is a special night out with friends, or there is a big presentation to make at work and we want to look our best, or the family are getting together from far and wide for a cousin's funeral and you have to stand up and do the eulogy. Whatever the reason, the shirts we already have just will not do.

How are we going to choose a shirt? It is likely we will have a price in mind. But then there is colour, pocket(s) or not, sleeve length, buttons, branding, style of cuff, fit, material, ease of ironing, durability, washing characteristics, material, sustainability, fair-trade, animal welfare, and probably a few more factors – let us call them variables, and there might be twenty variables that are important to somebody if not everybody. Some of those variables will be more important to one

280

person than they are to the next person. It is very unlikely we will all want the same thing in a shirt.

Then there is where we can buy a shirt from. It is likely that with local shops and online retailers we can easily consider 16 shops or websites. We might have some preferences from where we might want to buy a shirt. If we have had previous good experiences with one retailer or perhaps just one bad experience with another, we will bring that to the decision making too. And each of those retailers is likely to have at least 10 shirts that we might consider. So that is 16 shops x 10 shirts x 20 variables. So that is 3,200 pieces of information to potentially inform our decision making if we are to pick the best shirt. At best, it's a large spreadsheet. Is that how we make decisions? Of course not.

Try this exercise.
Read the following list of words once. Then turn the page.

- Seek
- Apparatus
- Disorder
- Approval
- Arrow
- Rain
- Welfare
- Language
- Petty
- Portrait
- Country
- Lamp
- Pudding
- Flock
- Transport
- Deck
- Cream
- Basket
- Professional
- Struggle

Please do not turn back to read the list of words again.

Find a piece of paper and something to write with.

Please write down as many words as you can remember.

How did you get on? Five maybe? A few more or a few less perhaps? Check if you misremembered a word. It's quite common and normal to do that. Were you better at remembering words from the beginning of the list, or the end of the list, or were the words you managed to remember scattered randomly? In the population about a third of people prefer remembering early items in a list, a third prefer late in a list, and a third do not have a preference. So, there is another difference between people.

But unless you are a savant with a photographic memory you will not have correctly remembered anywhere near 20 words. Imagine trying to remember and recall in context 3,200 pieces of information about shirts to make the optimum decision. That just is not how human decision making works. Even if we like to think of ourselves as rational and putting a lot of work into important decisions, not many people will have made a logical list of the pros and cons of marriage on a spreadsheet. As an aside, Charles Darwin – famous for describing the theory of evolution – did do just that, married his cousin, and they had ten children.

It still comes as a bit of a shock to be reminded that 40-80% of medical information provided by healthcare practitioners in consultations is forgotten immediately by the patient.[ccxi] The greater the amount of information presented, the lower the proportion correctly recalled, and almost half of the information that is remembered is incorrect.

Human beings have "bounded rationality". The term was coined by Herbert Simon – and yes, he is another Nobel Prize winner. After studying social science as an undergraduate, he began his research with a doctorate in political science - in organisational decision making.[ccxii] In his doctoral thesis he asserted that *"if there were no limits to human rationality administrative theory would be barren. It would consist of the single precept: Always select that alternative, among those available, which will lead to the most complete achievement of your goals".*

Simon argued that alternatives and consequences may only be partly known, and means and ends imperfectly differentiated, incompletely related, or poorly detailed. It is now clear that this truth from organisational decision making is also true in healthcare – that is obvious from the examples of treating a UTI or trying to prevent heart attacks and strokes with a statin. Simon defined the task of rational decision making being to select the alternative that results in the more preferred set of all the possible consequences. Knowledge of all alternatives, or all consequences that follow from each alternative is impossible. He described the usual and preferred approach to decision making as being "Satisficing" – collecting sufficient information to reduce one's uncertainty to the point at which we are able to make a decision.

We were never going to attempt to create a shirt-buying spreadsheet with 3,200 pieces of information. Most people have an idea of what they are willing to pay, will check out a few of their favourite retailers that have provided satisfactory shirts previously. If they find something they think fits the purpose, can afford, and they like the look of, they have probably reduced their uncertainty to the point they are able to make a decision. Only if the first strategy draws a blank is the search widened into less familiar retailers or shirts less typical than were originally under consideration.

Even then, that is not how it works all the time. We might have some money gifted to us at Christmas or had a modest tax rebate, and decide we will "go crazy" and get a shirt with what is for us an atypical design from the wacky retailer we have never bought anything from before. People make different choices in different ways, at different times.

Bounded rationality and satisficing shed light on the Gabbay and le May "mindlines" findings where doctors would base their approach on trusted sources of information and their own and their colleagues experiences. There are also strong links with the Information Mastery work of Slawson and Shaughnessy where we saw brief reading, talking to other people, and a variety of truncated approaches to looking for evidence were prefered to looking for the entirely of the published evidence on Medline.

In our patient with the typical urinary tract symptoms, it would be considered reasonable by most people in most circumstances not to pursue further investigations looking for alternative diagnoses before starting treatment. We can accept satisficing as a reasonable approach. There is residual uncertainty of course and some inexperienced diagnosticians find it difficult to come to terms with that, but it would be unreasonable in many circumstances to delay antibiotic treatment whilst, say, organising an abdominal ultrasound looking for, perhaps, appendicitis. The ultrasound, if requested routinely, would also be regarded as an inappropriate of use of limited health recourses - if lots of people gets scanned when there is a low probability of the diagnosis being something other than an uncomplicated urinary tract infection, the scanner is not available for other patients with a higher probability of more serious conditions.

Simon pursued these ideas in his research, exploring residual uncertainty and probability through computer simulations. As such, he developed expertise in computer science and he became a pioneer in artificial intelligence. But it is for bounded rationality and satisficing that he will be most often remembered, not least because it laid some of the foundations for the largest part of the jigsaw of human decision making – dual process theory.

Imagine you see a picture of someone famous, but who you haven't seen for a long time. President Kennedy, Marilyn Monroe, George Best would be examples for my generation. I am sure you can think of your own icons. You have not seen a picture of this person for a long time, and you have never met them in person, but you have no difficulty in recognising them very quickly when you see their picture. How do we do that?

Imagine you are driving along with the radio on, and on comes a song that was a favourite when you were 15 years old. The song was played at parties /dances / discos / clubs depending on your generation. You played it endlessly on whatever music system you had, and you and your friends would sing it together often. It is now many years since you heard that song. Do you have any difficulty in singing along accurately both with the words and the tune? Of course not. But that is a remarkable thing too. How come we can do that?

And if we are at a cousin's funeral and we see in the distance a woman walking with her back to us, even though we cannot see her face and she is wearing clothes we have not seen before and we have not seen her for some years, we still know that person is step-cousin Jill, three times removed who used to be in the diplomatic service. How do we do that?

Ask someone near you the answer to this sum:-

$2 + 2 =$

I would be pretty sure they could give you the correct answer "four" without any hesitation. They will have required little time and effort to make that decision. Indeed, they have made that decision so many times that the answer occurs automatically; they cannot prevent the answer "four" popping instantly into their consciousness.

Now give someone near you this sum:-

$464 \times 631 =$

I guarantee, unless they are a mathematical savant, that they will not be able to give you a quick answer. They will almost certainly need some paper and a pen to perform long multiplication, and even then they may need a calculator to give

285

you the answer or check their on-paper working. That decision making will be longer and effortful and is more prone to error.

And yet the human brain can perform feats which when considered rationally would appear to be magical. Read this text:-

Wehn Nael, the msot amzanig wirter, chgnaes teh letetrs ronud in tihs setcion of txet, msot cna stlil raed tehm becusae we cna reocngise patetnrs

Or even this:

7H3 M345UR3 OF 1N73LL163NC3 I5 7H3 481L17Y 70 CH4NG3

4L83R7 31N5731N

These exercises illustrate that there are two processes used in decision making, and which is used depends on our ability to recognise a pattern.[ccxiii] Hundreds of thousands of years ago when there were a few thousand human beings on the planet it was important to be able to quickly recognise a plant that could be eaten from one that would make you ill, to recognise a friend from an enemy, an animal that you could chase catch and eat from one that would chase catch and eat you. Pattern recognition has a survival advantage, and it is in our genes to use patterns when making decisions whenever we can. So, the song on the radio is a pattern, the famous face not seen for years is a pattern, the constellation of symptoms indicating a urinary tract infection is a pattern learned through formal education and training. Even the sum $2 + 2$ is a pattern, learned in the early years of school.

Fast, pattern-based decision making is called System 1 thinking. The patterns are created by repetition. Humans almost always must repeat new information a few times before it sticks in our memory. Revising for some critical test at school almost always involves a learn, test, relearn, retest, relearn cycle until the new information sticks and we can recall it when needed – at least long enough for a satisfactory score in the test. If I meet someone new and they tell me their name I have to consciously repeat it in my head a few times and when I get the chance, I might even write it down quickly so I don't forget. But after I've met them a few times I don't need to make that effort anymore.

For an undergraduate health care professional learning about urinary tract infections, a few supervised consultations with people with typical urinary tract infections and they are going to feel more comfortable with at least the technical aspects of the consultation when faced with the next person with typical urinary tract symptoms. Repetition drives the development of fast, intuitive, and often accurate decision making.

But if there is no pattern that we can rely on, or there are atypical features alongside a pattern we think we might be recognisable, then we are into slow, effortful and conscious decision making. This is System 2 thinking – hence the famous book by Danny Kahneman "Thinking Fast and Slow". The 464 x 631 sum is System 2 thinking. If I show health care professionals a picture of a characteristic rash of herpes zoster (shingles) on someone's chest, the learners who have been taught about shingles and seen it many times are able to use system 1 and quickly state the correct diagnosis and treatment. They have developed patterns – what we might call "illness scripts". However, those learners who usually work in a different area of healthcare and do not usually encounter shingles are slower, less accurate and less efficient system 2 decision makers.

Now try this exercise:

How many giraffes did Noah take into the Ark?

Most people have come across the story of Noah before. They know the animals "went in two by two" and if they remember the song will add "Hurrah, hurrah". This is System 1 thinking, it comes quickly and effortlessly, and usually gives the right answer. Does it in this case? Let's check what the guideline says.

The modern English version of the Bibles says in Genesis:-

"The Lord said to Noah, "You and your entire household go into the ark, for you alone I have seen to be righteous before Me among this generation. Take with you seven each of every clean animal, the male and its female, and two each of every unclean animal, the male and its female, and seven each of birds of the air, the male and female, to keep offspring alive on the face of all the earth."

If we cross reference to Leviticus it says:-

"You may eat any animal that has divided hoofs and chews the cud."

Giraffes have divided hooves and chew the cud. The correct answer is 7 or 14 giraffes depending on how you interpret the passage from Genesis. But the answer is not two.

That may seem disconcerting. So strong is most people's "pattern," that "the animals go in "two by two" pattern dominates decision making even when credible contrary information is provided. We have an explanation now for the difficulties faced when the evidence base changes and we need to prescribe ibuprofen or naproxen and not diclofenac.

Humans are cognitive misers and prefer System 1 decision making to System 2 decision making. They may continue to use System 1 when making decisions even in the face of a considerable amount of information to the contrary. I have had people in workshops checking Google and searching an online Bible to make sure I was not inventing something that undermined their belief that the animals went in two by two. A friend of mine who is a keen cyclist would not believe the widespread evidence of highly successful cyclist Lance Armstrong being a drugs cheat – until they heard Lance himself make a televised admission. The same friend has personally seen inefficiencies in a small number of NHS infrastructure projects, and strongly believes the NHS wastes lots of money. They find it difficult to accept that historically and in many much more costly aspects, the NHS is one of the most efficient of health systems.

Once we are aware of the importance of ingrained patterns and dual process theory it becomes more than a theory - it becomes reality, and we see it everywhere. In general, using patterns serves health care professionals well. We learn a constellation of symptoms and signs which are typical of a known condition, see a few real patients with that condition and, providing that the next patient with that condition has typical symptoms and signs then we can usually recognise the pattern and get the diagnosis correct. The same process works for technical aspects of the treatment of the condition - once the standard management is learnt, the technical aspects are mastered. However, novice diagnosticians are able to function only if symptoms and signs are typical – and especially in primary care and other "first contact" settings where patients are usually seen early in their illness, patients may often present with atypical symptoms.

However, pattern recognition can lead us astray. When people struggle with accepting that the animals go in 7 by 7 (or 14 by 14) that is conservatism bias – a tendency to insufficiently revise one's belief when evidence to the contrary is presented. That is the explanation for some of the delay in changing clinical practice when the evidence changes – diclofenac is a good example of conservatism bias.

As a medical student I was told very firmly by a very senior professor that I should never prescribe a medicine called a beta-blocker to a patient with heart failure. Beta-blockers were new medicines then and the professor believed that they would slow the heart rate and reduce the cardiac output, hence causing heart failure. Imagine my discomfort when some years later the treatment for heart failure changed and the NICE guideline made beta-blockers one of the most important treatments for heart failure. I suffered from a conservatism bias. Actually, I also suffered from authority bias which is the tendency to attribute greater accuracy to the opinion of an authority figure (unrelated to its content) and be more influenced by that opinion.

A large number of cognitive biases have been identified. A few examples from health care settings will illustrate the problem:-

Anchoring bias occurs when an individual's decisions are influenced by a particular reference point or "anchor". For example when a group of people were asked to estimate the correct answer to this sum − 8 x 7 x 6 x 5 x 4 x 3 x 2 x 1 − the median estimate was 2,250. When a group of people were asked to estimate the correct answer to this sum − 1 x 2 x 3 x 4 x 5 x 6 x 7 x 8 − the median answer was 512. The bias occurs because human beings "anchor" their answer to information early in the sequence. Car buyers are prepared to pay more for a car if it displayed next to another much more expensive car than when the same car is placed next to a cheap car. In health care an impressive symptom recounted by a patient early in a consultation may bias the eventual diagnosis even though the patient goes on to provide plenty of other information in the consultation which would make the original diagnosis improbable.

Selective perception is the tendency for expectations to affect perception. It is 3am one Sunday morning and I am driving home after an emergency visit to a patient. My route home takes me past where the night clubs are and a man emerges from the doorway of one of the clubs, staggers across the pavement into the gutter, falls, and I very nearly run him over. I stop and see if he needs help. What was the diagnosis I made? Well, my expectation was that he had consumed a considerable amount of alcohol, and he was probably drunk. That expectation could easily have led me astray because it turned out that he had actually had a stroke.

Availability bias occurs when immediate examples come mind. If something can be readily recalled, it must be important, or more important than alternative solutions not as readily recalled. Decision making is inherently biased toward recently acquired information. Health care professionals who have recently prescribed an evidence-based, guideline recommended medicine and have had the patient develop a serious and

290

unpleasant side effect will find it difficult for some time to prescribe the evidence-based, guideline recommended medicine for future patients even though the probability of any significant side effect is very low and that particular side effect they will probably never see again in their professional lifetime. Severity and frequency were two factors we identified when considering risk; to those we should add recency.

The **bandwagon effect** is the tendency for people to adopt certain behaviours, styles, or attitudes simply because others are doing so. This can be an explanation for variations in health care performance, and the bandwagon effect may accompany conservatism bias in delaying the wider implementation of better clinical practice.

Gambler's fallacy is the incorrect belief that, if a particular event occurs more frequently than normal during the past, it is less likely to happen in the future (or vice versa), when it has otherwise been established that the probability of such events does not depend on what has happened in the past. Such events are referred to as statistically independent. In the gambling game roulette, if the ball has gone onto a black number the last three times, one might think that on the next turn a red number has become more likely. This is, of course, nonsense. Where the ball landed last time can have no influence on when it rests the next time.

As a GP I might see less than four people in a year with a heart attack. If I have seen four people with chest pain in just the last two weeks and they all turned out to be having heart attacks, and now here is yet another patient with chest pain, I need to work hard try to suppress the thought that "This can't be another person with a heart attack". The truth is that this person's symptoms and them having them today cannot be connected in any way with the other four patients. The clustering of the chest pain patients in the last two weeks is just down to the play of chance.

Search Satisficing is the tendency for the clinician to call off the search once they have identified a cause of the patient's complaint or condition. This tendency can be responsible for an error in the diagnostic process known as premature closure. In premature closure, the clinician ends the decision-making before collecting enough data to support or refute the working diagnosis. Professor Pat Croskerry, a now "retired" academic Emergency Medicine specialist from Nova Scotia has written extensively about decision making in health care in general and about dual process theory in particular.[ccxiv ccxv ccxvi] He has been kind enough to come over to the UK many times and help with our thinking about decision making. He tells a great story against himself involving search satisficing. It is possible for search satisficing to occur when looking for fractures on x-rays. The patient's hand hurts. When a fracture is found, further investigation is stopped. The result of calling off the search is that a second fracture is missed. Except that in Pat's case there were no fewer than four more fractures. I very nearly made the same error myself a few weeks ago. Patients with a single hand fracture are assessed and generally need treatment less urgently and less intensively that someone with multiple hand fractures. No harm resulted, but the point is that even experts who know lots about decision making and biases are susceptible to biases.

Vertical Line Failure occurs when routine, repetitive tasks lead to thinking in silos. Because of the efficiency of the pattern recognition, the approach carries the inherent penalty of inflexibility. In contrast, lateral thinking styles create opportunities for diagnosing the unexpected, rare, or esoteric. An effective lateral thinking strategy is simply to pose the question "What else might this be?" or "What would be the worst-case scenario here?". As an example, consider the risks inherent in there being a high incidence of influenza in the community and a GP is seeing lots of people with high temperatures and feeling as if every muscle in their body is aching. A 15-year-old presents with high temperature and aching. How tempting is it for a human being seeing lots of people with influenza to jump to the conclusion that here is just one more patient with influenza. Except the 15-year-old turns out to have meningitis.

Blind spot bias is recognising the impact of biases on the judgment of others, while failing to see the impact of biases on one's own judgment. This might be linked to overconfidence bias – far more than 50% of people rate themselves as an above average driver. The point is we are all human beings, we all use System 1 preferentially, and because we are relying on patterns, we may all be led astray into one or more cognitive biases. No one is exempt.

Even when we know about cognitive biases, decision making does not get any easier, because in addition to cognitive biases there are affective biases. Our judgement is impaired when we are hungry, angry, late, tired or lonely.[ccxvii] There are theoretically easier means of avoiding or rectifying affective biases than there are for avoiding cognitive biases. However, given the current pace of clinical practice and a shortage of health care professionals in many organisations, affective biases as a cause of decision errors are not so easily prevented.

Nevertheless, a recent systematic review provided some evidence that teaching health care professionals and the general population about how they think and how they may be led astray by cognitive biases improves their decision making.[ccxviii] Because I knew about the Pat Croskerry search satisficing story about hand X rays, I managed to stop myself making the same error. The review found 67 papers which reported 87 studies. In 60 studies the intervention - directed at making health care professionals aware of how they make decisions - was beneficial. Strategies used included encouraging thinking "consider the opposite" and technological interventions such as the visual aids produced to inform decision making for cardiovascular risk and statins.

Attempts have been made to "debias" doctors to reduce the number of diagnostic errors. Results have been disappointing. It does not seem to work, and this is not surprising. The human preference for pattern recognition is part of being a human, baked in by hundreds of thousands of years of pattern recognition. And such doctors have considerable personal experience of pattern recognition mostly proving a pretty good way of making decisions, even if there are occasional, dramatic exceptions.

It seems better to encourage what the cognitive psychologists call "calibration". Calibration is really a "Stop and Think" moment, a technique often deployed nearer the end of a consultation than the beginning. Examples of calibration thinking would be "Am I being led astray by a cognitive bias here?", or "What are the possibilities this could be something else?", or "What is the worst-case scenario to rule out here?". In psychology, calibration is the human ability to resist the first impression that comes to mind. Most patients would quite like their doctors to be able to do that I reckon. There are some well-known Calibration Tests which seem to improve our self-awareness of the usefulness of stopping and thinking, and evidence that our innate ability to calibrate can be developed and become part of routine thinking in consultations.

Many people associate Daniel Kahneman with dual process theory, but he was not the only one nor the first to recognise two ways of thinking. We all stand on the shoulders of giants. William James described two ways of thinking - associative and reasoning - and he wrote his huge text "The Principles of Psychology" in 1890. William James's brother was the novelist Henry James and his godfather was Ralph Waldo Emmerson.

Certainly, Kahneman has made huge contribution to dual process theory, usually in collaboration with others. His major and most productive collaboration was with Amos Tversky with whom he developed Prospect Theory which itself strengthened dual process theory. It was that collaboration which introduced the term cognitive bias, and they described a number of the biases described above.   Kahneman's story is riveting.[ccxix] Michael Lewis wrote a best-selling book "The Undoing Project" which details the partnership between Kahneman and Tversky. Sadly, Kahneman won the Nobel prize but Tversky did not; Tversky died from cancer of the pancreas before the Nobel Committee announced its decision, and the rules are that Novel Laureates must be alive.

From fifteen years of personal study and teaching, I am convinced that an understanding of decision making helps health care professionals with their decision making. This is not least because once they realise patterns and System 1 decision making dominate their decision making, they then go on to realise that in consultations the patient also has their own patterns. The fact that there are two people who will usually have two completely different patterns driving their decision making helps them understand what is going on in consultations while it is going on. One contributor to the consultation has their patterns based on science and technical knowledge, the other contributor has their pattern based on past or current lived experience of their condition. As one patient put it, "Don't confuse your expertise based on a one hour lecture at medical school about my condition with my expertise based on living with it for the last twenty years".

But before we come to the consultation, there is one more cognitive bias to explore. Prevention bias.

CHAPTER TWENTY

Prevention, Testing and Screening

"Prevention is better than cure" is sometimes attributed to Erasmus, the 16th century Dutch philosopher. Benjamin Franklin said "an ounce of prevention is better than a pound of cure". The context seems to be that Franklin, impressed with the city of Boston's fire brigade, was proposing the first fire brigade in Philadelphia.

Early attempts at preventative medicine can be traced back to the waves of bubonic plague that swept across Europe from 1347 until the late 1700s. The word "quarantine" comes from the Italian "quarantena" meaning forty days; travellers and merchandise that had potentially been exposed to disease were isolated for that period to ensure that they were not infected.

Previous chapters have recounted the evolution of the understanding of the causes of disease and their prevention – John Graunt and his Bills of Mortality, John Snow and the pump handle, James Lind and scurvy, the tragic story of Ignas Semmelweis and puerperal fever. Edward Jenner's work with cowpox was taken on by Louis Pasteur in the late 1800s to generate vaccines for anthrax, cholera and rabies. Diphtheria toxin initially trialled in Copenhagen - the list goes on and on. Vaccination to reduce epidemics of infectious disease are one of the greatest achievements of medicine.

In the second half of the 20th Century, we have seen better and more options for contraception. That is important prevention too – of unplanned pregnancies. There have been successful interventions to reduce smoking thanks to Richard Doll's work which identified the risks. Motor vehicle safety has been greatly improved thanks to seat belts, air bags, better design features and safety improvements to road infrastructure. Fluoride in toothpaste has improved dental health. These are all now disasters that largely do not happen, and so we risk taking them for granted.

After the second World War, as epidemiology began to get to grips with risk factors for the development of disease using cohort studies such as Framingham, different types of prevention started to develop. Universal prevention still had a big part to play - clean water, vaccination programmes and so on. As late as the 1950s, polio killed or paralysed over half a million people every year worldwide. The first successful polio vaccine was created by US physician Jonas Salk. Salk tested his experimental killed-virus vaccine on himself and his family in 1953, and a year later on 1.6 million children in Canada, Finland and the United States. The results were announced on 12th April 1955, and Salk's inactivated polio vaccine was licensed on the same day. By 1957, annual cases dropped from 58,000 to 5,600, and there was little interest in Albert Sabin's oral, attenuated vaccine. He managed to run trials in the USSR and - overcoming opposition from some quarters because of the Russian collaboration during the Cold War - one of the last great epidemic diseases was on the way to being controlled across the world. Vaccination in the UK against polio began in 1956. I remember vividly being taken by Joan for a painful polio vaccination at our village health centre that year as a surge in cases occurred. Avoiding paralysis or death was difficult to explain to the snivelling young me as we waited to catch the bus home because one of us had a very sore arm. An oral vaccine initially given to children on sugar cubes did not become available until 1962.

But as the causes of non-infectious diseases became clearer, there arose the possibility of screening for diseases before they developed, or even identifying risk factors for such diseases and modifying them, thereby preventing the development of the disease. The notion was, and is, very attractive. Prevention sounds great. Who would rather wait for a disease to develop than have it detected early?

Here is a real story. It happened in the United States more than twenty years ago and is courtesy of Dave Slawson of Information Mastery fame. Names and details have been changed, but permission of those involved was given in the interests of educating health care professionals and the public about screening and its problems. There is a warning here – understanding this involves some numbers.

Jeff and Rosie were in postgraduate training as doctors. But they were also patients because they were faced with infertility. Eventually, after many struggles, Rosie became pregnant. Great joy, and Rosie was safely delivered of a son, Baby Jeff. Even greater joy.

In their hospital there was a renowned paediatrician with a special interest in a condition called Duchene Muscular Dystrophy (DMD). It is a horrible disease, caused by a genetic mutation. It almost always occurs in boys and results in a significantly reduced life expectancy. Some children die before they reach the age of ten, others in their teens. A few with good supportive care now make it to their forties or even fifties. One in 5000 male births develop DMD. There is no cure, treatment is only supportive.

The paediatrician had developed a screening test for DMD based on a tiny speck of blood from a heel prick, and asked Jeff and Rosie if he could include Baby Jeff in his evaluation programme. He already knew that his screening test identified correctly 100% of babies who would go on to develop DMD, and 99.98% of babies who did not have DMD.

Rosie and Jeff, still euphoric at the safe delivery of their much-longed for son, did not give the test much thought to their colleagues' request, gave consent, and Baby Jeff had the test performed. The next day the test came back positive, and Jeff and Rosie and all of their family and friends were devastated because they knew the prognosis all too well. Fortunately, one of their colleagues had been to McMaster and had learned a few evidence-based medicine skills. He drew up what is known as a two-by-two table (see Figure 21.1)

Figure 21.1.

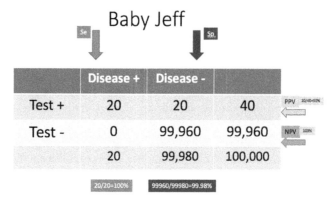

In this table we have calculated how the test performs in 100,000 male babies. We know that DMD occurs in 1 in 5000 male births; since a rate of 1 in 5000 is the same as 20 in 100,000, that is why we have 20 babies and children at the bottom of the 'Disease +' column.

Look first at the rest of the column headed 'Disease +'. All the babies and children who eventually are diagnosed with DMD are in this column. We know the accuracy of the test in those with the disease is 100%. That is called "sensitivity" and the column is labelled "Se". All 20 people with the disease test positive – and if the test is performing well the box 'Disease +, Test +' should be a much bigger number than the number in the box 'Disease + Test –' . In this case the test gets it right 20 times out of 20 in those with the disease, and never gets it wrong.

If we have 100,000 babies in total and 20 of them have the disease, that means there are 99,980 without the disease. That is the number at the bottom of the 'Disease – column'. We know that the test correctly identifies 99.98% of those without the disease. We call that "Specificity" and the column is labelled "Sp". We can calculate how well the test performs in people who do not have the disease: it is 99,980 x 0.9998 = 99,960 people who do not have the disease and test negative. Again if the test is performing "well" the 'Disease -, Test –' box should be a big

300

number and it is. That leaves 20 babies who test positive but who do not have the disease and they go into the box "Disease -, Test +".

Now let us look at what this means in consultations. Because positive tests come back and negative tests come back it is the rows, not the columns, that tell us what to tell patients with positive and negative results. If the test comes back negative, the test gets it right every time. We can tell all the parents of babies with a negative test result that they do not have DMD. But look at the positive tests. There are 40 of those, but only 20 of them truly have DMD. The other 20 are false positive tests. To use the technical terms, the negative predictive value (NPV) is 100% (99,960 / 99,960) but the positive predictive value (PPV) is only 50% (20/40).

Taking that news to Rosie and Jeff helped them a lot, as you can imagine. There was now some hope, because they now realised that there was now a 50% chance that Baby Jeff's test result would turn out to be a false positive. Baby Jeff went on to have the definitive test for DMD – a small piece of calf muscle was examined under a microscope - and was normal. Baby Jeff did not have DMD and the positive test was a false positive.

Almost all human beings start with the intuitive notion that early detection and prevention of disease are "good things". Was the screening test for DMD a good thing to be doing? Did it help Baby Jeff or his parents? If the test had been a true positive would it have helped Rosie and Jeff to know the diagnosis earlier? Is it possible that if the result of the screening test had been a true positive, all the screening test could have done would be to have given them more time to worry over their baby? There is, after all, very sadly no period in which early treatment improves the outcome for boys with DMD. Is screening for disease always a good thing? Arguably, with no treatment that alters the course of the disease, screening for DMD could only do net harm to the population.

The book 'Screening: Evidence and Practice" is one of the definitive guides to the complexity of screening for diseases.[ccxx] Its authors Muir Gray, Anne Mackie and Angela Raffle have been at the forefront of achieving improvements in UK screening over many years. Its first sentence reads, "All screening programmes do harm". Its second sentence reads, "Some do good as well, and, of these, some do more good than harm at reasonable cost."

Rushing enthusiastically into screening programmes is very unwise. Instinctively seen as a "good thing", they are very popular but they can also do harm - as Rosie and Jeff can testify. Whole body CT scanning to "pick up disease early" sounds worthwhile to many people. The reality is that there is a big dose of radiation from the scan which is potentially harmful, and there is a good chance of an abnormality being found. Yet most of those abnormalities will be incidental findings.[ccxxi] Quite a lot of individual patients who pay for such screening privately then find themselves having to undertake a whole host of unpleasant further tests and procedures to find out whether an abnormality is something or nothing. That eats up already scarce capacity within the health system. And of course, all the time they are worrying that it is something. Yet most times it turns out to be nothing.

But there will be a small number of people who have an early, important abnormality detected by the CT scan. Then the question is whether that cancer will grow or spread and do harm or be non-progressive and do no harm. These are not easy things to make definitive judgement calls on, and in the UK we are fortunate to have a National Screening Committee full of experts who know all the pitfalls associated with screening tests. At the time of writing, they have looked at 108 screening programmes or tests and have recommended just 32 of them.

Sir Kenneth Calman, Chief Medical Officer for England, said in the National Screening Committee's first annual report in 1998:

"We need to be sure that the new technologies for screening are effective; that they will not cause more harm than good; that the health needs of people determine the necessity to screen; that false hope is not raised by screening for conditions where an effective cure or treatment is unavailable, and that people's experience informs the continued improvement of screening services.

Early identification of a disease is important to the patient. As new technologies are discovered so people's interest is raised in the possibilities for new programmes. However, the promise of new screening technologies must be looked at carefully if the major undertaking and investment of a new programme is to meet all our expectations. It is therefore vital that before proceeding there is careful development and discussion with the service, the professions that would provide the screening service and the potential users of the service and consideration of whether this is the best use of resources."

Around the same time as the UK National Screening Committee was established, when the pitfalls of screening were being identified and debated, the World Health Organisation asked JMG Wilson from the Ministry of Health in London and G Jungner from Gothenburg, Sweden to produce a report setting out the principles and practice involved in screening programmes.[ccxxii] The "Wilson and Jungner" report has stood the test of time and the preface is deserving of a substantial extract:-

"In theory, therefore, screening is an admirable method of combating disease, since it should help detect it in its early stages and enable it to be treated adequately before it obtains a firm hold on the community.

In practice, there are snags. In developing countries there is as a rule such a vast burden of overt disease that the medical services are overwhelmingly occupied with the treatment of patients coming to them with often advanced stages of communicable disease. With so much curative work to do, they have little time, let alone resources in manpower and money, to spend on looking for disease in its incipient stages, and their preventive work consists largely of attempting to improve environmental conditions.

In the developed countries, the communicable diseases have become less important as killers than chronic diseases, often of insidious onset, such as cancer and the cardiovascular diseases. The developed countries have much greater resources than the developing countries, and can call on more qualified staff. And the diseases that have now come to the fore are of such a nature that, if detected early, they stand a reasonable chance of being cured, whereas if not diagnosed until the patients come to the doctor with clear-cut symptoms they may be incurable. In developed countries, therefore, it would seem that the practice of screening for disease should be widespread. That it is not so to the extent that might be expected is due to a number of factors, among them the cost of screening and the tendency in the medical profession to wait for patients rather than actively to look for disease in the population. Another factor undoubtedly is inadequate knowledge of the principles and practice of screening for disease."

Wilson and Jungner then came up with ten criteria for screening programmes which they considered should be taken into account when planning screening programmes:-

(1) The condition sought should be an important health problem.

(2) There should be an accepted treatment for patients with recognized disease.

(3) Facilities for diagnosis and treatment should be available.

(4) There should be a recognisable latent or early symptomatic stage.

(5) There should be a suitable test or examination.

(6) The test should be acceptable to the population.

(7) The natural history of the condition, including development from latent to declared disease, should be adequately understood.

(8) There should be an agreed policy on whom to treat as patients.

(9) The cost of case-finding (including diagnosis and treatment of patients diagnosed) should be economically balanced in relation to possible expenditure on medical care as a whole.

(10) Case-finding should be a continuing process and not a "once and for all" project.

Not all screening programmes will fulfil all ten criteria, nor do they need to. Judgements are required about whether for an individual screening programme the benefits are greater than the harms, and whether it would be cost-effective. There is inevitably a balance to be struck, and as we have seen before it is impossible to foretell what will be the outcome of screening or not screening in an individual case. Given the usual rule that human beings prefer certainty to uncertainty, and it is difficult to be certain in advance whether having screening is a good thing for an individual, simply informing people about what the uncertainties are with screening programmes does not solve the dilemma about whether to attend for screening. Better informed individuals can find it difficult to make decisions about whether to go for screening.

Let us use an example screening for breast cancer using mammography. The benefits and risks have been very carefully studied. Individuals may wish to look rationally at the numbers, and they can be provided. The Harding Centre for Risk Literacy[ccxxiii] have produced some of the best representations, based on a Cochrane systematic review.

Much to many people's surprise, four women die from breast cancer if 1000 women begin screening from the age of 50 compared to five women out of 1000 who are not screened. Humans often over-estimate benefits of medical interventions and under-estimate risks. But then in the screened population there are 100 women who have false positive results and who then need additional tests including biopsies. There are also five women who have operations to remove non-progressive breast cancers which were detected by screening, but which would never have harmed the woman.

When we study how women decide whether to have mammography or not, the numbers are of very little help. Their own mental pattern or mindline based on their own knowledge, past and imagined experience of hospitals and tests and diseases plays the major part in most people's decision about whether to go for screening or not.[ccxxiv]

There is no UK screening programme for prostate cancer, but men may request a prostate specific antigen test (PSA) test after informed discussion. The Harding Centre have also produced a representation of those numbers based on the best available evidence but again they do not solve the decision making.

If men are screened for prostate cancer there is no difference in overall mortality based on a large randomised controlled trial, although it may not have been big enough to show a difference if one truly existed. We know again that these numbers, even if they are known to an individual, are not what surfaces when men are faced with the decision about whether to have their prostate checked.

Men make decisions based on what their own mindline already is, and that might include strong messages in the general media from well-intentioned celebrities who have themselves had cancer of the prostate detected, often by having it "checked". What does not appear frequently in the media are the best available numbers which, according to the Harding Centre are that no fewer than 155 out of 1000 men having a PSA test get a false positive test and need further tests, and that an extra 51 men out of 1000 have a cancer detected that was never going to progress and which they would have died with rather than from. A number of those 51 opt for treatment up to and including surgery to remove the prostate, some of them have significant side effects from that treatment, and in my own experience they all understandably get very worried. At six months after radical prostatectomy 19% of patients report moderate to severe urinary incontinence and 66% report erectile dysfunction. This compares with 4% and 29% respectively in patients who do not have surgery.[ccxxv]

What also does not often appear in the media is the sort of patient story I heard recently. A 60-year-old man had a PSA test and it was raised. He went for further tests of course, in this case an ultrasound guided biopsy taken via his rectum using a wide needle to "suck out" samples of prostate tissue. About 6 people in 100 get an infection after such a procedure and it usually resolves relatively easily with antibiotics. However, in this case it did not. The infection caused septicaemia, kidney failure and heart failure requiring several days in intensive care. The kidneys started working again and the heart recovered, but it is still a long road back to the healthy man there was before the PSA test was done. And the prostate biopsy showed no signs of cancer, as 60% do in people with a "raised PSA" – they are the false positive tests. Suffice it to say that he will not be having another PSA test anytime soon. Difficult decisions all, and to repeat, with no ability to predict the future outcome of having the test in an individual.

The same issues with false positive and false negative tests apply to tests being used for to diagnose conditions rather than screen for conditions.

Imagine you are a keen rugby player. You wake up the day after a particularly fierce match with a sore, swollen calf. It was fine when you went to bed, but now you are in some pain, and it is difficult to walk without limping. You do not remember any injury during the match but could not rule out getting kicked in the calf in the previous day's hostilities. Never having had anything like this before you seek advice and are told to go to the local Accident and Emergency Department. There is apparently a need to rule out a clot in the leg, called a deep vein thrombosis (DVT).

The doctor you see at the hospital examines your leg carefully. She thinks there is only about a 10% chance that your problems are due to a DVT but she says will do a blood test called a D-dimer on the basis that "you can't be too careful". The blood test is sent off and you wait for the results. The doctor you have seen is going off duty but he says he will hand you over to her colleague who is just coming on shift.

The new doctor arrives. She says she agrees with the assessment that there is only about a 10% chance this is a DVT and she will return when she has the result. Eventually, after several hours, your blood test result is back. The new doctor comes to see you and she sits down and draws out this table and starts to explain the result (see Fig 21.2):-

Figure 21.2.

	Disease +	Disease -	
Test +	9	54	63
Test -	1	36	37
	10	90	100

She starts by saying "If there were 100 people like you, and about 10 of them eventually turned out to have a DVT, then the bottom row of this table would look like this. There would be 10 people with the disease – in the Disease + column on the bottom row, and so there are 90 people in the Disease – column on the bottom row.

"The test we have just done – the D-dimer – gives the correct result 90% of the time in people with a DVT. So out of the 10 people with a DVT, 9 of them will have a positive D-dimer test, but 1 will not. That's the left-hand column.

"D-dimer is a less helpful test in people who do not have a DVT. It gets the result right only around 40% of the time. So out of the 90 people without a DVT, only 36 of them properly test negative. There are 54 people out of the 90 who test positive, but still end up with a diagnosis of not having a DVT. That's the right-hand column.

"Now let's look at the rows. In your case the D-dimer test is negative so let's look at the bottom row. If there were 100 people like you, we would get 37 people with negative tests. The test isn't perfect but if it is negative, it is a very good guide. Only 1 person in 37 will get a negative test and eventually come back and be re-diagnosed as actually having a clot. It's possible but unlikely. The NICE guideline[ccxxvi] says we can send you home to rest and take painkillers, but you must come back if your legs get worse or if you get any pain in the chest or shortness of breath.

"If your result had come back positive, you would have been one of 63 people with a positive test. We would have done an ultrasound on the leg to see if there was a DVT, but we would only have found a clot in 9 out of the 63. The other 54 people would have had a false positive D-dimer test."

Not every patient would want an explanation in such detail, but some would appreciate a little more than "Your test is negative and you can go home" or the arguably even less desirable "Your test is positive, we need to send you for a scan". Particularly when the D-dimer test is positive, if there is not some qualification regarding false positives with a reasonable estimate of the chances of the scan showing a clot in the calf veins, then that seems much less desirable care.

I use this example a lot in my teaching of UK doctors. Despite the DVT and D-dimer example being a familiar one, it is very rare to find someone who has these consultation skills – before I start the teaching, obviously. They have all heard of the terms sensitivity and specificity, but most cannot accurately describe what they mean. It is the same as when we explore treatment benefits such as the statin examples we looked at in Chapter 19. The skills of evidence-based medicine are taught at UK medical schools, but they are not explicitly used routinely to aid decision making in consultations. There seems to be even less understanding of these basic evidence-based medicine skills if doctors have done their undergraduate training overseas.

Knowing what a guideline recommends for a population and following may often be technically correct, but for great care we need both an understanding of some basic evidence-based medicine skills with numbers, and great consultation skills involving probability and uncertainty.

It seems as if quite often some medical graduates have experienced a culture that was present in the UK fifty years ago – one of apprenticeship and blindly following what the expert said was the appropriate management plan. It is a lot easier cognitively to do what others tell us or do what the guidelines say.

It is a lot more cognitive effort, at least to start with, to think explicitly about probabilities and then use them in decision making with and for patients. But it is worth it, because a probabilistic thinker also makes better decisions in many other aspects of life, rather than muddling through relying on gut instinct or the last thing we read or heard.

The 2x2 tables are examples of an approach called Bayesian reasoning. Thomas Bayes was a Presbyterian Minister born in 1701 who studied Logic alongside Theology at Edinburgh University. Late in life he became interested in the mathematics of probability. However, he died 1761 and his papers on the subject were given to his friend Richard Price. It was Price who presented "An Essay towards solving the Doctrine of Chances to the Royal Society" in 1763 after Bayes' death and ensured its publication in the Philosophical Transactions of the Royal Society of London the following year.

The mathematics of Bayes theorem is fierce, but the principles are more easily explained. Let us use the lottery example again:-

1.   My neighbour tells me he is going to win the lottery tonight. How likely is it that he wins the lottery tonight?
We know the prior-probability – his chances of winning are approximately 1 in 14 million.

2.   The next morning, he tells me he has won the lottery. What is the probability he truly has won the lottery now?
Well, the probability has gone up, obviously. But I know he is a bit of a joker. So whilst him having won the lottery is a bit more likely, it is far from certain.

3.   A few days later he asks me to keep an eye on his house because him and his family are going on holiday. I get pictures sent of him on a three-week Caribbean cruise and he's staying in the Presidential suite. What is the probability he truly has won the lottery now?
Well, I am now thinking that the probability has gone up. He's still a joker, and this might be an elaborate ruse for some reason

310

I cannot yet work out, but I am really starting to think there's a good possibility he really has won the lottery.

4.   He comes back from the holiday. The next day a Rolls Royce and a Bentley are parked outside and within a few weeks he is no longer my neighbour because he has moved to a £5million house in the countryside with 10 acres, a wood, a trout stream and two swimming pools. What is the probability he truly has won the lottery now?

Ok, I know now about bounded rationality. Now I have sufficient information to reduce my uncertainty to the point at which I can make my decision. I have not seen the winning ticket but now I believe him. It looks like he really did win the lottery.

What's going on in this example? We start with a baseline probability, and then with each extra piece of information we end up with a changed probability. In this example all the additional pieces of information were positive, increasing the probability of the original "diagnosis" - which originally was very unlikely - to the point where it is highly probable that the original remote probability was true. But we have been here before, and we know how this story ends.

5.   A few nights later and I am watching the evening news on the television. I see my former neighbour being arrested on suspicion of a £50million bank robbery. What is the probability he truly has won the lottery now?
Here is an additional piece of information and this time it is strongly negative – the probability of him having won the lottery has once again become remote.

What has this got to do with decision making in health care? Let us illustrate that with this exercise:-

1.   Outside my consulting room is a 3-year-old girl. What is the probability of her having an infection of her middle ear (otitis media, or OM)?

311

Very low actually. Children get lots of diseases, perhaps somewhere around 10,000 different possibilities, so despite OM being one of the commoner reasons for children coming to see me, the initial or "prior-probability" of it being OM is pretty low.

2. She comes in to see me and I am told by her parent that she has been up all night with a raised temperature. What is the probability of her having OM now?

Well, the probability of OM has gone up a bit. Children with OM quite often have a raised temperature, but there are also lots and lots of other reasons why her temperature could be up. There is a higher probability of OM now, and we've narrowed it down from 10,000, but we cannot possibly conclude it is OM yet.

3. Then I am told that she has been crying and tugging at her ear. She is miserable, and I cannot get much response from her, but she does say "My ears hurt". What is the probability of her having OM now?

The probability of OM is now quite a bit higher. It's on my list and probably somewhere near the top.

4. I look in her ears and with difficulty I can see that both of her ear drums are very red. They are not bulging with pus behind them, and they have not perforated and let the pus escape. What is the probability of her having OM now?

Higher again. It's a pretty good bet she does have OM and I'm thinking painkillers for a few days and perhaps a delayed prescription for some antibiotics to start in a few days if she does not improve. All that is in line with the NICE guidance.[ccxxvii] Of course, her parents' values and preferences will influence the approach to treatment in this individual patient.

What is going on? Again, we start with a remote possibility. Each new piece of evidence – every single symptom or sign can be seen as a separate test – points towards or away from the diagnosis currently in mind.

5. Something makes want to just quickly check a few more things. Perhaps I am thinking of "calibration" or "rule out the worst-case scenario". I get permission to listen to her chest and feel her abdomen. I lift her dress and spot a purpuric (purple) rash on her abdomen. Her parent says it was not there when she was dressed an hour ago. The rash does not blanch when I press on it with a glass tumbler.

This is the equivalent of seeing my neighbour arrested on the TV news. This is a big negative for this being an ear infection. That now is a remote probability again. Until proved otherwise, this child has meningococcal septicaemia. She is given an immediate injection of antibiotics and rushed to the local hospital. There she makes a full and quick recovery with no long-term health consequences. Closing my mind to other possibilities early – a well-known cognitive bias - could have been disastrous.

Bayesisan reasoning is arguably a natural approach for clincians.[ccxxviii] Certainly it offers a useful insight into one approach to the acquisition of the difficult skill of diagnosis. The alternative approach is the often-unconscious acquisition of patterns through repetitions of different consultations – each one of which is unique, so it is not true repetition – or at least it does not feel like it at the time. As we shall see in a later chapter, it is a long journey from apprentice to expert and understanding what went on in a consultation framed by dual process theory, by an awareness of cognitive and affective biases and calibration, and by examining it within a framework of Bayesian reasoning might accelerate that process.

Before we leave tests and prevention, there are a few more difficulties that still need airing.

Firstly, test results are often central to monitoring health and informed decision making. Has the serum cholesterol concentration come down since starting a statin? Is the dose of thyroid medication correct? Has the HbA1c (the measure of how well controlled diabetes is) come down? Even when the laboratory has optimised their diagnostic testing processes to

313

minimise inaccuracies, there always remains an error in any clinical measurement due to unavoidable, naturally occurring variability. This comes as a shock to many doctors and their patients.[ccxxix]

Because test results are typically reported as a single static number without any statement of uncertainty, and often to more decimal places than appropriate, clinicians and patients may fall into the erroneous assumption that laboratory results are exact. This can lead to over-interpretation of an apparent change in what was measured, which, in turn, leads to potentially unwarranted intervention and feelings of fear, happiness, frustration, and confusion - both for patients and health care professionals.

The uncertainty arises from different causes of variation involved in measurement. There are human and other "preanalytical" sources of variation - the manner in which a specimen is collected, handled, or shipped and the storage conditions to which it was exposed - and these can lead to either random or systematic variation. Even when these are eliminated, there is always persistent analytical variation or imprecision ("instrument" variation). Finally, and most importantly, there is biological variation. At a given moment our blood glucose or our cholesterol will be higher or lower than at other moments. And when we get a result we do not know whether we were having a high moment, an average moment or a low moment when that sample was taken.

This is not just a theoretical worry. As a single example, let us consider the monitoring of diabetes control in a patient taking medicines to lower her blood glucose. Her baseline HbA1c level is 64 mmol/mol and she and her health care professional agree to add an additional medicine to lower her blood glucose and improve the control of her diabetes. This should be able to be demonstrated in a lower HbA1c result sometime after the additional treatment is started.

Typically, medicines for diabetes will lower a baseline HbA1c level of 64 mmol/mol by about 8 mmol/mol to 56 mmol/mol. This 12% drop (from 64 to 56 mmol/mol) in HbA1c is less than the calculated reference change value for HbA1c which is 17%. In other words, when the follow up blood test is done and the result comes back with the expected 12% drop to 56mmol/mol as a result of the additional medicine, both patient and their health care professional are likely to think "job well done". Except the change between the two measurements could be entirely due to measurement imprecision and biological variation. The patient could potentially have left the medicines in the bathroom cabinet and never taken a tablet and still got the 12% drop.

This is a hugely important yet under-recognised problem in decision making in health care. It should make a big difference in consultations, but there is usually an assumption of precision in test results which is not justified. The reference change value ranges from 2% to 50% for commonly reported tests used for diagnosing and monitoring common diseases. It's a brilliant paper from James McCormack and Daniel Thomas in Vancouver.

Then, given the common inclusion within guidelines of new recommendations it seems astonishing that only recently there has been described an approach which calculates how much good is done for the effort made, and whether the recommendations are feasible within the available capacity within the health system.[ccxxx] To be fair we have known for a while there were problems. A simulation study applying all guidelines for preventive care, chronic disease care, and acute care to a panel of 2500 adults representative of the US population estimated that US primary care physicians would require up to 27 hours a working day and to work 7 days a week to implement (and document) all applicable guidelines. To fully satisfy only the recommendations from the US Preventive Services Task Force would require 7.4 hours a day.

Similarly, to implement just the European hypertension guidelines in Norwegian adults, Norway would need more general practitioners than are currently in practice.

One potential approach to address this problem would be for guideline panels to estimate the time needed to implement an intervention when determining the direction and strength of their recommendations. A recent review of all lifestyle interventions recommended by NICE found that clinician time was not considered or estimated for any of the recommendations, and there were 143 of them.

The paper takes one NICE guideline as an example - "Physical activity: brief advice for adults in primary care." This guideline recommends general practitioners use questionnaires to screen all adults for physical inactivity and record the outcomes. For those not meeting the recommendations on physical activity, the clinician should give "brief advice" tailored to the individual, discussing motivation and goals; current level of activity and ability; circumstances, preferences, and barriers to being physically active; and health status. The brief advice should contain information about local opportunities to be physically active for people with a range of disabilities, preferences, and needs. The guideline encourages a written outline of the advice and goals, recording the outcomes of the discussion, and follow up in subsequent appointments.

Studies cited by the guideline suggest that offering this advice would take at least 10 minutes a patient. All adults from age 19 are eligible for screening, and roughly 40% of screened adults (the proportion of adults who do not meet the UK recommendations on physical activity) would then be eligible for brief advice.

Based on the NICE evidence review underpinning the guideline, 14 people with a sedentary lifestyle need to get brief advice on physical activity for one more person to report an increase in physical activity (the review found no significant beneficial effect on cardiorespiratory fitness, mental health, or other outcomes). Given that clinicians need to screen 35 people (which takes a minute per person or 35 minutes) to identify 14 people with a sedentary lifestyle, and then spend 10 minutes with each one giving brief advice (total of 140 minutes), it takes 175 minutes or 3 hours of GP time for one more person to increase their self-reported physical activity.

To implement this recommendation in a general practice of 2000 adults (the average population per full time GP in England), it would take 1 minute per person to screen all 2000 adults eligible for screening, for a total of 2000 minutes. Eight hundred adults (40% of 2000) would be eligible for brief advice, which at 10 minutes per person would require a total of 8000 minutes. The absolute time needed to treat (TNT) in a practice of 2000 adults is thus 10,000 minutes, or 167 hours, of GP time a year.

The practice TNT can also be expressed in relative terms by dividing the absolute TNT by the total time available for direct patient care per GP per year. A GP who spends 60% of their 40 hours a week in face-to-face patient care and who works 47 weeks a year in the practice will have a total time for direct patient care of 1128 hours. The 167 hours needed to implement just the NICE physical activity guideline will thus represent 15% (167 of 1128 hours) of the GP's yearly total face-to-face time with patients.

It seems obvious that a rapid review of preventative activity, the frequency of disease monitoring, and the ways that the results of such tests are communicated in real world consultations might form part of rebalancing medicine.

Finally, there has recently been reported a new cognitive bias – prevention bias.[ccxxxi] Researchers at the Bloch School of Management at the University of Missouri used a behavioural decision making approach to investigate factors causing possible inefficiencies of information resources security spending decisions. They performed a series of "economic games"- a standard approach in this field pioneered by Kahneman, Tversky and used now by many other researchers - featuring the key characteristics of a typical Information Technology security problem. They found several biases in investment decisions.

For budgeting their investment between major classes of security measures, decision makers demonstrated a strong bias toward investing in preventive measures rather than in detection and response measures, even though the task was designed to yield the same return on investment for both classes of measures. The researchers termed this phenomenon the "Prevention Bias." Decision makers also reacted to security threats when the risk was so small that no investment was economically justified. For higher levels of risk that warranted some security investment, decision makers showed a strong tendency to overinvest.

Now information security is a long way from health care but cognitive biases are not usually present in one domain of human decision making and absent in another. Might a prevention bias be responsible for some of the health care decision making we see? Is there another explanation for the popularity of PSA testing and mammography? Are the recommendations for the frequency of tests for disease monitoring the result of a "prevention bias"?

But then prevention does do a lot of good. Detection of high blood pressure, statins for some people for cardiovascular risk reduction, a steady continuing fall in cigarette smokers – all these are good things, even if some of them seem to require skills development from our current position to achieve fully informed consent. The issue is one of capacity in the health care system, or alternatively finding ways of achieving such prevention safely and effectively outside of traditional settings and with different approaches.ccxxxii

There is much complexity in thinking about how we might do prevention, testing and screening better as we rebalance medicine. But one theme is a constant – we could undertake better decision making if we had just a few more skills, thought a bit more about both why we were thinking in a certain way about the best decision for this individual, and finding out what the

318

patient knew already and preferred. Making decisions better with patients rests not only being better at understanding numbers and communicating risks and benefits, but also on our ability to have great consultation skills in order to have these better discussions with our patients.

And it is to consultation skills that we turn next.

CHAPTER TWENTY ONE

Words Matter

I am always a little cautious when discussing consultation skills with health care professionals. It is a very personal matter, and sits close to how health care professionals see themselves and their world. I have made the mistake in the past of being unreasonably defensive myself.

In the 1980s a technical revolution was about to transform the teaching and learning of how to have skilled conversations with patients. My response and that of my colleagues was not our finest moment. But of course, I now know there was a legitimate excuse. Thanks to a better understanding of cognitive psychology, I now can recognise that since we were seeing something that challenged our existing mindlines, and human beings often find it difficult to readily change their mindlines, a less than positive response is probably the norm. But it was still incorrect.

As I wrote in a blog for the British Medical Journal some years after the event,[ccxxxiii] I was lucky enough to be a young GP trainer when David Pendleton brought us the first videos of real, live consultations. David was then a young psychologist on a fellowship with the Royal College of General Practitioners and working on consultation skills with some equally innovative GPs in the Oxford region. The memory remains vivid so many years later.

Emulating James Herriot on his way to a cow's bottom, I drove for miles across North Yorkshire in the pouring rain very early one Saturday morning to David's workshop. It was video technology that had transformed our world, if only we knew it. As when Charles Fletcher first went onto national television with pictures of real operations for the first time, seeing other doctors' real consultations with real patients was fascinating, pioneering and transformative.

The technology filled a small van, and the tapes might have been Betamax. The audience was all people like me, GP trainers - people charged with the responsibility of developing the GPs of the future. We should have offered a standing ovation and a brass band — or at least hearty congratulations, a pint of Tetley's, and a pork pie. What David got was "We haven't got the time for this," "The patients will never consent to being videoed," and "You can't really teach consultation skills."

What should have said was: "This is new, it exposes our consultation skills in ways we've never seen before, and we need time to get used to the idea." A few years ago, David and I had the chance to have a beer and I got the chance to apologise in person. David was very generous but still, mea culpa.

Fast forward to the present and I am still worried about consultation skills. Their presence on the undergraduate curriculum of future health care professionals is ubiquitous, but I don't hear the students enthusing about the importance of the subject. Quite the opposite. In postgraduate training, the focus on the topic is strong in some specialties and settings - notably UK general practice - but looks much patchier in others. And after training is finished, how much continuing professional development is devoted to consultation skills? In many specialties, very little.

Do consultation skills matter? The evidence says "yes, a lot".[ccxxxiv] If we had an intervention that helps regulate patients' emotions, facilitate comprehension of medical information, and allow for better identification of patients' needs, perceptions, and expectations - we would want to be using that in medicine, wouldn't we? And if with the same intervention patients were more likely to be satisfied with their care, to share pertinent information for accurate diagnosis of their problems, to follow advice, and to adhere to prescribed treatment - we would want that too, wouldn't we? Patients' agreement with the doctor about the nature of the treatment and need for follow-up is strongly associated with their recovery. A better probability of recovery or a faster recovery? Who would not want that? And if studies of that intervention showed correlations between an improved sense of control and the ability to tolerate pain, decreased tumour growth, and daily functioning, together with enhanced psychological adjustments and better mental health – well, this is now starting to sound to be too good to be true.

But there is more. Some studies have observed a decrease in length of hospital stay and therefore the cost of individual medical visits, fewer referrals, better patient AND doctor satisfaction, less work-related stress, and reduced burnout, fewer formal complaints, and a reduction in patient litigation against care providers.

The intervention is, of course, better doctor - patient communication. And I am afraid that the evidence from patients is that communication is not always as good as the health care professional thinks it is. In 1998, the American Academy of Orthopaedic Surgeons conducted a national survey to which 807 patients and 700 orthopaedic surgeons responded. Patients rate technical skills as important but valued communication skills equally. According to this survey, 75% of the orthopaedic surgeons believed that they communicated satisfactorily with their patients, but only 21% the orthopaedic patients reported satisfactory communication with their surgeons.[ccxxxv] The defensive response is perhaps "That's in America" and "it was more than 20 years ago". Quite true, but a much more recent review for the Royal College of Surgeons of England found evidence that communication remained a serious problem – a third of patients think a "fractured bone" is a less severe injury than a "broken bone" when of course the terms are interchangeable.[ccxxxvi] Words matter.

Then there is the inspirational story of a young doctor, Kate Grainger. She became ill on holiday in California and flew home to be further assessed. She wrote:-

"If you can put yourself in my position – I'm 29 years old, I know I've got cancer, I think it's confined to my abdomen so I'm expecting to have an operation, maybe some chemotherapy and possibly a cure. I'm in a side room. I can hear everything that's going on outside. I'm in pain and alone. A junior doctor comes to see me to talk to me about the results of the MRI scan I'd had earlier in the week. I'd never met this doctor before. He came into my room,

he sat down in the chair next to me and looked away from me. Without any warning or asking if I wanted anyone with me he just said, "Your cancer has spread". He then could not leave the room quick enough and I was left in deep psychological distress. I never saw him again. I am a little bit psychologically scarred by that experience."

Dr Grainger died in 2016, but her campaign to improve the start of consultations with something as simple as introducing oneself being the norm #hellomynameis lives on.[ccxxxvii]

Whilst this was terrible for Kate Grainger, it was also terrible for the junior doctor tasked with that consultation. Communicating such devastating news to a fellow health care professional is the combined World Championships and Olympic Games Final of consultation skills. It may not have been appropriate to give that consultation to a fellow doctor in training, and it is no great surprise that it did not go well. Someone with demonstrably excellent communication skills is needed for such consultations. And if formal training in consultation skills had taken place some years earlier during the undergraduate course and there had not been ongoing or recent opportunities to refresh or upskill, then potentially those are important problems with an obvious remedy.

A few years ago, I was asked to lead a lunchtime session introducing some of the theories and practice of decision making to the clinical staff at a large hospital. Afterwards one of the doctors in training asked to speak with me. He told me he identified two broad categories of specialists. The first group were the ones who he would be very keen to sit with as they spoke with parents of children with very serious diagnoses. He would soak up their skills at communicating the technical aspects of the diagnosis, what it meant, what the anticipated treatment plan might look like, and what the eventual outcomes and their probabilities might be. At the same time, he recognised the incredible communication skills displayed by this group of experts as they tailored their explanations to that individual family, explored their understanding and feelings, and offered empathy and emotional support as well as the best that science and technology could offer.

The other category of specialists he described were those whose consultations he and his colleagues tried to avoid sitting in on. Those consultations did not contain anything technically incorrect, but they omitted the individualisation of care, the tailoring of the conversation to this family at this time, and most importantly, the emotional support. What he and his colleagues did was to make a note for themselves to go back later and attempt to compensate for the communication omissions of their more senior colleagues. That is not good enough, is it?

One last bit of data about consultations before moving on to more positive aspects. The Care Quality Commission, the independent regulator of health can social care in England, undertakes a big survey of patients who have spent at least one night in hospital in the last year. The survey has taken place every year for more than a decade and samples around 70,000 people each year. For many years the survey asks this question: "When doctors/nurses spoke about your care in front of you, were you included in the conversation?" Just let that sink in. If you were running this huge survey to assess the quality of care, would you think there was a need to check if health care professionals were doing things with and to patients without communicating with the patient at all? It seems to me that if the CQC has to just ask the question, there is a real problem with communication skills.

But they do, and when they do, more than a 20% of patients say they are never included in conversations about their care either by nurses or doctors.

This data could be framed as "three quarters of people say they were always included in conversations about their care". Whilst that would be factually correct, it would be to distort the importance of the findings. Not including the patient in conversations about their care should, in my view, be a "never event".[ccxxxviii] "Never Events" are important safety issues, as defined by NHS England, and include for example wrong

325

operations being performed, overdoses or underdoses of insulin being given due to abbreviations on drug charts, or incompatible blood transfusions being given. The General Medical Council in its key guide to the duties of a doctor says, "You must listen to patients, take account of their views, and respond honestly to their questions."ccxxxix Care being delivered or planned without the involvement of the patient should never happen. And yet just less than a quarter of NHS patients in hospital experience that at least sometimes during their illness. That is not good enough either, is it?

And yet having optimal conversations is a tricky business. Try this question. Having listened to the patient's opening statement outlining the reason for today's consultation, which is the better choice when attempting to find out whether the patient has additional items for today's consultation? Should the health care professional say:-

A.   "Is there something else we could usefully discuss today?"

Or

B.   "Is there anything else we could usefully discuss today?"

There are only three options. The answer is either A is better, or B is better, or there is no difference. You might be uncertain. When I put this to doctors roughly a third say A, a third say B, and a third say it doesn't matter. But when this was tested in a randomised controlled trial the answer was clear.ccxl Saying "Is there something else we could usefully discuss today?" uncovered 78% of additional patients' agendas. Swopping "anything" for "something" stopped these important disclosures. "Something else" seems to be a permissive phrase, and "anything else" in the health care setting seems to close down conversations. Who knew? In the same area of research it looks like with parents of sick children the health care professionals should say "Did that concern you?" rather than "Did that worry you?".ccxli What other routinely used phrases are inhibiting open conversations about very important matters?

326

When I was at medical school there was no teaching of communication skills. I learnt and was then examined on my competence at "taking a medical history". The initial approach has hardly changed - history of presenting complaint, past medical history, drug history, family history, social history, and finally "systems review".

Whilst this process might have begun with an open question – for example, "What brought you to the hospital today?" – it very rapidly deteriorates into an interrogation of almost entirely closed questions. "Where is the pain?". "How long have you had it?". "Did it start suddenly or gradually?". And so on. Social history would cover "Who do you live with?", "What is your job?", "How much alcohol do you drink?", "Do you smoke?" and the like.

And it did not end there. "Systems review" would cover almost all the common symptoms that any human being might experience. "Have you had any significant weight loss?" "Have you had any fevers or night sweats?" "Have you had a reduction in your energy levels?" "Has your appetite changed?" And then a whole series from head-to-toe – headaches, vision changes, hearing problems, swallowing problems, chest pain, cough, shortness of breath, abdominal pain, urinary symptoms, bowel symptoms, skin rashes, joint pain. And so on.

We were expected to learn these lists of questions, to ask every patient every question by rote, and of course for us that was a real struggle because our rationality was bounded and we needed lots of repetition to become competent at "taking a medical history". We observed our teachers performing their own inquisitions – either gruffly or kindly - and copied them. It was a system of enquiry that we all believed would mean we had collected every single piece of relevant data, and more data meant we could solve the diagnostic puzzle the patients had set for us more accurately. It was thought that maximising the information would mean fewer errors in diagnosis. The utility of bounded rationality and dual process theory in relation to health care were far in the future. Woe betide the student who omitted some apparently key part of the fixed interrogation. There was little concern for how the process felt to the patient, who was of course in hospital and therefore unlikely to be feeling their best. It was an entirely technical, and allegedly scientific process.

Before we move on, the true problem from the undergraduate health care professional's perspective is not in starting with this interrogative approach of how to take a medical history. Starting with a structured approach is probably needed as a starting point. Just as the chess grand master must learn the chess piece moves before being able to increase the degree of complexity as a player, repeated exposure to lots of patients helps the developing clinician to explore the ways that individual symptoms were often associated with other symptoms and findings on clinical examination. In such ways do clinicians progress from the learning and knowing the basic sciences into creating patterns which represent a diagnosis or an "illness script" – a key step on the road to expertise which we will turn to in the next chapter.

The true problem is not progressing from "taking a history". My generation's undergraduate training in how to listen and talk with patients stopped at interrogation stage. The situation today is rather better, with some time on the curriculum allocated to more advanced consultation skills. But the rest of the huge undergraduate medical curriculum is dominated by science and knowledge. Current data on undergraduate medical curriculums are elusive, but a 2001 survey of 24 UK medical schools found that the number of teaching hours dedicated to communication skills ranged from 18 to 91 hours. If the entire taught curriculum occupies 30 hours a week, 40 weeks a year, for five years, only 0.3% - 1.5% is allocated to teaching such skills. Undergraduate communication curricula are extensive and almost certainly difficult to cover in such limited time.[ccxlii ccxliii]

There was, and still is, some talk of the mysterious and quaint term "bedside manner". It was somehow associated with the confidence the patient had in the doctor, but I do not recall anyone properly explaining it or how to acquire the necessary skills to generate the required confidence. We were focussed entirely on knowledge, science, and collecting data. The measured outcomes were generating reasonable diagnostic probabilities and sound management strategies. As an old Punch cartoon put it, "Oh, well, I don't know much about his Ability; but he's got a very good Bedside Manner!". But we were different. We were scientists, and our self-worth was science and knowledge based. Our reliance on science meant that medicine was certain to be better than it had been for previous generations of patients. In some aspects it is. But in other aspects, we have lost a great deal.

Things started to change in 1976. Professors of General Practice are a relatively new thing. One of the first was Pat Byrne at Manchester University. In the early 1980s I once sat in a very small workshop in a very small room between Professor Byrne and Marshall Marinker, the first Professor of General Practice at Leicester. I was completely intimidated - not a frequent occurrence - and said almost nothing, and certainly nothing coherent, for the entirety of the discussion. Both Byrne and Marinker recognised the need to develop the theoretical educational framework for general practice and they were both among the authors in 1972 of what became one of the first academic "must read" books about general practice – "The Future General practitioner – Learning and Teaching".

However, it was in 1976 that Byrne published "Doctors Talking to Patients", written with his friend Barry Long, a psychologist. In the 1960s Michael Balint at the Tavistock Clinic in London had begun the modern era of studying the doctor-patient relationship. Working with his wife Enid, he applied psychoanalytic thinking to the understanding of the dialogue between doctor and patient.

Balint was a pioneer in this field and some doctors still find his approach helpful in supporting them but, echoing Archie Cochrane's doubts about psychoanalysis, his work is also widely criticised because of its lack of scientific objectivity.

With developments in the methods of studying human behaviour, and especially the development of portable cassette recorders, it became possible for Byrne and Long to make audio recordings of real consultations for the first time, and then develop tools for measuring aspects of the interaction between doctors and patients. That hidden part of medicine which we as students patronisingly dismissed as the "bedside manner" could be scrutinised in the same way as doctors scrutinised the patient's symptoms and physical signs. With the data of the audio recordings, a search could be made for patterns and meanings, some judgements made about what worked well in consultations and what might be better, and initial thoughts constructed about how to teach and learn consultation skills.

Byrne and Long produced a scientific analysis of an astounding 2114 consultations from 71 GPs of real consultations in real general practice. Marshall Marinker reviewed the book for the Journal of the Royal College of General Practitioners. Interestingly, he noted that with the growth of science and technology since the 18th century *"the doctor-patient relationship came to be seen not as the active ingredient of medical care, but rather as a vehicle or base in which the active ingredient, technical manipulation, could be made available. The growing realisation over the past few decades that the engineering approach to medical problems has a defined and limited success has led to a reawakened interest in the doctor-patient relationship."* He concluded *"Byrne and Long have, here, quite simply uttered some of the first words in a new field of exploration. It will be a long time before their successors write the last ones."*ccxliv

Marshall Marinker was very smart. He recognised the limitations of science and technology long before most of us did. That prediction has certainly came true. David Pendleton and the Oxford group followed not long afterwards with video recordings, and with video technology both widely available and affordable, research into the consultation flourished.

Over the next fifteen years many models for the consultation were proposed. These models are hypothetical descriptions of a complex process. They are not scripts to be learned and followed slavishly in the hope of the perfect, or even better, consultations. Each consultation is unique, and it is estimated that doctors will have 200,000 consultations in a professional lifetime. The interaction between patient and health care professional happens like a rapid, verbal tennis match. Neither participant knows what the other participant will say next, and then there is the often-unconscious response to unconscious non-verbal communication. When teaching and learning more advanced consultation skills than "taking a medical history" it should be recognised that the development of skills builds on the intuitive and personal communication skills that all human beings acquire from birth. The way we communicate with another human being is unique to us as individuals and is shaped by the way we see others communicate and our own experiences. But communication is a skill, and new skills can be learned.

Suppose you we were going for an important conversation – for example: a job interview, a first date, or Sunday lunch with prospective parents-in-law. Would you go armed with an extensive framework for the conversation created in advance, committed to memory by lots of repetition, and follow that framework slavishly, fully expecting that with that rigid approach the conversation was guaranteed to be a success? Of course not. You would, I hope, pay attention, ask lots of open questions, show interest in the other participants as people, and try your best to find out lots about them. No doubt you would be alert and "present"; these are not situations to be day dreaming.

So, there is not one single best way for all human beings to conduct these important conversations. The aim of improving our conversation skills in important situation is to do a bit better incrementally than our natural skills would do. If it were "Strictly Come Dancing" we would try and score a 7 instead of a 6, and then in time an 8 instead of a 7. Aiming for the perfect 10 in a single consultation, never mind every consultation, is pretty much unattainable. Consultations about health are the height of conversational complexity. There is often concern present, at least in the patient, and consultations can be or become very emotionally charged. Big decisions may be made and there is

331

apprehension. There is a power imbalance with the greater technical knowledge usually resting with the health care professional, even if the patient has greater lived experience. Both participants have their own unique and very different mindlines, and without very skilled explorations neither of them becomes aware of the other's thinking. Therefore a consultation is not something that can be "fixed". But in complex situations some things are better than others.

Consultation models emerged from this research. They are not the real world, but a human construct to better help us understand the real world. Here are a few examples:-

Byrne and Long (1976) [ccxlv]
1.   The doctor establishes a relationship with the patient.
2.   The doctor either attempts or actually discovers the reason for the patient's attendance.
3.   The doctor conducts a verbal or physical examination or both.
4.   The doctor, doctor and patient, or the patient (in that order) consider the condition.
5.   The doctor, and occasionally the patient, detail further treatment or further investigation.
6.   The consultation is terminated usually by the doctor.

This was the first consultation model to explicitly include the task of introducing and finishing the consultation. The introduction is especially important. First impressions in any interaction count for a lot. And if for whatever reason there is a difficult, awkward, or dysfunctional start to a consultation then the rest is less likely to go smoothly. Hence the "hello, my name is…." campaign. This was also the first time the task of considering the problem with the patient was described.

Byrne and Long found that the style of the consultation often reflected the personality of the doctor; at other times, but less frequently, it reflected that of the patient. Sometimes consultations were doctor-dominated (where the patient said little), and in others there was a virtual monologue by the patient (where the doctor became a passive listener). They found that dysfunctional consultations more often resulted from a lack of attention being paid to Phase 2 (not discovering reason for attendance) and Phase 4 (not considering the condition with the patient). Importantly, they found that doctors who asked more open questions tended to see their patients less frequently. Open questions, finding out what the patient thinks and expects, and and then being attentive and listening carefully to what is said and what is not, are three of the keystones of better consultations.

Subsequently they described Phase 7, which they called the Parting Shot - where the patient reveals the real reason why they have come just as they are about to leave.

The Health Belief Model (1975) ccxlvi

The model was first developed by a group of American psychologists – Irwin Rosenstock, Godfrey Hochbaum, Stephen Kegeles, and Howard Leventhal - from the 1950s onwards. They were working for the US Public Health Service and were concerned that few people were getting chest X rays to screen for tuberculosis even if mobile X Ray vans went to local neighbourhoods. From a purely rational perspective this made no sense, given the prevalence of TB and, even in the 1950s when antibiotics were available, its risks. The psychologists developed six constructs that they proposed varied between individuals and would predict their engagement or otherwise in health-related behaviours.

1.   Whether they think they are susceptible to a particular illness.
2.   Whether the consequences of the illness could be serious, physically or socially.
3.   Whether the 'treatment' would confer benefit.
4.   Whether there are barriers e.g. costs outweighing the benefits.
5.   Internal factors such as worrying about symptoms, and external factors such as media campaigns, or advice from family

and friends. These triggers that make a patient seek help are called "cues to action".

6.   Whether they have a strong internal or external controller.

Patients vary enormously in the way they accept responsibility for their health. Those with a strong internal controller seek to control their own health destiny. They see their doctor merely as an aid to achieving the treatment, prescriptions or referrals that they need. They have a firm idea of their own diagnosis and an equally definitive expectation of what the doctor should do for them.

Those with a strong external controller are more "fatalistic" - their likelihood of developing illness is totally out of their control and they cannot do anything about it. A third group still regard their health destiny rests externally to them, but accept it can be influenced by particular individual - a health care professional for instance. The locus of control, or at least some of it, rests with the notionally powerful, influential other.

This model, although originally published a year before Byrne and Long, only slowly became assimilated into most people's thinking about the consultation, perhaps because the authors continued to develop it over the years, and perhaps because it is entirely patient-focussed. It took a while for the dominant, doctor-centred approach to consultations to open up and incorporate the important patient perspective.

The Health Belief Model influenced the Oxford GPs working with David Pendleton, especially Peter Tate who went on to have a glittering career including being Chief Examiner for the Royal College of GPs.

Exploring the patient's Ideas, Concerns and Expectations (I.C.E.) has become a centrepiece of modern thinking about the consultation.

• Patient's ideas – For example, "Had you any thoughts about what might be going on?"

- Patient's concerns – For example, "And what concerns do you have about that?"
- Patient's expectation – For example, "And what were you hoping we might be able to do for this?"

McWhinney's Disease-Illness model (1986)

This divide between the doctor-centred, disease-orientated, scientifically based and technology-orientated view of the purpose of health care and consultations on the one hand, and the patient's view of their illness on the other, was first bridged by McWhinney and colleagues from the University of Western Ontario.

Their approach, later revived in 1997 by Stewart and Rotter,[ccxlvii] has become known as "patient-centred clinical interviewing". In this approach (see Figure 22.1), whilst the doctor's agenda is important (blue arrow in the diagram), so too is the patient's (green arrow). Therefore, a consultation weaves between the doctor's agenda and that of the patient's (purple arrow). In this way, agreement is reached about the problems or diagnoses, and an agreed management plan is formulated which includes the patient's ideas, concerns, and expectations whilst at the same time conforming to technical aspects considered "good clinical practice".

Figure 22.1:

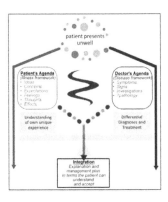

The Inner Consultation. (1987) ccxlviii

Clinicians seeking to improve their consultation skills sometimes struggle to manage the two agendas, the doctor's and the patient's. Roger Neighbour, a former President of the Royal College of General Practitioners, described the two different heads of the health care professional in the consultation. One is called the Organiser. This doctor-centred head is busy trying to manage the organisation of the consultation, asking questions, and deciding to examine, planning and negotiating clinical management, time keeping – slowing and speeding consultations, and making records.

The "other head" - operating simultaneously - is called the Responder. This patient-centred head tries to make sure that they are being attentive through listening properly, taking time to think and process information, creating and testing ideas, and being empathic.

This model emphasises that the aim of the health care professional is to find the fine balance between Organiser and Responder modes whilst journeying through the consultation. It is a bit like driving a car whilst explaining something technical to a passenger. The Organiser pays attention to the steering wheel, pedals and gears whilst the Responder maintains the conversation. When the traffic is busy or the road layout is suddenly complex or unfamiliar, the Organiser head takes over and you temporarily stop engaging with the passenger. But when things are calm again and easier, the Organiser will relax allowing the Responder to come back in and maintain the conversation. The Organiser continues to lurk in the background, and if things get more technically complex again, comes back in and takes over at short notice. These are not easy skills to develop, and we shall return to that.

The other very important contribution that Roger Neighbour brings to the key concepts of the consultation is "Safety-netting". We have previously explored uncertainty and probability, and the impossibility of a scientific approach delivering certainty either in the diagnostic process or a guarantee of treatment always delivering a good outcome. It therefore becomes obligatory that every consultation includes a back-up process for when even the best of consultations gets it wrong. This applies even when health care professional and patient share their different agendas optimally and agree together on diagnosis and treatment. No patient is safe unless the consultation includes safety-netting.

Technically, the safety-netting process requires three questions:-
1. If I am right, what do I expect to happen?
2. How will I know I am wrong?
3. What would I do then?

The process fits very well with the calibration "stop and think moment" from cognitive psychology. We all have a natural ability to resist the first thoughts that come to mind and consider alternatives. Health care professionals and patients can further develop that innate ability and use safety-netting routinely.

More difficult is determining how much detailed safety-netting should be shared with the patient. By its nature safety-netting requires thinking ahead and envisaging the worst possible outcomes. Well-intentioned transparency can turn readily into crippling anxiety as the patient feels the need to ask for reassurance time and time again to query minor deviances from a normal recovery. Patients differ in the level of explicitness and the nature of the uncertainty that they are comfortable with, and that level may differ in the same person in different circumstances. But despite these dilemmas, an indication from the health care professional that they are already looking ahead, and the patient should do so too is an absolute requirement.

It might be general – for example, "I'm happy with all that. Are you? We can always think again if things change. You know where we are."

337

Or it might be a bit more specific – for example, "We've effectively ruled out a clot in your leg for now. But there's still a possibility….. about 3 people in 100 might need to come back for reassessment, but for now we're good. If pain and swelling worsen or you get short of breath or get chest pain don't hesitate to ask us to take another look sharpish. But if you follow the plan we've agreed, then I'd expect your calf to slowly improve and be much better in 2-3 weeks at the most. If it doesn't, then do seek help".

Or it might be very specific – for example, "I think we're both happy that this is just a non-specific virus with a rash. But you're obviously going to keep an eye on the rash. If the colour of it changes from pink to a red or purple and when you press with a glass it doesn't go pale, you know to get back to us without any delay because that might mean something much more serious such as meningitis. There is nothing to indicate anything serious like that at the moment, but we've always got to sensibly monitor the situation and think about even the rarest of events. Yes? (pause) Are sure you are ok with that? (pause) I'll ring you first thing in the morning and see how you both, and especially the temperature, are doing."

5. Calgary-Cambridge (1996) [ccxlix ccl]

In the 1990s as the consultation models research continued to expand, so did the evidence about:-

- how consultations actually happened for real.
- that it really was possible to teach consultation skills and improve performance in the long term.
- which teaching and learning methods work best for most people.
- the patient-centred behaviours were just as important as the clinician-centred tasks in optimising decision making for individuals.

Over twenty years, gradually the consultation models moved away from a list of tasks for the clinician to complete, to at best a

338

combination of technically-focussed tasks and an exploration of the patient's ideas, concerns, expectations, values and preferences. All this was pulled together in a remarkable piece of work covered in two books by Jonathan Silverman from Cambridge, Suzanne Kurtz from Calgary and Juliet Draper from the Eastern Deanery in the UK. (See Figure 22.2).

Figure 22.2.

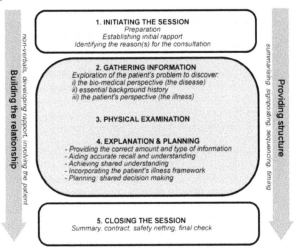

Since its publication it has become the most well-known consultation model internationally. It is the only comprehensive model which marries each of its components with the available research evidence on the skills that aid doctor-patient communication. Its five steps capture the disease and illness frameworks illustrated in McWhinney's Disease-Illness model, and combine process with content in a logical schema. Alongside this, the model impresses the importance of the need to provide structure to the interview and to build the relationship with the patient as the consultation progresses through the five steps.

Whilst the comprehensiveness of the Calgary-Cambridge (C-C) model is one of its many strengths, its apparent complexity can be daunting – especially to learners coming to it having worked for some time in a predominantly bio-medical model and more used to consulting in a "taking a medical history" style. In its full form the C-C has 78 items – some of the detail is expanded upon in Figure 22.3.

Figure 22.3: Skills in the Calgary Cambridge Model (truncated)

1. Introduction & Orientation.	•Greetings • Introduction - self, role, nature of interview, requests consent • Respect - demonstrates interest, concern and respect, attends to patient's physical comfort • Opening question to identify problem that patient wishes to address • Listening without interruption • Screening - checks if other problems patient is concerned about • Agenda setting negotiates agenda taking both patient's and physician's needs into account.
2. Gathering Information.	• Encourages patient to tell story chronologically • Question style open to closed • Listening attentively, not interrupting, allowing patient time • Facilitation – use of encouragement, silence, repetition, etc. • Cues • Clarifies – statements that are unclear / need amplification • Summarisation to patient - at intervals to check own understanding
3. Understanding Patient's Perspective.	• Ideas/Concerns/Beliefs/Feelings • Effects • Expectations
4. Providing Structure	• Summarising • Signposting

5. Developing Rapport	• Sequencing – logical sequence • Timing & keeping to task • Non-verbal behaviour • Appropriate level of note taking • Not judgmental • Empathy & support • Sensitive
6. Involving the patient	• Explaining thinking/rationale • Explaining examination
7. Explanation	• Comprehensive & appropriate information according to each patient's needs. • Correct type, amount & level of information • Clear information – avoid jargon • Timing of information • Avoiding premature reassurance
8. Aiding Recall and Understanding	• Emphasis and use of aids • Prioritising information • Asking patient to restate ("Teach back")
9. Achieving a Shared Understanding	• Explanations linked to patients' views, problems & requests for information • Invites questions • Sensitive to patients' signs of puzzlement, overload, etc. – picks up cues
10. Planning	• Shared decision making – team talk (decide together), option talk (comparing alternatives), decision talk (expertise combined with values and preferences) • Negotiates, offers choices, encourages patient to contribute ideas and preferences, checks patient's acceptance and decisions
11. Closure	• Summarises, agrees next step, any final questions.

Some of these items may come very naturally to some human beings and not actually require any adjustment in conversational approaches, but the same skills may be very unfamiliar approaches in a conversation for others. Even though not all items in the C-C model are needed for each consultation, there is such a lot going on in a real consultation at a very fast pace - with the next thing in the conversation being completely unpredictable. Given the complexity of the skills required, there are some questions to ask about the most successful learning and teaching strategies to improve communication skills.

We have previously discussed how the evidence-based movement ignored for at least twenty years the complex question of how to incorporate the best available evidence into consultation. This complex question was by-passed and instead those involved with EBM, including me, answered the less-complicated question, "How do we compile all the best evidence so it is together in one place?". We have ended up with hundreds of guidelines and thousands of systematic reviews, and only now have we turned to the original question of how to have those evidence-informed consultations.

In the same way, those involved with teaching consultation skills to actual and prospective health care professionals also to some extent not fully addressed the complex problem of how to optimally teach consultation skills. There has been more effort and energy put into the merely complicated question which described models of the consultation. To be fair, both Pendleton et al and the Calgary-Cambridge team have described their traditional methods of teaching consultation skills. But we reviewed current performance in communicating with patients at the start of this chapter, and no one could claim there is not more to do

Consultation skills are a skill. That sounds pretty obvious, right? But the "it's a skill thing" is actually very important. No one could expect to be able to act brilliantly by reading even the very best book about acting and memorising the key points. To become a competent actor you have to try it yourself and then practice doing it better. If you wanted to play tennis well, you would not expect to become a good player just by going along to Wimbledon and watching the players. Millions of people watch Strictly Come Dancing every Saturday night for weeks every autumn, but most of us are still terrible at dancing.

Most of us have learned to drive a car, and that's a skill too. If we think back, the one thing that made us good enough to pass our driving test it was having the opportunity to practice. To acquire skills, some **instruction** is useful – "this is the clutch pedal, this switches on the windscreen wipers" and so on. Then **demonstration** can be helpful. If you have never paid attention when seeing someone reverse into a parking space, then a formal demonstration with perhaps a running commentary of what the key positioning requirements are as the manoeuvre takes place is going to give you some insights.

But the thing that really accelerates progress is experiential learning. Skills require **practice**. We will probably be very disappointed with our first efforts, but with repetition we get better. Many of us could be passable dancers, or tennis players, or artists, or speakers of a foreign language. We could need some instruction and demonstration. But mostly, we need to practice, and to put some cognitive energy into that practice.

When we are trying to learn a new skill we are in System 2. With driving, there are all sorts of new knobs, switches, pedals, and we do not know how far or how fast to turn the steering wheel. But with repetition we slowly get some familiarity with a few of the multiple tasks, and they become a bit more automatic. It still is not easy, but if we concentrate hard, we can just about manage to carry out the required piece of driving.

The final thing that helps us accelerate our progress with skills is **assessment with supportive feedback**. In general, it helps most people to have a softly spoken, kind, and relaxed driving instructor who observes our learner driving attempts and then gives a few key pointers for us to work on next. It probably helps that he or she is in their car which they have chosen especially for its learner-friendly features and characteristics, and they have fitted dual-controls so there is an additional safely net for the instructor to bring the car to a halt if the learner gets into difficulties.

Those characteristics mean that a well-trained, highly competent, professional driving instructor is generally much better than a stressed parent who is tired after a busy day at work, and who has no experience of teaching anyone to drive. Then they are using their own beloved car which has not been selected for having learner-friendly features, has no dual controls, and they are attempting to teach a complex skill to a teenager who is normally resistant to taking parental advice on any topic most of the time. If one scrapes beneath the surface, quite a few teenagers have real problems with not being able to do something that his or her parents can apparently do very competently and apparently effortlessly. A supportive and skilled tutor for consultation skills who can do the assessment and supportive feedback is an important part of the jigsaw.

Because consultation skills are highly personal to health care professionals, in some groups not used to such personal exposure and experiential learning, approaches may need to be based on pre-recorded consultations by others rather than real or role-played consultations by group members.[ccli] Mindlines which have become strongly embedded by years of apparently successful clinical practice (all be it with an emphasis on mostly technical aspects of care), may generate considerable defensiveness when challenged by the externally-introduced concept of the patient's expertise and their values and preferences. The thorny topic of giving learners feedback on their consultations has been addressed in detail by both the Pendleton group and the Calgary-Cambridge group.

Other traditional approaches to developing consultation skills involve non-videotaped role plays - either with actors or with learners taking turns to play the role of patient learner and observer, or direct observation of real consultations, all followed by feedback and discussion. The constant limitation is that both of these approaches do not allow for sufficient **practice** so that the complex requirements can be slowly assimilated from System 2 into System 1 by **repetition**.

It may be that another technology-based revolution is about to happen to take the teaching and learning of consultation skills on to the next level. With colleagues at Keele University, we have been pioneering the use of avatars in teaching consultation skills.[ccli] [cclii] [ccliv] Here are a couple of examples which are freely available:-

- Discussing a statin for primary prevention of cardiovascular disease
  https://www.keelevp.com/virtual-patient/eidm

- Reviewing a patient with osteoarthritis
  https://www.keelevp.com/virtual-patient/shared-decision-making

Avatars address several weaknesses in the use of video consultations for skill acquisition Most importantly they offer endless opportunities for practice. The avatar never gets tired, and it never deviates from the designed consultation, even though there are multiple routes through the consultation which the health care professional can explore for themselves – uncovering which responses from them produce the more optimal outcome. For the acquisition of new skills this seems to be a big advantage. Assessment and feedback are built in with the avatar-patient providing feedback to the clinician after each consultation. The current design offers multiple choices for the health care professional to select as their next contribution to the discussion. This meets the requirements for **instruction** and **demonstration**.

Interestingly, we commonly get feedback on the avatars along the lines of "none of the multiple options is exactly what I as the health care professional would want to say next". This illustrates that these conversations do indeed use the individual, System 1-based conversational skills acquired during our lifetime, and also

345

demonstrates the over-confidence bias that says "My individual approach is better than the other options the avatar programme is providing". Very rarely is that the case, because the avatar is built using the best evidence available distilled from years of research into optimising such consultations using models such as Pendleton's and Calgary-Cambridge.

It is still early days for avatars, but it may be that their development will be as big a step forward for consultation skills as portable cassette recorders and video cameras were in the 1970s and 1980s.

In our own teaching we have also found it helpful to learners to provide some guidance as to how to truncate consultation models such as C-C into something more cognitively manageable. A model with 78 items inevitably triggers cognitive overload. These models were never intended to be lists of questions to ask in sequence as in "taking a medical history".

One way of approaching the topic of consultation skills is to focus on one important aspect of the consultation – the beginning. David Haslam, former Chair at NICE, says this is very simple.[cclv] Learner-clinicians do not need long checklists of consultation actions taped to their computer terminals. Actors would never learn to act by simply learning skills mechanistically. They would try and get inside the skin of the character. They would need to understand both how their character feels, thinks and reacts, and how the characters they are interacting with feel and think. David says the start of the consultation should be "Shut up and listen".

And yet we don't do this enough. Important aspects of the opening of the consultation would be eliciting the patient's agenda and doing so without interruption. A recent analysis in the US produced findings typical of previous research internationally.[cclvi] In primary care clinics, the agenda was elicited in 49% of encounters compared to 20% in specialty care clinics. Of the primary care encounters where the agenda was elicited, physicians interrupted the patients in 63%. Of the encounters in specialty care where the agenda was elicited, physicians interrupted patients in 80% of consultations. The median time to interruption was 11 seconds, and when not interrupted patients completed their agenda in a maximum of 108 seconds; the average was 6 seconds. And remember that this data was obtained in the period after consultation skills became ubiquitous in undergraduate teaching. Undergraduate teaching of consultation skills is necessary, but it is not sufficient for there to be great consultations happening everywhere and all the time.

David goes on to add two more items to form a six-word consultation model; "shut up, listen, know something, be kind". For me, those six words are the essence of an approach the encapsulates both the clinician's agenda and the patient's agenda.

Gradually, as the work on consultation models progressed and the assessment of whether that good practice was being enacted showed disappointing results, the twin aims of the consultation have become much more formalised. High level health care policy now defines being "patient-centeredness" as being focussed on the needs of the individual, and describes a culture where a partnership exists between health care professionals, patients, and their families, the aim being that decisions respect patients' wants, needs, and preferences, and that patients have the education and support they require to make medical decisions and participate in their own care.^{cclvii}

Shared decision-making (SDM) is the outcome of being patient centred. It is a joint process in which a healthcare professional works together with a person to reach a decision about care. It involves choosing tests and treatments based both on evidence and on the person's individual preferences, beliefs, and values. It makes sure the person understands the risks, benefits, and possible consequences of different options through discussion and information sharing. Patients and clinicians who engage in SDM work together to understand the patient's situation and determine the best course of action to address it. In this process, an important first step is for patients and clinicians to determine which problems require attention through collaborative conversations.[cclviii]

The UK's General Medical Council is very clear on the approach.[cclix] Great, patient-centred consultations are not just good practice, they are a professional obligation. It says:-

"If you assess, diagnose, or treat patients, you must work in partnership with them to assess their needs and priorities.

"You must recognise a patient's right to choose whether to accept your advice, and respect their right to seek a second opinion.

"All patients have the right to be involved in decisions about their treatment and care, and be supported to make informed decisions if they are able to.

"The exchange of information between medical professionals and patients is central to good decision making. You must give patients the information they want or need in a way they can understand. This includes information about:
(a) their condition(s), likely progression, and any uncertainties about diagnosis and prognosis
(b) the options for treating or managing the condition(s), including the option to take no action
(c) the potential benefits, risks of harm, uncertainties about, and likelihood of success for each option.

"You must listen to patients and encourage an open dialogue about their health, asking questions to allow them to express what matters to them, and responding honestly to their questions.

"You must treat each patient as an individual. You must not rely on assumptions about the treatment options or outcomes a patient will prefer, or the factors they will consider significant."

There is also case law which makes person-centred care and shared decision making not just good practice, but a legal obligation.[cclx cclxi]

In March 2015, the Supreme Court decided unanimously in favour of Nadine Montgomery in the Montgomery v Lanarkshire

Health Board case. For Mrs Montgomery, this was the culmination of a 16-year battle.

Nadine Montgomery was pregnant, had Type 1 diabetes mellitus, and was of small stature. Diabetes increases the risk of a large baby and women of short stature have an increased probability of having s small pelvis through which the baby must pass if the delivery is vaginal. Mrs Montgomery expressed concerns throughout her antenatal care, asking her obstetrician if the baby's size was a potential problem – the alternative to vaginal delivery being caesarean section. This would reduce some of the risks of delivery, notably the large baby's shoulders becoming stuck during delivery - a term called shoulder dystocia.

Mrs Montgomery's obstetrician did not discuss the increased risk of this complication in vaginal delivery. Mrs Montgomery delivered her son vaginally but there was a twelve-minute delay between delivery of his head and his shoulders. This resulted in the blood flow through the umbilical cord being compressed, resulting in a lack of oxygen to the baby's brain with consequent cerebral palsy, and there was also a significant permanent injury to the nerves to one arm.

Mrs Montgomery sued for negligence, arguing that if she had known of the increased risk, she would have requested a caesarean section. The judgement in her favour established that a patient should be told whatever they want to know, not what the doctor thinks they should be told. In technical terms, this ruling supported the concept of material risk. Material risk is a risk that is deemed to be of significance by an individual patient rather than by a body of doctors. The judgement established that doctors need to find out what concerns an individual patient; a snooker player may have different concerns regarding a hand operation when compared with someone else whose livelihood does not rely on dexterity. There can be no "one fits all" approach. Importantly, shared decision making is most definitely not properly represented by a consultation in which the health care professional sets out the options and asks the patient to choose. The aim is a discussion in which both parties actively collaborate. Documentation of the discussion and the options offered is also a GMC-standard professional obligation.

The Montgomery judgement means that the law on consent has progressed from doctor-focused to patient-focused. The practice of medicine has moved significantly away from the idea of the paternalistic doctor who tells their patient what to do, even if this was thought to be in the patient's best interests. A patient is autonomous and should be supported to make decisions about their own health and to take ownership of the fact that sometimes success is uncertain, and complications can occur despite the best treatment. Importantly, this ruling requires both the exploration and discussion of risks and options, not just risks alone. As the ruling stated, *"it is not possible to consider a particular medical procedure in isolation from its alternatives. Most decisions about medical care are not simple yes/no answers. There are choices to be made, arguments for and against each of the options to be considered, and sufficient information must be given so that this can be done."*

Today, patients should expect a more active and informed role in treatment decisions. But the evidence shows that does not happen everywhere and consistently. A key part of rebalancing medicine is to reduce the variation in the way decisions are made, and to gradually shift the focus of the conversation towards shared decisions. This is not easy. The current environment in most health care settings is hectic with high demand for care and in the NHS, rising waiting lists for elective care. It is hard to ask some of the tired and demoralised workforce, worn down by austerity and the demands of the coronavirus pandemic, to change their current approach to consultations. And yet not meeting the professional and legal obligations are a serious issue and one that must be faced.

Anyone who reads a little of the evidence on changing clinical practice knows that the alternatives are "help it happen" and "make it happen". This is not the time for the latter - for coercive approaches. At any time, they are, overall, likely to be less successful than educational approaches that support change rather than force it. At this time, clumsy attempts to address a lack of person-centred care and shared decision making are likely to be counterproductive. How such things are achieved matters as much as what is achieved, and it seems very important to remember that there will not be a single person working in health care who would not want the better outcomes that improving clinician-patient communication brings.

But we must do better with consultation skills. As Don Berwick, Emeritus President of the Institute for Health Improvement puts it, "Everyone in the NHS has two jobs: doing the work and improving it".

And words really matter.

CHAPTER TWENTY TWO

Expert

The well-honed skills and extensive knowledge of experts allow them to perform the most complex tasks with a graceful ease and extraordinary proficiency.

We have already discussed how we expect health care professionals to be great at decision making and yet there is comparatively little effort made to teach them how they make decisions and how they might do so better. The undergraduate and postgraduate curricula for health care professionals is dominated by knowledge and science, with communication skills being largely confined to the undergraduate course for most specialties. Yet we should expect great person-centred consultations with shared decision making - and those approaches are mandated by the health care regulators and the law. So, it will not come as any surprise that despite developing expertise being an inherent requirement of a healthcare practitioner, it is very rare for there to be any item in their undergraduate or postgraduate curricula which covers the pathway to expertise. There are some still early attempts to teach clinical reasoning in undergraduate courses, but with that exception it seems that just like cognitive psychology and, in much postgraduate training, consultation skills, health care professionals are expected to somehow catch on to what is required.

Personally, I am powerfully convinced by the argument that it helps learners if they can appreciate what is going on while it is going on. The psychologists call this metacognition. Learners can become more efficient and more effective learners if they understand what approaches in general help human beings learn. Knowing something about study skills and then finding out what approaches work best for them as an individual makes them better and less stressed students. Similarly, it is helpful in consultations for health care professionals to be able to recognise what thoughts or feelings may lay behind their own and their patients' responses as the conversation proceeds. Knowing oneself better helps in understanding others. And therefore, in the search for expertise it helps learners to have spelt out what the route to expertise is, what the stages are and what it is likely to feel like as the hard work to independent practice as a health care professional looks like. If that map is not laid out and used to empathetically emphasise key aspects required for progression, then it is more likely that frustration at the apparent lack of purpose and direction in day-to-day work will be accompanied by suboptimal progress.

Thanks to cassette recorders and video recordings we now have a good understanding of better consultation skills. But until recently there has been limited research into how health care expertise is acquired and even less covering how the route to expertise can be made easier or accelerated. What evidence we have reveals that expertise is developed through long years of effort and experience. Yet, effort and experience do not alone lead one to become an expert. What do we know about how expertise is developed?

Experts possess characteristics and qualities that set them apart from the rest. Roger Kneebone is a former surgeon, GP and now Professor of Surgical Education and Engagement Science. He wrote in his magnificent 2021 book[cclxii] "Expert: Understanding the Path to Mastery":

"The most skilful GPs I ever met seemed able to put their finger on a patient's problem with no apparent effort. They weren't displaying medical knowledge, they were just listening – and maybe doing a little talking. They didn't drive things or insist on asking questions in a specified order. They didn't show off. They seemed to be able to crystallize any problem without effort.

"But ask them afterwards what was going on and their language would switch in a flash. They would describe how they had been considering this diagnosis or that, and weighing up the chances that it might be something serious. They'd talk about recent papers they had read, or how they were thinking about referring the patient to one specialist or another.

"They would have made contingency plans and put safety nets in place in case they had got things wrong. Yet none of this was obvious. For their

patients, the consultation was just something natural: a conversation that helped."

Observing an expert, however, does not get us very far in understanding how that expertise was acquired. We are back watching the best tennis players in the world at Wimbledon and then expecting to be able to translate their expertise onto our own home-grown efforts. The end point after improving is different from, say, tennis too – in health care we are interested in the largest possible number of competent practitioners and none who are incompetent. Extrapolating principles for improving the development of performance of health care professionals from studies of the development of elite, world class performance in tennis, chess or piano playing may not provide the whole story. But it is the philosophy and cognitive psychology literature that first gives some insights.

The 3rd and 4th centuries BCE were the golden years for Greek philosophy. Plato followed Socrates in thinking of wisdom as being anything that could be spelled out as explicit principles and definitions. This thinking has flowed through Western philosophy and natural sciences to the present day. At the end of the 20th Century "In God we trust, all others must bring evidence" was a mantra in the evidence-based medicine movement.

After all, when there are important life or death decisions to be made it would be better not to base those on hunches or doing what other people thought was the right thing to do, but on principles that can be laid out and justified to one's peers. Aristotle was Plato's famous student and agreed with that general approach but thought that there was more to it. His conclusion was that in addition to the *techne* (knowledge) there was a need for *phronesis* (wisdom), and the *phronesis* involved a judgement that allowed experienced practitioners to apply their principles to particular cases.

Aristotle's view was if you had a serious problem, you were better asking a wise old person what to do rather than looking to a philosopher and their principles and rules. I get as frustrated as anyone by the slow progress in moving from population-based medicine with its guidelines, rules, and pay-for-performance to individualised, person-centred, shared decision-making health care. But perspective helps. Human beings prefer certainty to uncertainty, so have a natural preference for rules-based decision making, even if they might, at least sometimes, realise that a rules-based approach is not optimal. The arc of history is indeed long; human beings have been grappling with this for more than two millennia, so it may take a little longer than we might hope to get to shared decision making being the norm everywhere.

The debate flowed backwards and forwards. Galileo and Descartes were in the rules and definitions camp. Pascal, despite being a great mathematician, believed in trusting emotions and intuitions when it came to decision making. Liebnitz, another mathematician, believed in the rational, writing down of best practice. David Hulme, a contemporary of Liebnitz in the 18th Century, held that knowledge was not grounded in theories and principles, but was based on habits formed by successful coping - heralding repetition and system 1 decision making by almost three centuries.

In the 20th Century several influential philosophers rejected both sides of the traditional debate. Martin Heidigger and Maurice Merleau-Ponty simply tried to describe everyday experience. They concluded that human perception could not be explained by a set of rules. Human understanding is akin to a skill. Applying knowledge is what counts - knowing how to find one's way around in the world, rather than just knowing a lot of facts but not knowing how to apply them for good for oneself and for others. Many people know how to ride a bicycle. A book about riding a bicycle does not help others much to learn how to ride bicycles. Experiential learning is required – even if it is sometimes painful. But that lifelong experiential learning means most people know how to flexibly adapt a conversation depending on the circumstances - talk will flow differently with friends in the pub on a Friday night than it will in the office having your annual appraisal with your boss. This level of expertise is only acquired after years of having many different types of conversations, and undoubtedly reflecting most on the conversations that did not go well.

Practice is required even for maintaining know-how. I recently undertook a self-assessment test on writing prescriptions for controlled drugs - medicines such as morphine which are subject to special rules. I used to write such prescriptions many times a week and could do so without much cognitive effort. Now I do not write such prescriptions at all and have not done so for some time; unsurprisingly my test result reflected my lack of practice.

Some of the GP registrars I help with their examination preparation have worked in other specialties for some years before entering GP training. The examination they are preparing for tests, in part, their knowledge of rare but important conditions - diseases which they will perhaps have last studied in detail in their final year at medical school. For some doctors who have worked for a time in other specialities before beginning the switch to general practice, their final year at medical school may be a decade or more ago. This means that, for example, it can be difficult to remember in a pressurised and unfamiliar examination situation when you have less than one minute per question what happens to the biochemistry of the body in hyperparathyroidism, especially when you have not even thought about it in the last 10 years. A little practice - refreshing those older memories with some brief and recent reading - can transform performance in a career-critical examination.

The 20th Century philosophers approach laid the groundwork for cognitive psychology. For example, Merleau-Ponty described what became analogical reasoning – human beings can read across from one problem that they successfully solved and use the same approach applied flexibly to a similar but not identical problem in the future. This is a feature of experts' decision making, based on long experience and many cases.

We are not born with the skill to drive a car, ride a bicycle or be a health care professional. We must learn. Some simple tasks we can learn from trial and error, others from imitating those already proficient. More complex tasks involve written or verbal instruction, often in the role of formal education. What observational research shows is that learners do not suddenly jump from having factual knowledge (knowing what) to experience-based, individually-tuned, applied knowledge (knowing how). "Knowing what" is back or white. "Knowing how" is multiple shades of grey.

If the expectations of what a GP registrar's good performance looks like in undergraduate and postgraduate education is shaped by prior experience in which regurgitating facts based on what the textbook says or what the professor does and that gets them good marks, all they have achieved is "knowing what". UK medical practice is about "knowing how", and it takes time to appreciate the difference, learn even more new skills - perhaps when far from home and family, shift their approach to consultations, and incorporate high level consultation skills and shared decision making. It is often not easy to acquire such expertise..

That progression occurs in stages. Just as with consultation skills models, there are a number of different constructs that describe these stages, but they all have a great deal in common. At their core are five principles:

(i)   practice leads to faster and

(ii) more efficient uses of knowledge, which enables faster performance and

(iii) results in less demand on mental resources. As a result, the performance of what have become low-level tasks becomes second nature, and

(iv) this frees up mental resources that can be utilized to attempt higher level behaviours. Ultimately

(v)   skilled performance reflects the development of many component processes.[cclxiii]

The dominant model was developed over many years by two brothers, Herbert and Stuart Dreyfus.[cclxiv] Hubert came from a philosophy background and Stuart was a mathematician and early computer programmer. They both ended up working at the RAND corporation on computers and the early days of artificial intelligence. They were for a time in the same research group as Herbert Simon, though their ideas did not always coincide, and relationships were at times strained. However, like Simon, it is fortunate for us that their work on determining how computers could store and use information to make decisions led them into studying how humans made decisions. Their model for the development of expertise has five stages – novice, advanced beginner, competent, proficient, and expert.

1. Novice.

Novice learners need to acquire information as a first step, and so spend a lot of time learning and remembering basic science. The is absolutely - the science is a necessary component even in the context of a modern curriculum based on problem-based learning. Discretionary judgement is not yet developed, novices need to "follow the rules", and learning is context dependent.

Their learning is helped by working with basic and straightforward cases, the provision of structure and direction including concept maps, emphasising the basic science knowledge that underpins the clinical situation, emphasizing the features that discriminate in situations, and helping learners prioritise the importance of some information over other information. Small changes in instruction and study habits can yield significant benefits in terms of retention and recall of information and higher order thinking.[cclxv]

At this stage the novices judge their performance largely by how well they follow the learned "rules". However, after learning many facts and rules, cognitive overload means significant concentration is required to remember those basic principles consciously, and unless rules become more automated further development is impaired. It is important to recognise that individuals may be novices for some topics and much more advanced practitioners for others.

Novices can also be helped by gaining an appreciation of more effective and more efficient learning strategies. Spaced learning, interleaving, learn – test – relearn – retest cycles, learning in the context of daily experience with patients, using flash cards, mind maps or visual representations as well as plain text, and using materials which are at a complexity which challenge just sufficiently to encourage rather than discourage learners – all these help.[cclxvi] It may seem crazy to suggest that undergraduates and health care professionals, who by definition are good at learning and passing examinations, can benefit from additional understanding of how to optimise learning, but believe me – it can be very helpful to explore the topic with them, because many of them actually have little or no theoretical understanding about how they have become so good at acquiring knowledge.

And because some people are not using some of the optimal learning techniques which suit them as an individual, they are might – perhaps for the first time ever - begin to struggle with assessments. Previously their examinations have largely tested knowledge, and their whole time was spent studying; studying and passing examinations was their job. They now must undertake further study in addition to working long hours in very demanding jobs, and their examinations now test the application of knowledge rather than largely remembering facts. It is often helpful to introduce the concepts of bounded rationality and dual process theory so that postgraduate students are reminded why repetition is required for both technical knowledge and consultation skills to become largely automated. System 1 means they can gradually adapt to and survive large cognitive loads, and eventually function efficiently and effectively in their field of work.

2.   Advanced Beginner.

Seeing similar situations on several occasions means the advanced beginner begins to recognise familiar aspects of common, if straightforward, situations. Basic science knowledge is broader and less fragmented. Nodes of knowledge become compiled and as a result some essential information is retrieved automatically and therefore with less effort. However, learners still need assistance making meaningful connections between familiar and less familiar nodes of information. There are still difficulties in differentiating important from less important features, but advanced beginners can start to produce partial solutions to unfamiliar or complex situations. "Rules" can now involve recognising the presence or absence of key features; experience is becoming more valuable than written or verbal descriptions. They should not be over-confident about decision making and will still often seek rules-based goals when reflecting on their approach.

The learning of advanced beginners can be helped by explicitly making connections between cases and other course work, and by reviewing and reflecting on more subtle technical points and communication approaches with some specific and targeted feedback. Peer-peer and near-peer coaching can be helpful and reduce learner anxiety about their pace of progress. A focus on "why" decisions are made and "talk aloud" sessions by experts about what they as experts were thinking as a debrief after consultations can be useful strategies. However, they should be actively discouraged from attempting to blindly emulate the approaches of experts who still have very different approaches from advanced beginners.

3.   Conscious Competency

By the early postgraduate years the learner has developed "illness scripts". Learners have assimilated lists of features that characterise the disease including temporal features. Based on repeated experience with patients, system 2 thinking begins to be replaced with system 1, and the illness scripts generated are sufficient to diagnose, or at least consistently generate reasonable differential diagnoses, and create sensible management options.

Learners work with increased autonomy and remaining gaps are attenuated by ongoing preceptor oversight. At this point, the learner is on the way to mastering the science and technical aspects of their work. Though still requiring conscious effort, if they are exposed to the importance of consultation skills acquisition and have the opportunity to practice different ways of consulting, for straightforward problems they begin to develop approaches to consultations that are more patient-centred with decisions based on a shared approach. The learner starts to develop a their own "voice" and sees their role in relation to the patients' clinical outcomes including individual preferences rather than merely "being safe" or "doing the right thing".

Coaching, encouragement of reflection, exploration of thought processes and emotions during the consultation are now helpful approaches to further development. "Asking" the learner rather than "telling" is a key difference. Preceptors must strike a difficult balance between supervision and encouraging autonomy.

4.   Proficiency

The health care professional now has an increased sense of responsibility and confidence. The earlier stages of rule following, and effortful and conscious choices are usually set aside, save for very complex or unusual situations. They quickly see what is relevant and less relevant and recognise when there are appropriate deviations from normal rules and patterns. They are more comfortable with unusual presentations of common conditions, because they have wider experience. Decision making is less effortful, rather it just seems to happen. They solve new problems in the context of prior experience using analogical reasoning. Decision making is quicker, more automatic, and more intuitive. Patient-centred consultations with shared decision making should be the norm. Further development is dependent on identifying and using teachable moments, self-reflection, teaching others, and peer support.

5. Expert

The usual mode when problem solving is System 1, with System 2 used occasionally in novel situations or when problems occur. The health care professional no longer consciously recalls rules, guidelines or principles, and has the cognitive capacity and skills to routinely individualise care. Decision making has become part of usual life and most of the time technical aspects take no more conscious cognitive effort than routine walking or driving. In terms of their approach to consultations, they are involved rather than a technical participant. They do what usually works - not in terms of rule following - but in terms of their approaches to a consultation. Calibration - a conscious reflection on what system 1 has determined - is also automatic. "Is there a need to reconsider the first impression that comes to mind?" "Is there something here that is leading me astray?".

The expert is largely self-directed with continual, specialty-specific development. They will have a focus on teaching others or discovery of new knowledge. They share experiences with others, seek a deeper understanding of their work, and learn from being challenged by others.

The downside to increasing expertise is that being an expert in a domain does not necessarily mean they are inherently proficient in teaching those less expert. The decision making that experts have developed can make identifying the exact process that they go through difficult to articulate since the thinking process itself has become intuitive. Experts can hurt learners because experts may forget what is easy and what was difficult to learn. Expert teachers not only have their domain specific expertise, but have also dedicated time and energy to acquiring knowledge about teaching in order to become not just an expert but an expert teacher.

These stages of development are dependent on progressively more complex problems to solve. These need to be aligned with the learner's stage of development, and of course individual learners progress at different rates, and may be in one stage of development for some problems and at another stage of development for other problems. Learners also have individualised approaches to their own development, and that can make a difference to the pace of development. In 1993 Anders Ericsson and colleagues described "deliberate practice".[cclxvii] This term has been widely taken up by others interested in the development of expertise, but unfortunately it has frequently been misrepresented.

Ericsson et al found that many characteristics once believed to reflect innate talent are the result of intense practice extended for a minimum of ten years. This has been distorted into the notion that expertise development requires 10,000 hours practice. There is no question that in health care and many other fields the process takes many years. This can be dispiriting for learners unless they are given information not only about the process they are undertaking and its length, but also about the approaches they themselves should take to accelerate their development.

Imagine two basketball players who are both seeking to improve their scoring – getting the ball through the hoop. Player A takes 200 shots in a practice session and takes the trouble to personally analyse errors as they occur. In addition, s/he has a colleague or coach make a note of success and failures and the apparent reasons for unsuccessful shots – do the misses go left, right, long or short, for example. After the practice session s/he reviews the notes and determines the skill elements requiring particular attention in the next session. Player B takes 100 shots in the session, spends time dribbling the ball aimlessly, does not systematically analyse the reasons for errors and does not have anyone to record them. Which player do you think is more likely to improve quickest? Pretty obviously, it's Player A.

In deliberate practice it is more than the number of hours of practice. More important is the quality of practice that supports the development of expertise. In my work with GP registrars, they are able to perform in some areas at stage 3 (competent) and in others at stage 2 (advanced beginner) depending on their prior experience. Until recently their development was in protected time, at high school or university. Now they are workers and must blend their development into their supervised service role. This may require some adaptation of their usual approaches to learning.

Those learners who progress more rapidly and with apparent ease are those who carry a notebook routinely. As their day at work proceeds, they use the notebook to record knowledge gaps or skills which they need to still develop. They diverge away from just about managing to handle today's problem with this patient safely and most of the time; rather, they look for wider aspects of caring for people with that condition or seek to increase their skills in preparation for consultations like the one they have just had. They do not necessarily spend a lot of time working through every point in the long lists in their notebook of every potential learning point, but steal a few minutes during their busy day to quickly look things up and makes some notes. If the same topic crops up several times in a short period or they receive some impactful feedback, or experience a stimulating teaching session, they prioritise that learning. They routinely make notes, flash cards or mind maps based on what they have looked up – preparing revision and self-test materials. Their learning may be compressed into ten minutes here and there, but they cover at least a few points every day.

They also regularly spend a little of their own time after work looking up information and making notes about that day's consultations, but they do not need to extend the working day onerously by cramming for several hours. Rather, they mostly progress by squeezing every moment of time out of a working day. This means they still have time for family, friends and fun. That is not to say that this approach to the development of expertise comes easily. Maintaining deliberate conscious effort helps to refine the cognitive skills required to exceed a current level of performance. This conscious effort will at times cause discomfort and requires consistent work on the part of the learner, especially if this has not been their natural approach to learning up in the past.

When it comes to summative examinations it appears to their peers that these consistent learners usually achieve a pass with ease. They themselves may not consciously realise that their natural learning approaches give them an advantage over those who have different strategies. For examination preparation all they need to do is check their learning by testing themselves against a commercial question bank, find that they are on largely track, take the examination and pass. They then tell colleagues who have not been continuously, conscientiously learning in the context of the patients that they passed the examination "just by doing a few practice questions". Unsurprisingly, that approach does not work well for learners who have been just about getting by in consultations but have not been advancing their knowledge and developing their expertise by looking things up and preparing for future consultations as they go along. Player A almost always outperforms Player B.

In the last ten years there has been interest in accelerating progress through the initial stages of expertise development by teaching undergraduate healthcare students clinical reasoning. This seems to have been stronger in medical student teaching than in those of other health care professions because the focus has largely been on improving the rates of diagnostic error. Most diagnostic errors are not due lack of knowledge. It is cognitive failures, such as failure to recognise cues, or synthesise all the available information correctly, or failure to use the physical examination findings or test results appropriately, that to contribute to most diagnostic errors.[cclxviii]

The research mirrors my own experience - undergraduate and postgraduate trainees largely learn the knowledge, skills and behaviours required for effective clinical reasoning implicitly, through experience and apprenticeship.[cclxix] Accurate interpretation of diagnostic test results is universally poor,[cclxx] and shared decision making is not routinely used in the US as well as in the UK.[cclxxi]

In the UK in 2020 members of the Clinical Reasoning in Medical Education group (CReME) met to discuss what clinical reasoning-specific teaching should be delivered by medical schools (what to teach).[cclxxii] I should declare that two of this group are former colleagues of mine at Keele University, and we first met to explore decision making in 2008 when I was working at the National Prescribing Centre. Also a few years ago I gave a plenary session at the CReME annual conference.

A literature review was conducted to identify what teaching strategies are successful in improving clinical reasoning ability among medical students (how to teach).

In their literature search they found only 27 relevant publications that described a teaching intervention designed to improve the clinical reasoning ability of medical students.
Research in this area is far from mature.

Consensus identified five domains:-

1.   Clinical reasoning concepts.
•   Clinical reasoning theories; e.g. illness scripts, dual process.
•   How clinical reasoning ability develops.
•   The role of clinical reasoning in safe and effective care for patients.
•   Cognitive errors.
•   Other factors that may impair the clinical reasoning process/outcome.

2.   History and physical examination
•   Effective communication skills and purposeful interviewing.
•   History taking from all available sources when relevant

- Hypothesis-driven enquiry.
- Knowledge of epidemiology, probability of the presence of signs and symptoms in specific diseases, and likelihood ratios to estimate clinical probability.

3. Choosing and interpreting diagnostic tests
- Pre-test (clinical) probability and post-test probability.
- Sensitivity and specificity.
- Predictive values.
- Factors other than disease that influence test results
- Important characteristics of commonly used tests relevant to local context.
- Evidence-based guidelines.

4. Problem identification and management.
- An accurate problem representation or problem list.
- Use of semantic qualifiers and precise medical terms.
- Prioritised differential diagnosis, including relevant "must not miss" diagnoses.
- Safe actions when a diagnosis is not possible.
- Management plans taking patient's preferences, co-morbidities, resources, cost-effectiveness and local policies in to account.
- Metacognition and critical thinking in decision making.

5. Shared decision making
The ability to make decisions with:
- Patients and carers
- Clinical teams
- Guidelines, scores and decision aids
- Evidence-based medicine applied to the patient's circumstances
- Professional values and behaviours that support decision making

That curriculum has been covered in its entirety by this book, which should be reassuring. Implementing a clinical reasoning-based approach in an undergraduate medical curriculum will be a significant undertaking and, as the authors of the consensus statement acknowledge, will require a significant programme of faculty development. Stand-alone modules teaching clinical reasoning are unlikely to be successful.

However, even if this curriculum were to be successfully implemented at the undergraduate level, there is bound to be a need for input during postgraduate training simply because of the strong evidence that the development of expertise is far from complete upon successfully completing an undergraduate course. Consultation skills, taught at the undergraduate level but then given little attention thereafter, do not result in uniformly good consultation skills. The danger is that undergraduate teaching in clinical reasoning is also seen as a complete solution.

That can never be, not least because the NHS is grateful for many international graduates coming to the UK to work and pursue their postgraduate studies. In many countries around the world, one or more of evidence-based medicine, consultation skills, and clinical reasoning are absent from undergraduate teaching. It seems inevitable that all three need to be established as a key part of undergraduate and postgraduate training for all health and care professionals across all specialties if we are serious about rebalancing medicine. That is a mammoth task.

CHAPTER TWENTY THREE

Crisis

"Predictions are difficult, especially about the future". This quote has been attributed to many people, from the Nobel prize-winning physicist Niels Bohr to legendary baseball player Yogi Berra. Whoever really got there first, it rings true, especially when it comes to medicine. Who knows what the impact of artificial intelligence will be, or whether the Galleri blood test will successfully transform screening for cancers, or whether we will get successful mRNA or DNA or adenovirus-based vaccines on the back of COVID vaccine research to massively impact cancer, heart disease and stroke, or whether one of many other science or technology developments in the coming years will be the next big stride forward, for health care - or not? If I knew I would invest all our savings in the big development of the future that saves us all, and I'll see you on the beach, drinking a cocktail.

The best we can do is to make as honest an assessment of where we are now in terms of health care, take the lessons of history fully into account, assess where there might be benefits in rebalancing some the current activity, and work towards that rebalancing. And even then, as Billy Connolly exhorted us in one of his famous monologues, we must "Stay awake, because it's all going to change"!

The next few chapters contains some suggestions as to how we can get medicine back into a better balance. These are not recommendations or "to do's". Collectively they might be a "Manifesto" - suggestions based on my reading of the past and the present which we have discussed in this book, and in the hope of a better future. But that is only a hope. Most definitely they should not be perceived as definitively "telling people what to do". It is not clear what the effects of making some of these changes might be. Health systems are complex, and it is highly likely that unintended, unhelpful consequences will arise from actions that are rooted in evidence and good sense, and attempts to do good.

But we need to do something. Health care systems around the world are struggling. Standing still and hoping things will improve is not an acceptable response. Thinking that simple, neat

371

20th century approaches are appropriate for complex 21st century health care problems is common but plainly wrong. In the UK many believe there is an existential threat to one of the great creations of civilisation – the National Health Service. Urgent action is required to stabilise health systems, and then changes are required. But structural changes to the health system – we have had plenty of those in the NHS and they have not delivered – and may even have been counter-productive.

We have also had 40 years of quasi-market structures introduced into other UK public services and that approach has not worked either. Most people would struggle to mention any UK privately owned, public service currently functioning well. Instead of focusing on structures, we need a radical review of how the health system functions, how people interact with the system, how the system works for them, what are the outcomes we should be measuring, and how we can afford a system that best meets the needs of the population and of individuals.

If we begin with William Kissick's iron triangle of health care which I mentioned earlier in this book, it describes how the three competing priorities of health care delivery - cost, quality, and access - are interdependent and form a zero-sum game.[cclxxiii] If costs are squeezed by fiscal austerity then either access to health care is more difficult for patients, or quality of care deteriorates, or both happen.

Where do we stand? There is so much disinformation and misunderstanding about what actually has happened to funding for the NHS that it is necessary to spell out in some detail what has actually happened in recent years. Using UK government data, the Health Foundation has calculated that growth in health care funding has been lower than the historic rate since 2008, artificially boosted since 2019 by the requirements of the coronavirus pandemic.[cclxxiv] If the iron triangle holds true then with lower increases in funding there should have been a reduction in public satisfaction with the NHS and an increase in NHS waiting lists, if we accept those indices as proxies for access and quality. That is indeed the case. The King's Fund has reported on the British Societal Survey of 2021 which showed high satisfaction with the NHS in the years when the NHS was funded to the point where it matched European levels of health funding, followed by a precipitous decline in satisfaction in the second decade of the century.[cclxxv]

Waiting lists were reported on at the end of 2022 by the Institute for Fiscal Studies.[cclxxvi] Comparable records began in 2007 and the improving position for many years was associated with a decade of increased funding. This was followed by a substantial rise in people waiting for treatment as austerity hit the NHS after the 2008 banking crisis; the twin effects of inadequate funding and the coronavirus pandemic have undoubtedly hit health care capacity.

Then, and this has happened quietly and with relatively few fanfares, the character of health care has changed. As previously described, the first half of the 20th century was broadly defined by advances in managing infections - thanks to improvements in general health with clean water and a better diet, and of course the wonderful twin discoveries of vaccination and antibiotics. The second half of the 20th century has been dominated by better options for the management of many common conditions – diabetes, heart disease, respiratory diseases, and some cancers – thanks in large part to the massive expansion of pharmaceuticals as an industrialised process mostly after the second world war, driven by science but also motivated by the prospect of large profits for successful companies.

But whilst science and technology and the commercial world concentrates on the next "breakthrough" test or treatment, healthcare in the first half of the 21st Century is now dominated by multimorbidity. Few players associated with the provision of care have fully adapted to that last change. The increase in the number of people in the population with a lot of birthdays is a triumph, and not a problem. I am personally delighted to have lived longer than most of my father's generation and will continue to attempt to do so for as long as possible. However, the proportion of the population over the age of 65 years was in 2016 three times that when the NHS was created. And health care spending is concentrated in the older age groups.[cclxxvii]

We are too often still treating older people with multiple conditions in the same way we treat younger people with single conditions. Someone in their seventies might be attending the diabetic clinic for their diabetes. Then there is another, separate trip to the hospital to the eye clinic for a glaucoma check. Followed a few weeks later to see the dermatologists about psoriasis. Then to another service for a retinal photograph to check whether the diabetes has damaged the back of the eye. And then the oncology department requires yet another trip for a follow up to a breast cancer a few years previously. And so on. Single disease-orientated health systems place inordinate demands on patients, their relatives and their friends just to get to appointments, to say nothing of the stress associated with sitting in multiple waiting rooms expecting what may be bad news on every trip to the hospital.

Without adaptations to care delivery systems or accounting for scientific and technology advances, a single disease-orientated health system looking after an aging population places increased demands on health spending of 1.3% per year and 3.7% on social care spending per year. An important measure is the proportion of life expectancy spent in good or ill health. *Compression of morbidity* occurs when individuals who are expected to live longer, spend the same amount of time (or less) in ill health. This could be driven by better preventative population health leading to lower incidence or later development of chronic conditions – diet, exercise, a reduction in poverty and income inequities ,and so on.

This would be a good thing, though with current approaches apparently elusive. But *expansion of morbidity* occurs when rising life expectancy is not matched by improvements in morbidity resulting in more time spent in ill health. This might be represented by a failure to address the social determinants of health, a focus on technology being used for prevention to detect disease early when such detection offers limited benefits on quality or length of life, and a single-disease focused health system

374

when people have multiple conditions. Currently we seem to be in the latter situation and not the former in many countries, and this is not being significantly adapted to and managed well by the health systems.

However, health spending patterns and demand are not explained purely by changing patterns of population growth, ageing, mortality and morbidity. Patterns of demand are influenced by public expectations, reflecting preferences for improvements in health care compared to other possible uses of public and private spending. As societies get richer, research suggests they prioritise part of that growing income and wealth for health care. This is known as the *income elasticity of demand*. Whether this growth will continue indefinitely is unclear, but all research so far shows that income elasticity continues to grow health care spending over time.[cclxxviii]

These fundamental drivers of health spending are the same in many countries. Most countries like the UK saw their health spending grow by more than inflation and economic growth in the 20th century, and that has continued into this century. One projection has spending on health and long-term care growing on average among the Organisation for Economic Co-operation and Development (OECD) countries (a collection of 36 countries) by between 3.3 and 7.7 percentage points of gross domestic product (GDP) between 2010 and 2060, depending on the extent to which countries are able to contain costs.[cclxxix]

Scientific and technological advances continue. In 2021 in the UK 35 new medicines were approved for use. This is a pretty typical year, so over a decade there are around 350 new medicines to be learned about by health care professionals, managed by patients into their daily routines, and paid for by the health system. More of the population using those medicines are older, and they live longer with long term conditions, and thanks to scientific advances health care professionals can do more to, in theory, better manage their conditions. But it all costs. And because of the design of health systems largely focuses on single-diseases, and the drive is for scientifically correct, evidence-based care as represented in clinical guidelines, many people end up with a cocktail of treatments comprising a large number of medicines, sometimes with no single person co-ordinating care. This is poor medicine, and expensive, and wasteful, and without great coordination risks patients becoming sick because of the side effects of the medicines and especially the interactions between them.

Since 2009, pandemic aside, the NHS has worked hard at increasing its delivery with a pre-pandemic NHS productivity growth of 1.7% per annum. However, spending growth since 2010 has not kept pace with demand and cost pressures. The Health Foundation and Institute for Fiscal Studies (IFS) estimated in 2018 that, in the next 15 years, real terms funding will need to grow by 3.3% just in order to maintain current levels of care given the increasing and ageing population, rising prevalence of multimorbidity and modest real wage growth and productivity.[cclxxx] That is 3.3% more than inflation. Since that report there has been no planned increase in health and social care expenditure of a magnitude that would ensure improvements in care.

We face a crisis. There are simply not enough doctors and other health care professionals to safely treat the volume of patients, and this will only worsen as demand rises and more people leave the NHS. Just to stand still, more health and social care funding is needed. If we want better care, we need more than 4% growth per annum. And if we do want that, in the UK system tax returns to the government must increase or there has to be a radical rethink of how care decision are made with individuals, or both. That can only come from a faster growing economy as a whole, or from higher taxation, and most importantly from a really serious look at how we truly begin to address shared decision making with individual patients.

Despite 40 years of introducing quasi-markets into health care in the UK no one could claim that policy, which remains current, has worked. Services have improved, but only when reasonably funded. But with ever more funding needed, reform is needed to.

Not in yet more structural reforms, which have delivered nothing tangible, But radical reform at the level in which care is provided for individual patients is required – not least because it is the sort of care that people want and deserve. It is inevitable that more money is required right now - but annual, big, incremental tax increases meaning health and social care consumes an ever increasing proportion of Gross Domestic Product is not a credible approach. Tax increases are popular with few people, and it follows that if we want to mitigate the rate of increase in taxation to create the necessary budget for healthcare we need imaginative, 21st century approaches to health care alongside a more realistic growth in the budget.

As if the complexity of these system-level issues were not enough, there are two pressing short-term problems affecting the delivery of health care. Firstly, there is no question that a significant proportion of NHS and social care staff are tired and feel undervalued. As the 2022 survey of staff by NHS Employers found, the proportion of staff that would recommend their organisation as a place to work was 57%. The percentage of staff that would be happy with the standard of care provided by their organisation fell to 63%. As NHS Employers themselves wrote in commentary, *"These scores reflect pressure on staff and concerns over quality of care. It will take overall improvements in NHS staff experience and resourcing to make significant shift to these scores."*

It does not help that the NHS has many unfulfilled staff vacancies. In September 2022 the total number of vacancies in was 133,446, a vacancy rate of 9.7%. This represented an increase from the previous year, when the number of vacancies was 103,809 and the vacancy rate 7.9%.[cclxxxi] There is currently no effective workforce plan for the NHS, and there is little visible evidence of concerted efforts to try and retain existing staff at any stage of their career. And incredibly, in 2022 the number of medical students was reduced from 10,000 per year to 7,500.[cclxxxii]

And then fiscal austerity has hit the pay of many public sector workers, as the Financial Times reported in January 2023.[cclxxxiii] Many groups of health care workers feel under-valued and under-rewarded, but I will mostly consider doctors here because they are the group I know best. Doctors have been particularly disadvantaged in monetary terms, seeing their average pay fall by around 25% in real terms between 2011 and 2020, with doctors who recently graduated seeing an effective pay gap of 35%. People in operating theatres assisting surgeons to perform major operations are being paid £14 an hour, when they have succeeded in an intensively competitive academic course and emerged with around £100,000 in student debt. These are the same people who put their lives on the line in the pandemic, worked outside their own specialties to offer care to the large numbers of COVID patients overwhelming their hospitals, and coped uncomplainingly about the disruption to their postgraduate training programmes. Towards the end of that training doctors personally take on considerable clinical responsibilities, the teaching of medical students, and teaching and supervising other doctors. And yet they are earning around £29 an hour.

It is not just the money. The body responsible for managing postgraduate medical training was until April 2023 Health Education England. In April 2023 they merged with NHS England and are trying their best to manage a 30% reduction in their budget, one that had already been drastically reduced over the last 12 years of austerity. It is not easy working for that organisation, and I know of many good people who do heroically good work supporting their colleagues through postgraduate training under very difficult circumstances.

In March 2023, to "celebrate" the end of the organisation, readers on Twitter were asked by Health Education England to post their experiences of postgraduate training. If anyone wants to understand a little more about how the current dire state of morale amongst these doctors arose they could do a lot worse than read the savage responses to this tweet using the hashtag #HEE10. A few highlights: "Job interviews scheduled less than 72 hours ahead, giving many applicants no opportunity to attend because they were scheduled for patient care". "The doctor who nearly died in a car crash after being told to attend a mandatory training day after finishing a 12 hour night shift." "The doctors who give up training because they cannot manage to move jobs and especially locations every 6 or 12 months for eight to ten years of postgraduate training." "The doctors who could not arrange to be off duty on the day of their weddings, despite giving many months' notice". And so on. As Charles Massey, Chief Executive of the General Medical Council said in November 2022, *"Doctors are not leaving UK practice because they have fallen out of love with medicine. Instead, it is because they can't tolerate the environments in which it is practised. The problem is not their work, it is their workplace."*cclxxxiv

In 2023, the year in which the 75th anniversary of the NHS should have been celebrated, the response of the General Medical Council, the regulatory body of the medical profession issued updated guidance on professional standards. This was the latest edition of "Good Medical Practice"cclxxxv which sets out how doctors should behave in all aspects of their work and life. Most of the changes related to the environment and culture of the workplace. It said:-

"You must help to create a culture that is respectful, fair, supportive, and compassionate by role modelling behaviours consistent with these values.

"You should be aware of how your behaviour may influence others within and outside the team.

"You must not abuse, discriminate against, bully, or harass anyone based on their personal characteristics, or for any other reason. By 'personal characteristics' we mean someone's appearance, lifestyle, culture, their social or economic status, or any of the characteristics protected by legislation – age, disability, gender reassignment, race, marriage and civil partnership, pregnancy and maternity, religion or belief, sex and sexual orientation.

"You must not act in a sexual way towards colleagues with the effect or purpose of causing offence, embarrassment, humiliation or distress. What we mean by acting 'in a sexual way' can include – but isn't limited to – verbal or written comments, displaying or sharing images, as well as unwelcome physical contact."

In every year of my long career as a doctor, it seems like someone would be claiming the NHS "was in crisis". There have been many times when providing good quality, timely care has been very difficult. Somehow the NHS survived - with its core values of universal access free at the point of need, general practice as the foundation of patient care, and NHS staff working for a common good being identified for the NHS's 70th anniversary as the NHS's three biggest successes. But only five years later, waiting lists are at an all-time high, it seems like it has never been more difficult to see an actual GP, people routinely wait many hours in A & E departments, nurses, junior doctors and consultants have been on strike over pay, and staff, patients and the public seem to have lost hope, confidence and trust.

And when the General Medical Council has to tell doctors that they have a professional responsibility to be civil to each other, to their colleagues and to their patients, nobody can deny there isn't a crisis.

CHAPTER TWENTY FOUR

Structure

To give some order to what would otherwise appear to be a disparate set of ideas and suggestions to rebalance medicine, I will turn again to Avedis Donabedian, who first wrote about his model for healthcare systems in 1966. He stated that it helps to consider healthcare systems in three domains – structure, process, and outcomes. Structure describes the context in which care is delivered and includes buildings, staff, financing and equipment. Process includes the transactions between patients and providers. Outcomes are the effects of healthcare on the health status of patients and populations. I will add one more item to the traditional list of Donabedian outcomes, the health of the people providing the care. It seems clear that especially after the coronavirus pandemic, we should actively consider the pastoral care of the people working in the NHS - for there are many problems there.

The crisis is health care centres on a lack of people to deliver care, the increased complexity of care due to multimorbidity, the relative underfunding since 2009, the fragmentation of care with the resultant loss of continuity of care, and several infrastructure issues including many aging and inadequate buildings and fragmented and poorly functioning IT systems. I wish that was not the case, but it is. And I am afraid that the unpalatable truth is that almost everywhere one looks in health systems in the UK or around the world, care for acute, serious, dramatic problems sometimes functions well, but routine care of ongoing, chronic, multiple conditions is often suboptimal.

What we can quickly and emphatically dismiss is the question of whether it is still the best approach to fund a health system out of general taxation. In short, yes it is. Multiple studies have examined this question and every one comes to the same conclusion. Insurance based schemes operate across most of Western Europe and whilst they too provide universal coverage, their management costs are higher. Most people who advocate a shift to an insurance based scheme are not 90 years old and struggling to manage everyday living, never mind negotiating insurance coverage and bargaining over premium costs. Some people who advocate an insurance scheme might stand to gain a lot personally if the NHS was sold off. The evidence is that the NHS works as well or better than any other health system when it is properly resourced.

But currently it has big problems. Crucially for the NHS, in the UK the number of fully qualified general practitioners is falling. The 2015 target of increasing the number of GPs by 5,000 by 2020 was missed. The 2019 target of increasing the number of GPs by 6,000 by March 2024 has also been missed.[cclxxxvi] The population has grown, the proportion of the population who are older and who have multimorbidity has grown, because of science and technology there are new things that can potentially help patients and they cost more and take time to introduce and monitor. And yet in January 2023 there were 2,087 fewer fully qualified, full time GPs than in 2015. This is a contrast with the growth in the number of hospital consultants – more than 150% increase in the last 25 years for consultants compared with 0% for general practitioners is a startling difference[cclxxxvii].

Since 1948 the number of GPs has doubled. But there are TWELVE times as many specialists as there were when the NHS was created. This is because over the last seventy years of the NHS the focus has been on science, technology and specialist care. That has brought us some spectacular successes. Who could not be impressed by the wonders of modern cataract surgery, or hip replacement, or transplant surgery, or the thousands of other modern medical miracles. Some years ago, when I needed Achilles tendon surgery, my consultant had specialised to the point where he only operated only on the back of the ankle. That was great for me because his expertise in relation to the back of ankles was very great indeed, and consequently the probability of my surgery having a good outcome was therefore very good. But it did leave me wondering about how easy it was to get access to similar quality care locally for hips, knees or even the front of the ankle.

We have not matched the energy, enthusiasm and funding provided for the science and technology inherent in modern, acute, specialist care with the effort and resources required to manage long term, multiple conditions. Just 9% of the NHS budget goes to primary care where the majority of the care is provided. The accumulated knock-on effect is a serious issue of access, especially to primary care, not only for those patients with several long-term conditions, but also patients with acute and more simple problems. William Kissick's iron triangle demonstrates that if the system is to offer access and quality then that can only be addressed via resources.

When a shrinking and exhausted workforce is challenged by a post-coronavirus rise in demand for care from the public it is not surprising that many patients report difficulties in making an appointment with their GP practice. And yet it seems to be an issue of rising demand. Despite many reports of post-pandemic difficulty accessing care from GPs, the number of appointments each month in general practice is continuing to rise to record levels.[cclxxxviii]

GPs do retire and many are, and many practices now report it is now difficult if not impossible to recruit a replacement GP. Record numbers of appointments being provided is taking a serious toll on those still working as GPs; on average they see 50% more patients than the accepted safe volume of clinical work. Unsurprisingly, the 11th biannual work-life survey of general practitioners in 2022 found 33% of GPs were likely to quit direct patient care within five years. In GPs over 50 the figure was 61%; among GPs under 50, one in every six (16%) said they were planning to leave.[cclxxxix] Some of the largest numbers leaving are GPs within five years of completing training.

This is a truly calamitous situation for any health system given the importance of primary care to the health of the population, and the importance of continuity of care with its many benefits including a reduction in premature mortality and a reduction in the use of other health care resources. More funding has been provided for more nurses, more pharmacists and controversially more physician assistants are working in general practices, but the evidence is whilst they do sterling work and can work well with patients within their professional competence, their presence does not actually reduce the load on GPs. In the short-term at least, new roles in general practice for other clinicians increases the time GPs spend delegating tasks and supervising, with a negative effect on continuity of care.

Funding has been provided for non-GPs in primary care but there continue to be real-world reductions in the funding for GP practices – the increase for 2024/25 was only 1.9%, a figure far below general inflation over the preceding 12 months. We have now reached the situation where many GP practices are unable to afford to replace GPs who leave or retire, and as a result newly qualified GPs are unable to find work – even temporary locum posts. The net result is that despite record numbers of appointments being provided, many people are unable to see any GP within a reasonable time frame, never mind a GP who knows them and can offer continuity of care. Instead, fragmented primary care is provided by the soonest-available person in the GP practice – commonly a variety of non-GPs with a shorter period training and usually less expertise than a trained GP, and their work should be supervised by one of the remaining GPs. This is about as far away from an optimally configured primary care system as it is possible to get. As the Mad Hatter in Alice in Wonderland said, "If I had a world of my own, everything would be nonsense". At best this is a collective failure of medical and political leadership. At worst it has been a deliberate attempt to undermine primary care – and if primary care fails the rest of the health system crumbles.

As GP retire or leave, and the number of GP partners in a practice shrinks, the spectre of being "last man standing" and being the one partner left who is then personally responsible for all the redundancy payments to every single member of the practice staff creates a domino effect. Sometimes, when facing difficulties such difficulties, a GP practice can very quickly change from being viable and thriving to being unsustainable and folding. Regrettably this happened to the practice in which I was a partner – all be it some years after I had left. It is now not at all uncommon for GP practices to simply hand back their contract

385

and walk away, leaving neighbouring practices who are already struggling with demand to take on even more patients.

Though this mirrors the problems in many other countries, it is incredibly worrying for the NHS. Extensive research describing the contribution of primary care to health systems and health by Barbara Starfield and others shows that in health systems when primary care is strong it helps prevent illness and death.[ccxc] The evidence also shows that primary care (in contrast to specialist care) is associated with a more equitable distribution of health in populations, a finding that holds in both cross-national and within-national studies. The means by which primary care improves health are also well established:-

• Primary care increases access to health services for relatively deprived population groups.

• Primary care physicians do at least as well as specialists in caring for common diseases. For less common conditions, care provided by primary care physicians with appropriate backup from specialists may be the best model; for rare conditions, appropriate specialist care is undoubtedly important, as primary care physicians would not see such conditions frequently enough to maintain competence in managing them.

• The impact of primary care on prevention, and this is not confined to purely "medically" provided interventions. One would expect immunisation rates to be higher, but in addition breast feeding, eating a healthy diet and even seat belt wearing are higher when there is more primary care.

• The impact of primary care on the early management of health problems. In 2002 in the United Kingdom, each 15 to 20 percent increase in GP supply per 10,000 population was significantly associated with a decrease in hospital admission rates of about 14 per 100,000 for acute illnesses and about 11 per 100,000 for chronic illnesses, even after controlling for the degree of social deprivation in the area in which people live, their social class, ethnicity, and multimorbidity.

• The accumulated contribution of primary care characteristics to more appropriate care. The beneficial effects of primary care on mortality and morbidity can be attributed, at least in part, to the focus of primary care on the person rather than on the management of particular diseases. Where general practitioners are the point of first contact and act as a "gatekeeper" to secondary care they protect patients against over treatment by specialists. The evidence is consistent that first contact with a primary care physician (before seeking care from a specialist) is associated with more appropriate, more effective, and less costly care.

• Continuity of care, as was described in detail an earlier chapter, is associated with greater patient satisfaction, better compliance, and lower hospitalisation and emergency room use. Previous knowledge of a patient increases the doctor's odds of recognising psychosocial problems influencing the patient's health. People who report a particular doctor as their regular source of care receive more appropriate preventive care, are more likely to have their problems recognised, have fewer diagnostic tests and fewer prescriptions, have fewer hospitalisations and visits to emergency departments, and are more likely to have more accurate diagnoses and lower costs of care than are either people having a particular place or people having no place at all as their regular source of care. And astonishingly, a systematic review of the effects of continuity of care found continuity reduced mortality.[ccxci] Of course everybody dies eventually, so it is more accurate to say continuity of care in primary care reduces premature mortality. Nevertheless, if continuity of care in primary care was a medicine it would have to be incorporated into every single clinical guideline.

The adverse effects of seeking care directly from specialists have a strong theoretical basis. Since these specialists are trained in the hospital, the patients seen by specialists are not representative of the way in which patients present symptoms in community settings; the latter have a much lower prior probability of serious illness requiring the services of a specialist. The properties of diagnostic tests (sensitivity, specificity, positive and negative predictive values) operate differently in populations with a high or low prevalence of serious illness. Therefore the same test is used very differently and has a very different utility in specialty and in primary care settings. And because specialists

387

have a high component of technical knowledge and skills in their training and in their daily practice, their focus tends to be on "doing things" rather than finding out explicitly and routinely what an individual patient's ideas, concerns and expectations are. I should quickly say that this is a generalisation – care of the elderly consultants, for example, are true expert generalists and fly the flag valiantly for patient-centred care in the face of complex multimorbidity.

The result is that most specialists when seeing patients "unfiltered" by a primary care generalist overestimate the likelihood of illness in the patients they see, with a consequent increase in inappropriate use of diagnostic and therapeutic approaches, both of which raise the costs of health care, increase waiting lists and therefore time to investigation for all patients (including those who have serious disease), and increase the likelihood of adverse effects from treatments that are sometimes not actually necessary. There is now a significant amount of research describing over-diagnosis and over-treatment. Proposals for self-referral by patients directly to specialists - outside of a few specific instances – are, based on very good evidence, a recipe for disaster, as are proposals for specialists to "plug the gap" created by falling numbers of fully trained GPs and directly provide services in the community.

If health care systems work best where general practice operates as the first contact point for people who are ill, then the evidence is that the health system needs adequately resourced general practitioners.

Other health care professionals can fulfil valuable roles, but the skill mix issues are more complex than many seem to realise. It is tempting to think that if there is a shortage of GPs then getting another healthcare professional to see the patients is better than no one. This is a good example of an apparently simple solution to a complex problem being attractive but quite wrong. Firstly, many health care professionals moving from treating patients in hospitals have distorted perceptions about disease prevalence. If they have done lots of hospital paediatrics, then their mindlines are likely to be heavily influenced by the very sick children they have seen. You have to be a very sick child to be in a hospital bed. When that individual health care professional transfers to primary care they see lots of sick children too. Except that very few of them get very sick and need lots of treatment, tests or even admission to hospital. In hospital, clinicians test for disease. In primary care, they test for normality. And of course, tests function differently in populations with a low prevalence of disease. In a low prevalence situation, positive tests are much more likely to be false positives. It all leads to over-diagnosis, over-testing and overtreatment – and all that eats up chunks of capacity within the NHS, it all costs money, it increases the fragmentation of care, and patients do not like it. Most people intuitively know the value of a known GP in who they can put their trust.

The long and short of it is that we know that a general practitioner's expertise is not quickly acquired. Minimum training time is five years at medical school, two years as a foundation doctor and then three years in a specialist training post. The role of Physician Associates, particularly in primary care, has become contentious. At first sight, offloading some of a doctor's work onto faster-trained Physician Assistants would free up doctors' time to concentrate on more skilled work. At least that is the theory. Physician Associates have a three-year science degree, which might be botany or zoology or computer science for example, followed by two years of supervised training. That is a very long way away from the length of time legally required to become a GP. The literature on the acquisition of expertise shows that seeing acute, undifferentiated cases in primary care requires lots of time training and lots of skills. It was always intended that Physician Associates would work under supervision of a doctor. However, whilst that happens often, a shortage of GPs apparently means Physician Assistants being recruited for clinical care where medical staffing is problematic. It is not surprising that there have been several tragic cases involving misdiagnosis or mismanagement involving Physician Associates working in UK general practice. If you are acutely sick, the best person to see is a GP, preferably a GP who knows you. Someone who may have had just two years of supervised clinical experience after a botany degree probably is not going to have the same level of expertise.

The delegation of a GPs work to others still might be a good thing if it could be managed safely, wouldn't it? Well, probably no, actually. Other health systems including the United States, have been down that route and evaluated the change. Disappointingly for the proponents of that policy, that data is in and substituting doctors with other clinicians leads to higher health service utilisation by patients and higher costs.[ccxcii] Less experienced clinicians with a reduced period of training make more mistakes, order more tests and bring patients back more often.

There is also the impact on the role of the supervising doctor when other clinicians see some of their patients. This also seems to be other an apparently simple efficiency gain which does not materialise. Simple, apparently obvious "solutions" to complex problems are usually wrong. In better-resourced times GPs enjoyed the variety of problems that presented. Some were simple consultations; some were very complex. It is a big part of the reasons many doctors opted to be GPs, alongside the continuity of care. As has been said many times, as a specialist the diseases stay the same but the patients change, whereas as a GP the patients stay the same but the diseases change. There is something very beneficial about seeing people and their families over time that produces the benefits from continuity of care for patients, but that continuity is also one of the most enjoyable parts of the role for the GP.

GPs now, without any discussion or choice, have become supervisors of other people's clinical work. Their own consultations consist unremittingly of the more complex cases, allocated to them by someone else. It is simply not what they signed up for, it results in fragmented care, a further loss of the important continuity, and increases the likelihood of GPs retiring early or reducing the number of days they can work – because the work has become so much more pressurised. The more primary care is dispersed to other health care professionals, there is a greater reduction in the willingness to tolerate uncertainty. Patients and their health system will end up burdened with more tests and more referrals to hospital. What might appear a sensible move to shift some simpler work of GPs onto others has serious unintended consequences.

More GPs, well-resourced and working in suitable premises are required, but it takes a minimum of ten years to get from A-level student to GP. A recently announced expansion of medical school places back to 10,000 per year from 2025 is a very small start. It doesn't help that after years of broken promises about "more GPs" and other false promises of "forty new hospitals", doctors are jaded and sceptical at best.

More money in the short term is going to be required to stabilise the NHS in general and general practice in particular. We are currently recruiting many more doctors from abroad to work in the NHS. They are properly called International Medical Graduates (IMGs). In some parts of the country where I teach, over 80% of the doctors training to be GPs there are IMGs. I love working with them. Many of them have overcome hardships that we can barely imagine. Even if life has not been completely traumatic, if for example you are born in Nepal, have gone to medical school in the Philippines where the teaching was in Spanish and not of course Nepalese, and you are now working in the UK in your third language and third health system there are a lot of challenges that UK graduates do not face and most people can barely appreciate.

I was struck recently by a UK A&E consultant who had emigrated to Australia and then returned to the UK for family reasons. He said he was surprised, even though there was no new language to learn, how hard it was to work in a different health system. Cognitively, because everything was unfamiliar, medical decision making was so much harder. It never felt familiar despite being in the Australian system for some time. His first shift back in A&E in this country, and it was like putting on a familiar and well-worn coat. Knowing about dual process theory and pattern recognition explains the difficulties doctors and other health care professionals face when they move countries. It is therefore no surprise that, on average, IMGs who come to live and work in the UK seem to need more educational support during their postgraduate training. I have no doubt that like previous generations of doctors from abroad who have come to the UK to work in the NHS, they will become very valuable to their patients and as colleagues. But in the meantime, because there are more IMGs, we are asking the GPs who are responsible for training them who are already at a low ebb and overburdened with many things, to step up and do more.

Experienced general practitioners are very good at managing uncertainty, safety netting, and negotiating management plans based on realistic assessments of probabilities with patients. But of course, even they do not always get it right. Rare presentations of common diseases and rare diseases themselves can mean those plans, even when well communicated and agreed between patient and clinician, can be viewed with hindsight as flawed.

And the key words are "with hindsight" because, as we explored in an earlier chapter, many decisions are made based on probability - and there is almost always some residual uncertainty. If a GP makes a little more than 200 important decisions a week – and that is probably a serious under-estimate - then that equates to around 10,000 important decisions every year. If that GP gets 99% of those decisions correct, that still means there are 100 decisions a year that, in hindsight, were "incorrect". If only 1% of those lead to serious adverse consequences, each GP on average and will each year experience making one decision which with hindsight could have been a lot better.[ccxciii] What can be done about that? There are only two alternatives.

One approach to coping with the residual uncertainty is for GPs or others taking their place to do lots more tests and referrals to specialists. That means more work for hospitals, worsens waiting lists and times, and exposes patients to all the damage done by false positive tests and potential treatment for conditions that might resolve without any hospital-based treatment. Over-diagnosis, over-testing and over-treatment again.

The other alternative is that the work of GPs is properly recognised and rewarded, and the number of GPs increases, so that the workload is more manageable. But there is more. In their primary care consultations the GP should routinely make the uncertainty explicit, and discuss the diagnosis in terms of probability. When that happens both the GP and the patient accept the probability that serious disease is unlikely, safety netting is in place and agreed, and subsequently fewer tests and referrals are made for fewer people. The threshold for doing tests or referring to specialists cannot be set arbitrarily; rather it should properly be individualised. If we are serious about rebalancing medicine and managing health and disease in an older population with affordable costs, reasonable access and sufficient quality then accepting uncertainty must be part of the rebalancing. That means a massive effort to revitalise, and then re-educate general practice and the rest of primary care. The chapter on "Process" will expand on this.

But because things will go wrong simply because medicine is predicated on probabilities, why do we still have the burden of adversarial medical litigation? For my entire career a "No Fault" compensation scheme has been suggested as a means of providing the necessary financial support to people harmed by their experience in the NHS. Is it not time to look at that again? If there were better consultations where explicitly discussing uncertainty and probabilities was the norm, and this was coupled with a no-fault compensation scheme, would that not make inroads into the current incredibly expensive NHS litigation bill which was £2.7billion in 2022/23.

The question of no fault compensation could occupy an entire book itself, but in essence the problems with the current prove-negligence based scheme is that it requires adversarial litigation. This can be difficult for those allegedly a victim of negligence to access, legal costs are high, cases usually take years to be resolved, proof of breach of duty is required, and proof of causation of foreseeable damage is required. Negligence-based schemes also claim to create a deterrent – so that individuals and organisations strive not to make damaging errors. I am not sure this is true because it does not seem to have deterred the well-documented multiple NHS catastrophes in the last twenty years. But even if it were true, the downside of the deterrent argument is that it induces defensive medicine – multiple tests and investigations being performed "just in case", so reducing capacity in the health system, reducing access for other patients and overall increasing costs.

Critics of no-fault compensation schemes largely worry about their costs. A scheme has operated in New Zealand since 1995, and also in Sweden. Those injured cannot sue for damages but can receive payments from the schemes for "unexpected treatment injury". This is defined as injury that is "not a necessary part or ordinary consequence of the treatment".

We simply do not know what will happen with complaints and litigation if consultations were routinely conducted in the context of uncertainty and probabilities, and if decisions were routinely shared decisions. But a no-fault compensation scheme is surely worth another serious look alongside a big push on consultation skills, because the other linked influencer on negligence and litigation is likely to be a big one – Artificial Intelligence (AI). AI is discussed in more detail in a later chapter. However, it is worth a mention here because of two potential uses of AI that impact litigation costs.

Firstly, AI has already been shown to perform well as an ambient listener in consultations. It can readily produce a draft summary of the matters covered in a consultation and of the decision reached, saving much time for doctors recording their notes. AI can also perform well as informed prompter – encouraging "stop and think" moments. Such calibration can suggest alternative diagnoses, or make alternative treatment suggestions, or simply suggest a more nuanced and shared decision be attempted before the consultation concludes. Or sometimes all three. Easier to compile and perhaps more comprehensive records of consultations, improved consultation skills with decisions and uncertainties routinely shared with patients, and an AI-induced increase in calibration might make a serious dent in complaints and litigation. There is of course good evidence that better consultation skills alone reduces complaints and litigation.

Such issues cross over the Donabedian distinctions between structure and process, but for me there is something important in signalling an end to defensive medicine with no fault compensation, if that happens alongside a big push to recognise uncertainty and improve consultations within the shared decision-making paradigm and the introduction of AI into mainstream healthcare. AI is going to happen anyway, and quickly, and it will be available to patients. If doctors don't use it with patients, patients will be back with their own refined probabilities informed by their own use of AI.

Turning back to the question of healthcare resources, whilst the picture now is desperate in primary care, it is far from wonderful in secondary care. In a 2018 report by the Royal College of Physicians[ccxciv]:-

- 45% of advertised consultant posts went unfilled due to a lack of suitable applicants.
- 53% of consultants and 68% of trainees said rota gaps occurred frequently or often, with significant patient safety issues in 20% of cases.
- Trainees reported that a fellow junior doctor was absent due to sick leave in 46% of their on-call shifts.
- Both consultants and trainees estimated that they worked on average 10% more than they were contracted to work.
- 59% of trainees would not train in general internal medicine if they had their training period again. 27% of trainees reported that if they could turn back time, they would take a medical job outside the NHS and 31% a job outside medicine. When trainees were asked what would improve the quality of their training 87% said no rota gaps, 82% a better balance

between service and training, and 72% protected time for professional development.

Nevertheless, the number of staff working in hospitals has risen substantially whilst the number of GPs has fallen.[ccxcv] [ccxcvi] How is it possible to ensure that if the number of doctors graduating in the UK does increase in 2030 and beyond that enough of them will eventually enter specialist training to be GPs and eventually take up a post as a GP? Historic data says the expansion in specialists is largely where UK doctors have ended up. We are out of balance between primary and secondary care, and without a renaissance in primary care, secondary care's struggles will only worsen. Whilst GPs are providing more appointments in response to demand for access, it is clear that secondary care is struggling to return activity to pre-pandemic levels. Early in 2024, heroic efforts in secondary care have reduced the number of people on waiting lists a little in the last few months, but there is still a long, long way to go.

Some of those difficulties have been in part due to a lack of suitable social care facilities into which hospitals could discharge medically "fit" patients who still need care, but not hospital care. Social care provision and quality of care are a well-documented part of the current difficulties. Spending on social care in England fell by 11% from 2009/10 to 2015/16.[ccxcvii] While other devolved nations have held or increased their spending on social care, the government in England has frozen the means tested thresholds in nominal terms, reduced funding, and access for those with limited financial resources, and as a result have shifted more of the cost of social care on to the individual.

Successive governments have shelved plans to reform and adequately resource social care - which is important for all vulnerable groups in our society, but especially in this context for the increasing numbers of older people with multimorbidity. The dedicated, even heroic, staff in care homes are too often working for minimum wage without an adequate training programme and progressive career structure. As I have personally witnessed in family members, a well-run, happy and stimulating care home

396

can be transformative for its residents. And the worst of care homes are a matter for national shame.

In 1997 when Frank Dobson was appointed, much to everyone's surprise, Secretary of State for Health, he had a full day of meeting with senior civil servants and people from across the NHS. At the end of it he said to the assembled crowd, "So, it's all about the dosh then?". This may be an apocryphal story, but it still holds true that a major role of government ministers is to extract as much money as they can from the dead hand of the Treasury for their department. Britain is a rich country. Even in the post-pandemic, post-energy crisis world there are choices that can be made about health and social care funding. Many governments seem reluctant to grasp the social care nettle especially, but there remains an inevitability about the demographics. As for healthcare funding, is it realistic to be looking for the generally agreed 4% real growth to be delivered?[ccxcviii]

It seems to me that to expect 4% real growth in the NHS budget year on year indefinitely is both unrealistic and unnecessary. But if the NHS and social care workforce is paid reasonably that would be a start. A 2024 survey by UK Universities and the Nuffield Trust found that an encouraging three out of four young people have considered a career in healthcare with "helping other people" the biggest reason. But most were put off by perceived low pay, poor work-life balance and job stress. The lack of bursaries and payments for placements during training leading to large student debts were also big factors.

Most people in the NHS did not go into it to earn lots of money and they are not motivated by it. But they are demotivated if they have fifteen years of austerity, they see their standards of living falling, they find their own lives are getting more difficult, and every day at work they have to apologise to patients and their relatives that they are unable to meet the standard of care it would be reasonable to expect. There is a real crisis with the numbers of vacancies, and massive efforts are required in the short and long term to plan as best one can for a workforce that is bolstered in the short term and enhanced in the long. Lurching from crisis to crisis is not acceptable.

The NHS is about looking after people, both those who are ill and those who look after those who are ill. In the last decade and a half, it does not feel as if there is a commitment to looking after the people who look after us when we are ill.

In 2012 a young psychiatrist, Dr Daksa Emson killed herself and her three month old daughter. Out of this devastating and dreadful event some good came. The difficulties doctors face when struggling with their mental health – stigma, feeling of failure, being treated by colleagues, and simply accessing appropriate services – were for the first time acknowledged. The outcome was "NHS Practitioner Health", which made a confidential source of support more readily available for doctors struggling with their mental health. In a very short time NHS Practitioner Health developed a reputation for providing great support. Testimonials flooded in from doctors who had used the service. Some of them had help with less than life-saving issues such as examination anxiety – but never the less an important and values source of help when doctors are struggling with difficult postgraduate examinations. Many other doctors reported being brought back from the point of suicide thanks to Practitioner Health, having reached that point at least in part because of the pressures of caring for others. Suddenly talking about mental health was permissible much more widely within the medical profession, barriers to seeking help were melting away, and I can personally testify to the quality of the service provided having advised a few colleagues to look up Practitioner Health and get in touch with them.

Most people would have thought the service was one of the jewels in the crown of support for NHS staff – troubled as many still are with their experiences during the pandemic. And yet, astonishingly, in April 2024 NHS England suddenly closed down the funding for secondary care staff to access Practitioner Health, and Practitioner Health issued a statement saying they were unable to accept new referrals with immediate effect. In just three days 16,000 doctors signed a letter to NHS England, and the decision was reversed by the Secretary of State pending a review. Perhaps the scenario of another doctor committing suicide in the run up to a general election after closing down the service and not responding to 16,000 health care professionals saying this was a terrible decision played some part. If one imagined the worst example of how NOT to value essential NHS staff it would be hard to come up with that scenario. In 2024 it really feels as if many decisions have been made to harm the service and the morale of those who work in the NHS deliberately.

NHS IT hardware and software, especially in hospitals, has been a tragedy of Shakespearian proportions.. NHS England's target for all trusts to have an electronic patient record (EPR) by March 2025 has been declared "unachievable". It aimed to have 90% of all trusts have an EPR of an acceptable standard by the end of 2023, and 100% by March 2025. In June 2022 it was revealed only 20% of all trusts (43) had an EPR in place that met NHSE's required standards. A further 138 trusts had an EPR which required an extension or optimisation, while 30 trusts didn't have any EPR in place.[ccxcix]

And we have all seen inadequate premises with leaking roofs and worse, and little long-term planning or progress to improve the NHS estate.

Without some pump priming and some visible progress on structural issues it will be difficult to begin the long process of the NHS digging itself out of the current situation. It can only be the NHS workforce that can do that, and they need to see and feel that they are supported. It is the role of governments and NHS policy shapers and makers, together with national and local NHS leaders and managers simply to support front line staff. If they see that they are being backed, then they are some of the best people in the world and they will be able to deliver a great service once again.

It is not just pay. For example, there needs to be a serious look at junior doctors and the organisation of their training. If someone gives a year's notice of the date of their marriage it doesn't seem unreasonable that they can plan their wedding secure in the knowledge that they will not be on call that day. The days of doctors being able to give their all to the NHS and just that have gone. People have lives and families, they have a busy, stressful job with lots of responsibilities, they are studying for their postgraduate examinations which have a significant failure rate, the GMC is on the record as saying that many workplaces are toxic, and some doctors have a daily commute of over two hours when it would be perfectly possible for them to complete their training in a GP practice much nearer to their home. In this day and age, it really is not on.

But if there is a recognition of an NHS crisis, and appropriate early measures are taken, it does seem as though, once morale improves, there is a real opportunity to do things differently. In medicine there is a growing realisation that science does not fix everything, that more is not always necessary, and that asking patients about what matters to them is a very important thing. In 2023 I was asked to give a keynote address on "Rebalancing Medicine" for the British Society of Lifestyle Medicine. There were over 1,000 people at the Manchester Conference Centre, and they were all committed to working in a new way.

In the future, the process of care could and should look quite different.

CHAPTER TWENTY FIVE

Process

Over the last thirty years, as illness patterns have changed from single, acute conditions in relatively younger people to multiple, chronic conditions in older people, there have also been significant and fundamental changes in the way health care is delivered in the UK. I have already described the 2004 GP contract changes moved 24-hour responsibility away from general practices, for example.

Both during the working day and especially out of hours, an increased number of first contacts with the NHS are via a dedicated telephone line now called NHS 111. The service uses clinical decision support algorithms which may recommend a range of responses from telephone advice, a call back from a GP, advice to attend an Accident and Emergency Department or the dispatch of an emergency ambulance. According to GPs who work shifts out of hours, the decision support system operates very cautiously and so many people with very minor problems have their level of contact escalated "just in case". Whilst this is understandable, there are significant adverse consequences of this approach. Algorithms are not calibrated to incorporate levels of uncertainty individualised to the tolerances of individual patients and their clinicians; those taking the calls must operate within the limits of the algorithm. In the past, in many circumstances, a GP, especially one who knows the patient and their family, would be able to agree with the patient a simpler approach to their problems. Now the computer algorithm says "just in case" and patients are advised to attend A&E or an ambulance is dispatched with paramedics to assess the patient.

Paramedics say their work has changed too. Instead of lots of major medical emergencies their work now is dominated by less serious cases - and their work is also now driven by protocol that means even simple cases take an hour or more, with lots of e-paperwork to document every detail of their assessment and management. Not realising that decisions in medicine are usually taken based on probabilities and that certainty is rarely possible, there is no tolerance by ambulance trust management of clinical "errors". Every "i" has to be dotted and every "t" crossed, and woe-betide the paramedics if that is not the case. Nurses in hospital say the same thing – and when they repeatedly get told off for looking after patients instead of completing the paperwork, they leave and that's another unfilled vacancy in the workforce. More of that later.

These are some of the reasons why ambulance response times have worsened and why sometimes elderly people with a serious hip fracture after a fall at home wait 10 hours,[ccc] 14 hours,[ccci] 25 hours,[cccii] and even an astonishing 40 hours[ccciii] for an emergency ambulance to reach them. I recently waited for an ambulance for six hours with a 91-year old relative of mine with an obvious fracture. The UK is the fifth (or sixth depending on when and how it is measured) richest country on the planet, and yet people can wait 40 hours for an ambulance when they have a life threatening fall? How can that be in any way acceptable? In December 2022 the average wait for an ambulance to reach a patient with a heart attack was 93 minutes. That is the average time – so 50% of patients waited more than an hour and a half for an ambulance when they were having a heart attack, and in that situation outcomes deteriorate with every passing minute.

And then, because Accident and Emergency departments are busier than ever with patients who self-refer because they have difficulty accessing their GP in-hours or waiting for NHS 111 to ring them back for a consultation out of hours, or because the patients they are assessing have multimorbidity and require more complex assessment, patients sit for many hours in an ambulance outside the A&E department. If they are "lucky" they spend time on a trolley in the A&E department before they finally get into a hospital bed, their clinical condition can be properly stabilised, and they can be prepared and scheduled for surgery.

A hip fracture is one of the most serious consequences of falls in the elderly, with a mortality of 10% at one month and 30% at one year. Only 50% of survivors return to their previous level of mobility after a hip fracture, and up to 20% of patients are unable to continue to live independently. NICE guidance is that surgery for hip fracture should be performed on the day of or the day after admission. The current UK incidence of hip fractures is between 70,000 to 75,000 per year. The Royal College of Physicians runs an almost real-time count of how well actual hip fracture treatment matches up with national guidance.[ccciv]

Some collections of data are helpful and this is one of them. Despite the increases in the number of specialists and no dissent about the importance of managing hip fracture well and quickly, the NHS only meets best practice in all key aspects for less than 50% of patients. Time to surgery, one of the most important determinants of the best recovery possible, is achieved for just 60% of patients, having been below that level for most of 2022. Hip fracture is one of the canaries in the coalmine for health care. These hips are broken, and whilst the NHS itself may not be quite broken, there are serious capacity and workforce issues.

The blunt truth is that 21st century problems are still being addressed with 20th century approaches that have demonstrably not worked, a number of these approaches have created significant adverse consequences, a decade and a half of austerity has reduced service availability, staff shortages have not been fundamentally addressed, and there remains a significant impact from the coronavirus pandemic on NHS staff. But there is another important factor. There is a whole generation of doctors now in post who have never experienced going to work, consulting with patients, finding out what matters most to them, and then looking after them to the best of their ability. The current generation of doctors is largely wedded to rigidly following the "rules" of guidelines because they see that as optimum care, and that means they are protected from patient complaints, litigation, and the General Medical Council. They wearily accept the drudgery of form filling and often pointless data collection, perhaps because they have known nothing else.

Here are a few snippets from a recent discussion I was part of – and the participants are those keen on avoiding overtreatment and overdiagnosis:-

"I had a complaint - and the Medical Defence Union (one of the organisations which insures doctors in case they are sued) spent some time

checking exactly what guideline was in place at the time of the consultation, to ensure they could check my management against the guideline at that time. Sadly, [this] does not allow for personalisation of treatment and the more this continues the less hope of the next generation ever moving out of tramlines - I have many such discussions with my GP registrars."

GP1

"I see litigation and threat of complaint letters as a driver against de-prescribing and doing less. We may have a shared decision about stopping statins or not bringing the blood pressure down any lower. That's fine. The patient has an MI. The family write a complaint letter 'how dare you stop a life-saving medication' etc. GPs practise in fear because patients have been given the idea that pills can save their life."   GP2

"It is not just GPs; consultants also fear complaints, litigation, coroner and not following guidance. It is all fine saying 'guidelines are not tramlines' but the trusts, courts and coroner will ask: 'were the guidelines followed'. I hear this all the time from hospital teams of all grades from F1 to senior consultants. [The] Joys of modern medicine."

Care of Elderly Consultant 1

But there are healthcare professionals who see the world in a different way. The British Society of Lifestyle Medicine are one group. The British Medical Journal has an overdiagnosis theme with numerous papers and articles. Even some health systems are encouraging, even enthusiastic, about a different approach. "Realistic Medicine" in Scotland and "Prudent Healthcare in Wales" do sterling work supporting the notion that science and technology is great, but it doesn't fix everything, that sometimes other approaches are what patients want and may even be more effective than prescriptions and hospitals. There is a recognition that often what the NHS has to offer has limited effectiveness in the face of the social determinants of health – poverty, poor housing, support for children in their early years provision, the unequal distribution of wealth and low educational achievement. Such doctors are increasingly advising social interventions – choirs, walking groups – and are mobilising the collective strengths within their communities to improve health and wellbeing.

Some doctors are trying to change their relationships with their patients. They are listening more carefully, asking about their ideas concerns, and expectations more often, sharing their uncertainties about diagnoses and offering treatment options instead of "fixes", and trying their best to offer personal care and support. But this isn't happening everywhere. In fact what we know is shared decision making is an innovation in need of a better implementation plan. The evidence is so strong about the positive benefits of better consultation skills that spreading best consultation skills is one of the best things we could do to rebalance medicine.

This emphatically is not just in primary care. In the last year I have personally experienced the NHS as a patient more frequently than for many years. I went for a screening test – I don't go to many because I know the risks and benefits of screening tests. But I did go for this one, and it was positive. And it was eight long months before I got a diagnosis. Heaven knows I'm not alone in experiencing delays in the NHS, but eight months living every day with a frisson of anxiety is too long. I got started on some treatment after my diagnosis and then my follow up appointment gets cancelled. I'm not on my own there either, but I am sitting there taking treatment and not knowing whether it is working, and I'm looking for the postman every morning for the replacement appointment. Finally the science and the technology kicks in and I get two operations either side of Christmas which technically seem to go well, though there was an absence of any caring other than the technical aspects.

In terms of the process, the healthcare providers introduced themselves about 50% of the time, and not once did anybody ask about my ideas, concerns and expectations. Nobody has spoken to me about probabilities. There has, however, been lots of me being told definitively what the next treatment is. There has never been a single discussion; and certainly none about when and why I think it would be good to have my follow up tests. I'm in a sausage machine that does things by rote, and it is very difficult even for me, even as a doctor, to challenge the system.

I'm not criticising anyone, other than those who took the political decisions which have resulted in this NHS crisis. Everybody in the NHS is frazzled, with too much to do and too few people to do it. But I can tell you, those consultation skills really do matter.

If we are serious about doing fewer tests, avoiding overdiagnosis, and reducing the burden of unnecessary treatment (medicines especially), then we must get serious about consultation skills. I don't have a problem with undergraduate courses being science-dominated. An earlier chapter has discussed the development of expertise, and we know that the higher-level consultation skills are difficult to master until the more basic building blocks of knowledge are in place. A bit more on consultation skills, perhaps revisited a few times during the course, would be great. Those teaching clinical reasoning to undergraduates are doing a great job – but that still needs to be evened up and everywhere. Uncertainty, probability, an insight into how one becomes and expert, and especially cognitive psychology would help knit together the consultation skills, the science, and the emerging illness scripts as the end of the undergraduate course looms.

Teaching consultation skills as a stand-alone topic without, say, cognitive psychology seems to me to be missing a trick. Incorporating cognitive psychology into my work with postgraduate doctors and many other health care professionals started 15 years ago. GP, palliative care, oncology, and psychiatry postgraduate training all major on teaching, practicing, and assessing consultation skills. For all other specialist training programmes, at best it is not well established. Sometimes I have conversations with people doing postgraduate teaching in other specialties and I come away thinking they really do not even understand the concept of shared decision making. And this is despite shared decision-making being a requirement by the General Medical Council and having legal precedent. It seems to me that perhaps many specialties need to be considering big changes in their postgraduate training programmes. Those specialties not currently delivering consultation skills as a strong element of their programmes should be getting a bunch of tips from those who do. The GMC could do a lot more here. They write and say all the right things and have done for years, but the rate of progress is demonstrably glacial.

Then there are the doctors who have completed their postgraduate training – the hospital consultants and the GPs. Some of them have brilliant consultation skills, but it is clear that a proportion do not. Fortunately there has been a great deal of research into the obstacles to shared decision making. The MAGIC academic consortium was funded by the Health Foundation and they summarised their findings in the British Medical Journal in 2017.

Changing attitudes is key. Many clinicians feel they already routinely undertake shared decision making when that is not the case. Others think they need more decision aids, when in fact, as the authors reported, "skills trump tools, and culture trumps skills". Then some doctors think patients don't want shared decision making. Some patients want different levels of involvement in decisions, but many patients (including myself) feel unable to participate in decision making. "We can't measure shared decision making" is then the next reason given. Undoubtedly knowing that a change in approach in consultations is making a difference can help embed a change in clinical practice. In better times, resources would be allocated to such a quality improvement project, and patients would be surveyed using validated tools for assessing their involvement in decision making in their consultations. Finally comes what I think is the main reason – "We are so busy doing other things and there aren't enough people". Remember this work was published in 2017 and before the coronavirus pandemic. I would judge that post-pandemic there are no reserves left for the big push on consultation skills that is needed until some of the current workload pressure is relieved.

But while consultants and GPs are important, they have a role that goes beyond being part of the workforce delivering lots of care. They are also the role models for doctors in training, and many of them have formal teaching roles. The hidden impact of ongoing doctor-centred, "paternalistic" consultations continuing as sometimes the norm should not be under-estimated, because it perpetuates the same approach to the consultation that the previous generations followed. It seems as if little will happen without something radical changing the fear of complaints and litigation. Perhaps a no-fault compensation scheme linked with uncertainty, probability and consultation skills might have something going for it after all?

CHAPTER TWENTY SIX

Artificial Intelligence

Alan Turing was a British mathematician, logician, and computer scientist who made contributions to mathematics, cryptography, and artificial intelligence (AI). His contribution to cracking the German Enigma code during the second World War was told in the hit film "The Imitation Game".

The Turing Test is a thought experiment outlined in his paper "Computing Machinery and Intelligence," published in 1950. In this paper, Turing sought to answer the question: "Can machines think?" He proposed that the ability of a machine to exhibit intelligent behaviour could be tested through a simple experiment involving human judges and a computer.

In the test, there are three participants: a human interrogator (judge), a human respondent (interlocutor), and a computer (machine). The interrogator is tasked with determining which of the two respondents is human and which is a machine. The interrogator communicates with both the human respondent and the computer through a text-based interface. The participants are not physically present, and the interrogator cannot see or hear them. The goal of the Turing Test is for the computer to generate responses that are indistinguishable from those of a human respondent. If the interrogator is unable to reliably distinguish between the human and the computer based on their responses alone, the computer is said to have passed the Turing Test.

Research into AI since 1950 has had many ups and downs. But in the last few years enthusiasm has been rekindled as natural language processing, conversational agents, and better human-computer interaction has developed. In 2023 I had several conversations with people I greatly respect who all urged me to look at the latest generation of large Language Models (LLMs) and to consider how they might fit into medicine. Long experience makes be sceptical. I have seen far too many scientific and technical developments in my career that have been heralded as "game changing" when they turned out to be nothing of the sort. "Prediction is difficult, especially about the future" applies, and it takes a lot to convince me that we are on the threshold of something very important. But with the most recent generation of LLMs, my goodness I am impressed. "We tend to overestimate the effect of a technology in the short run and underestimate the effect in the long run," was coined by Roy Amara, and I do just think that might be where we are with AI in medicine now - most people are probably underestimating how AI will change medicine.

I took at random a complex question from "GP Self-Test", a question bank of over 2,500 multiple choice questions used most often by GP registrars to test their progress during their preparation for postgraduate examinations.

Here is the question I posed to ChatGPT, one of several LLMs now available:-

"You are working an out-of-hours shift doing telephone triage. The carer of a 70-year-old man calls you – the man has run out of his immediate-release morphine sulphate. He has bowel cancer and currently takes sustained release morphine sulphate 30 mg twice daily. He takes immediate-release morphine sulphate for breakthrough pain, although the carer is unsure of what dose he has been taking.

What is the SINGLE MOST appropriate dose of immediate-release morphine sulphate for breakthrough pain for this patient? Select ONE option only."

A. 10 mg
B. 2.5 mg
C. 15 mg
D. 1.5 mg
E. 20 mg

I used version 3.5 of ChatGPT. Version 4 is available indirectly via the Microsoft search engine Bing, but I have found ChatGPT performs better when it is directly accessed via the www.ai.com website than when the later version is accessed via Bing. It answered immediately:-

412

"A. 10 mg. When managing breakthrough pain in a patient who is already on sustained-release morphine, a common starting dose for immediate-release morphine for breakthrough pain is usually around 10 mg. This dosage can be adjusted based on the patient's response and the severity of the breakthrough pain, but starting with a lower dose is generally prudent to assess individual tolerance and response."

According to the RCGP, and I have no reason to doubt them, Chat GPT got the answer correct. Their answer said "This patient is taking a total daily dose of morphine sulphate of 60 mg (30 mg twice daily). The standard breakthrough dose is between one-tenth and one-sixth of the regular 24-hour morphine sulphate dose. One-sixth of the total daily dose is 10 mg (one-tenth is 6 mg)."

Pretty impressive. Dosage calculations can be tricky and in mock examination settings I have found up to 10% of GP registrars make a dosage calculation error when under examination conditions and pressure. That is not to say that they would make the same mistake in a clinical situation where they can look at guidance in the British National Formulary or ask a knowledgeable colleague such as a pharmacist, or do both.

But perhaps Chat GPT got lucky. So I tried it again.

"Which ONE of the following drugs is the MOST LIKELY to be associated with neonatal toxicity? Select ONE option only."

A.   Carbamazepine
B.   Citalopram
C.   Lamotrigine
D.   Lithium carbonate
E.   Fluoxetine

ChatGPT says:-

"D. Lithium carbonate. Lithium carbonate is known to be associated with neonatal toxicity when taken during pregnancy. It can lead to a condition

413

called neonatal lithium toxicity, which can cause symptoms such as lethargy, poor feeding, hypotonia, and even cardiac arrhythmias in newborns whose mothers were taking lithium during pregnancy. Therefore, among the options listed, lithium carbonate is the most likely to be associated with neonatal toxicity."

And again, it agrees with the RCGP.

But it doesn't get everything right. I tried it with this question:-

"A 23-year-old man telephones you for advice. He contacted the out-of-hours service two weeks ago and was diagnosed with viral gastroenteritis following a telephone consultation. His condition deteriorated, and he was admitted to hospital three days later with acute appendicitis. He wants to make a complaint and demands financial compensation for his time off work.

What is the SINGLE MOST appropriate advice to give to this patient regarding his complaint? Select ONE option only."

A.   Advise him to contact the Local Medical Committee (LMC).
B.   Advise him to contact a solicitor.
C.   Advise him to contact the out-of-hours provider.
D.   Advise him that although it was unfortunate that he developed appendicitis, he has no basis on which to make a complaint.
E.   Advise him to contact the General Medical Council (GMC).

Chat GPT said:-

"D. Advise him that although it was unfortunate that he developed appendicitis, he has no basis on which to make a complaint. In this scenario, the patient's condition deteriorated after the initial diagnosis of viral gastroenteritis, leading to acute appendicitis. While the situation is unfortunate, it's not necessarily indicative of negligence or malpractice on the part of the healthcare provider. Therefore, advising the patient that he has no basis for a complaint is the most appropriate course of action."

This is not correct. The RCGP says the correct answer is C. "Every NHS organisation should have a complaints procedure. A complaint can be made to either the organisation that provided the care directly or to the organisation that commissioned that NHS service. In this example, it would be appropriate to advise this man to contact the out-of-hours provider directly to make his complaint, in writing, by email or by speaking to them. Many complaints may be able to be resolved successfully at this stage without having to go through a formal complaints process. If local resolution fails, the matter can be referred to the Parliamentary and Health Service Ombudsman."

I informed ChatGPT of its error, and it then said again incorrectly that the Local Medical Committee was the right answer. Finally, at the third attempt it gave the correct answer. That is a worry, but when I am using ChatGPT – just for fun – it really does feel like I am exchanging notes with another human. For me, it passes the Turing test. But are there additional risks with AI-induced errors? Does it sound so authoritative that questioning it is cognitively difficult?

Having tested out this particular AI platform more widely, it seems to me that the existing technical standard is at least as good as many of the GP registrars I teach – before I start the teaching, of course. The response to most of the trickier questions is truly astonishing but we should not be surprised. Without any specific training, GPT-4 (the latest iteration of ChatGPT) performed "at or near the passing threshold" of the United States Medical Licensing Exam, and passed three of four papers in the Faculty of Public Health Diplomate Examination, surpassing the current pass rate. When it was given 45 questions from the RCGP mock AKT examination which all GP Registrars have to pass, it scored 96.7%.[cccv] I spend a lot of time helping postgraduate doctors to achieve the usual pass mark of a little over 70%. Achieving over 90% is very unusual.

If that were not astonishing enough, ChatGPT4 was recently asked to answer database of 195 questions about healthcare from a public social media forum where a verified physician had already responded to a public question.^{cccvi} The original question along with both the anonymised and randomly ordered physician and chatbot responses were evaluated by three licensed health care professionals. Evaluators chose "which response was better" and judged both "the quality of information provided" (very poor, poor, acceptable, good, or very good) and "the empathy or bedside manner provided" (not empathetic, slightly empathetic, moderately empathetic, empathetic, and very empathetic). Mean outcomes were ordered on a 1 to 5 scale and compared between chatbot and physicians.

Of the 195 questions and responses, the evaluators (who themselves were physicians), preferred chatbot responses to physician responses 78.6% of the time. Chatbot responses were rated of significantly higher quality than physician responses (P < .001). The proportion of responses rated as good or very good quality (≥ 4), was higher for chatbot than physicians (chatbot: 78.5%, physicians: 22.1%). Chatbot responses were also rated significantly more empathetic than physician responses (P < .001). The proportion of responses rated empathetic or very empathetic (≥4) was higher for chatbot than for physicians (physicians: 4.6%, chatbot: 45.1%, The chatbot had a 9.8 times more empathetic or very empathetic responses than the physicians. The design of this study has serious limitations – the real doctors were responding to factual written queries on a social media platform and their responses may well have been very different and more empathic if placed in a professional setting - but the results should at least make us think that AI may have something very interesting going on.

If I were a patient with some symptoms, might it help me make sense of them? Perhaps. Would I try it if I couldn't readily get an appointment with my GP? Maybe. Does this need a lot more urgent thought and consideration by patients and the public, by the healthcare professions, and by those with responsibility for quality and licensing of medical devises? For sure, and quickly, because the pace of development is now so fast that the use of AI may only be constrained by our imagination.

If we are to understand how AI might help support human decision making and some of their limitations and how they might make errors, it might help to know a little about how LLMs work? In many ways, they emulate how we humans make decisions – repetition and probabilities play a big part.

Let us imagine we are a primary school teacher and we are teaching children to add up numbers. One of the ways we might help our pupils would be to create "flash cards". On one side of a card we might write "3 + 1 =" and other the back of the card we write "4". Pupils who are still learning addition might have to guess at an answer when the teacher holds up "3 + 1 =" and most times they get it wrong. The teacher shows them the right answer, reinforces this repeatedly with other teaching strategies, and they try to remember it. Perhaps with a second, or even a third, attempt at calling out the answer to "3 + 1 =" they get it right, and with further reinforcement they are never going to forget that the answer to that sum is 4. These learn – test – relearn – retest – relearn cycles are still useful later in life. I am often talking to GP registrars about creating flashcards to increase their efficiency and effectiveness as they seek to improve their knowledge for their postgraduate assessments.

The LLMs work in a similar way. There is an input – let's say we ask Chat GPT "What are the most important medicines a patient with heart failure should be taking?". The LLM will come up with a host of possible answers – let's say four of the answers it identifies are bananas, amoxicillin (an antibiotic), ramipril and bisoprolol. The latter two are medicines used extensively to treat people with cardiovascular conditions. The LLM then assesses the probabilities of those answers being the correct answer.

If you have ever played the word game "Wordle" you do the same thing. In "Wordle" the aim is to guess the five-letter word of the day. We start with five blank spaces. I have no idea of course what the word of the day is, so I might pick "ADIEU" as one tactical approach which will at least show me whether one or more of four of the five vowels are in today's word, or I might pick "SHARE" because that word contains some of the commonest letters in five-letter words, be they vowels or consonants. Both approaches depend on probabilities. I have only six attempt to get to the correct word.

Let's say today I use "SPARE", and the game tells me that the word does indeed begin with S, but none of the other letters are in the word. That information changes the probabilities. I am now thinking that the second letter might be an "H", a "T" or a "C". In many word S is followed by T, H or C, but I don't know which one is right in this case, and other letters might still be possibilities. It might begin "SM" as part of "SMOCK" or "SN" as part of "SNORT" for example, but H T and C have higher probabilities of following S in five-letter words. I try "SHUNT" and again I'm wrong, but the game tells me the S H and T are in the right place. Now the probabilities are settling out to the very few five-letter words that have "SH" at the beginning and T at the end, and don't have P A R E U or N anywhere in the word. On the next attempt I think the probability is the SH is followed by an I or an O. I rack my brains for a word that is SHI_T or SHO_T where the missing letter cannot be P A R E or U. In the end I try "SHOOT" and I am right. What my brain was doing was taking the inputs – the words on the screen – and running through the extensive body of knowledge I have in my brain about the spelling of five-letter words in English. Eventually there was an output – my next attempt - and that output is again displayed on the screen.

If we ask a LLM about the most important treatments for heart failure it can generate all sorts of possibilities, some of them with better probabilities than others. For example, "banana", "car" and "oceans" it can quickly dismiss because the LLM searches the body of knowledge it has been trained with. This body or "corpus" as it is called consists of thousands and thousands of textbooks, research papers, and many other sources of information and knowledge. The LLM then looks for "bananas" and all the other options in its corpus. It is looking for the word "bananas" close to the phrase "heart failure". It does not find any unless there is a discussion about the effect of potassium-rich bananas in people with heart failure. A medicine – any medicine - might have a higher probability, and it finds "amoxicillin" is a medicine but it is not closely associated with heart failure other than in the clinical setting where people with heart failure also have an infection requiring an antibiotic and a good choice for that infection is amoxicillin. Finally, the LLM finds that "ramipril" or the class of medicines to which it belongs (ace-inhibitors), and "bisoprolol" or the class of medicines to which it belongs (beta-blockers) are closely related in the text of many heart failure guidelines world-wide which have been incorporated into the LLM as part of its training. The probability is therefore strong that these are two of the medicines, perhaps the two most important medicines, to be considered in the management of heart failure, and the LLM uses that information in its output.

There's an awful lot of matching of patterns going on in LLMs, just as there is in decision making with our own brains. Unsurprisingly, pattern matching for real has been one of the first early applications of AI in healthcare. A large randomised study of mammograms in 80,000 women being screened for breast cancer, with or without AI support, showed improvement in accuracy with AI compared to radiologists alone reviewing the mammograms, and a 44% reduction of screen-reading workload for the radiologists.[cccvii] A systematic analysis of 33 randomized trials of colonoscopy, with or without real-time AI machine vision, indicated there was more than a 50% reduction in missing polyps and adenomas, and the inspection time added by AI to achieve this enhanced accuracy averaged only ten seconds.[cccviii] These results are almost too good to be true, but they are.

There is another attention-grabbing story from the United States.[cccix] A four-year old boy began to get headaches every day, and they seemed to start when his mother bought him a small "bouncy castle". He then seemed to be chewing inappropriately, and amongst many other theories an orthodontist thought teeth grinding might be part of the problem. Then his growth seemed to stop, or at least it slowed. Then he seemed to be using his left leg more than his right. A paediatrician sent him for physiotherapy, but it did not seem to help. After seeing 17 different doctors and no one able to provide an answer, his mother put her son's symptoms into ChatGPT. It suggested the diagnosis of spina bifida occulta and tethered cord syndrome. This is a rare condition, which should have been picked up on the tests and scans previously performed. She scheduled an appointment with a new paediatric neurosurgeon and told him her son's lengthy history of medical problems and what ChatGPT was suggesting. The neurosurgeon looked at an old MRI scan. "Yes, you're right" he said. "Here's the spina bifida occulta and here is the tethered spinal cord".

One anecdote does not equate to proof, but it should make us think as we evaluate the enormous potential, and it is currently only potential, of AI to help in healthcare decision making. There have to be several caveats. Obviously the LLM can only work with the information it has been trained with. Training LLMs is not instantaneous, and there are huge volumes of data to incorporate every time the LLM undergoes a training period. That means the LLM might be out of date – it simply won't have access to new research published after the last training. Then it is going to be dominated by the status quo. If information is new and radical but correct, and the dominant theory in the all the documents is the conventional one, what will be the output from the LLM? We might wonder how an LLM might respond to Barry Marshall and Robin Warren's discovery that many ulcers were caused by a bacteria called *Helicobacter Pylori*. All the conventional thinking at the time was that ulcers were caused by stress, or smoking or medicines, not this "innocent" bacteria. Marshall and Warren had a hard time with their fellow gastroenterologist and microbiologists, but eventually the quality of their research was recognised and they were awarded the Nobel Prize. Would a LLM mean quicker transference of brilliant, new, but unconventional thinking – or would it be because "the LLM says No", its presence would delay the adoption of important and correct new thinking. LLMs might turn out to be the modern day equivalent of the Catholic Church when Galileo reported on Jupiter's moons. Then LLMs will be dominated by what already exists, so the outputs will be influenced more by publications from Europe and North America and less by other parts of the world. Their outputs will also reflect the biases in the existing literature – there is already a study showing an LLM can perpetuate race and gender biases.[cccx]

We already know that individual human doctors respond in different ways, one from another, when LLMs are introduced to support their decision making. When radiologists had AI input into their task of interpreting chest x rays, some of them were overconfident in their own abilities and incorrectly ignored the AI suggestion. This is no surprise to anyone who has studied cognitive psychology. There's a well-known "overconfidence" cognitive bias, and since doctors are human beings it is not surprising that some are fallible to it in the context of AI support.

Then there are questions about acceptance of AI by patients and doctors. Will both parties be willing to have the computer listen to the consultation and then produce a draft set of clinical notes? Our response years ago to videotaping consultations was not uniformly welcoming, at least at first. For the most part doctors and patients have got used to it, at least for research, training and assessment. Routine "listening in" might be something else again, even if there were the prospect of time and effort being saved. We simply do not know how that might work out.

Many GPs might be very welcoming to some AI software that could quickly and accurately write draft referral letters or produce with a single voice command an email to inform a specialist of a request to expedite an operation date, or any one of the hundreds of other administrative tasks that currently have to be done at home in the evening and at weekends. Likewise, scheduling and rescheduling of appointments should be much less onerous once AI gets involved.

But for the clinical roles for AI, the AI must be able to do Information Mastery - discern valid and relevant evidence from poor quality evidence. We know already it can provide answers quickly and conveniently. The convenience part of the Slawson and Shaughnessy equation will be automated by the entrance of AI into producing summaries of research. The question is can it sort fake evidence from sound evidence? What if there was a malign organisation or individual that somehow managed to distort the AI process of pattern recognition and the output reflected untruths placed there with the intention of commercial gain or worse? Can we be sure that what we see in an AI-supported evidence summary is not distorted by vested interests?

Perhaps the biggest challenge for AI, certainly in primary care, is to bolster the holding of uncertainty. The danger is that AI drives even harder and faster the algorithmic care that has been so damaging. If the AI probabilistic approach is set to "just in case" that will led to more tests, more referrals and more unnecessary treatments. But if AI gives both clinician and patient a more realistic idea of probabilities as part of its "calibration" function and then supports individualised choices of the available options we might have something very valuable to aid the process of decision making.

There is a lot to debate, test, and try out in considered ways. And an early look at the legal implications. We know LLMs do not always get things right. Sometimes, for yet undiscovered reasons LLMs "hallucinate" – in other words they make things up. The output does not qualify or even identify when the LLM hallucinates – it gives the same clear , confident and positive outputs whether it is right, wrong or hallucinating.

What happens if clinical care is being decided the clinician is in favour of one diagnosis or treatment, and this is supported by the LLM, and then subsequently the diagnosis and treatment is incorrect. If we are in an adversarial, negligence-based legal system who is negligent? Is it the clinician or is it the LLM? To be decided.

But what if the decision was shared between the patient and the clinician, they took the LLM output into account of course, but in the end, it was their shared decision. If, with hindsight, the decision goes wrong, is there negligence, and if so who was negligent? Arguably nobody, and hopefully the ambient-recorded clinical notes would back that up. But wait a minute, the patient has still been harmed. Is that where a no-fault compensation scheme has advantages?

It does seem likely that teaching medicine, even the basic sciences, will look very different in an AI-era, and arguably will be more engaging. Whatever we do to rebalance medicine, AI is going to be part of it. And as we turn back to the last Donabedian theme of outcomes in the next chapter there is one last ChatGPT exercise to report. I asked it:-

"What will be the effect of giving GPs in England an annual increase in funds of 1.9%, when inflation is running at 4%?"

ChatGPT's reply was:-

"When GPs in England receive an annual increase in funds of 1.9% while inflation is running at 4%, it means that their funding is not keeping pace with the rate of inflation. Inflation erodes the purchasing power of money over time, which means that with a 4% inflation rate, prices for goods and services are rising at that rate annually.

Given that the increase in funds for GPs is only 1.9%, it effectively means that their real income, adjusted for inflation, is decreasing. In real terms, their purchasing power is diminishing because the cost of living is rising faster than their income.

This situation could lead to several potential effects:

Financial Strain: GPs may experience financial strain as their income fails to keep up with the rising cost of living. This could impact their ability to maintain their standard of living or invest in practice improvements.

Recruitment and Retention Issues: The reduced real income may make general practice less attractive to healthcare professionals, potentially exacerbating existing recruitment and retention challenges within the healthcare system.

Quality of Care: Financial constraints could impact the quality of care provided by GPs. Practices may struggle to invest in necessary resources, technology, or staff training, which could affect patient care and outcomes.

Workforce Morale: The perception of being underfunded relative to inflation may lead to decreased morale among GPs and healthcare staff, potentially impacting job satisfaction and performance.

In summary, while an annual increase in funds for GPs is generally positive, failing to keep pace with inflation can have significant implications for GPs, their practices, and the quality of care provided to patients. It underscores the importance of ensuring that healthcare funding keeps pace with the rising costs and demands of the healthcare system."

Sometimes AI might get very close to the truth.

CHAPTER TWENTY
SEVEN

Outcomes

Don Berwick is president emeritus and senior fellow at the Institute for Healthcare Improvement. President Obama appointed him to be the administrator of the Centers for Medicare & Medicaid Services. A paediatrician by background, Dr Berwick has served on the Faculty of the Harvard Medical School and Harvard School of Public Health, and on the staffs of Boston's Children's Hospital Medical Center, Massachusetts General Hospital, and the Brigham and Women's Hospital. He served two terms on the Institute of Medicine's (IOM's) Governing Council, was a member of the IOM's Global Health Board, and served on President Clinton's Advisory Commission on Consumer Protection and Quality in the Healthcare Industry. Recognized as a leading authority on health care quality and improvement internationally, Dr Berwick was appointed an Honorary Knight Commander of the British Empire by Queen Elizabeth II in recognition of his work with the NHS. When Don Berwick writes or speaks, it is usually worth a listen or a read. I once heard him give a keynote address at a Royal College of General Practitioners annual conference. He got the biggest, loudest, and longest standing ovation I have ever heard for any speaker at any health care professionals conference, and I can go back 50 years.

In April 2015 Dr Berwick wrote about the "three eras of medicine".[cccxi] As we think about how we ended up with QOF and the numerous other number-counting outcome-describing exercises in health care, we should consider what we have lost because of it. Don Berwick's paper is - at this point in the narrative - worth a substantial summary.

Don Berwick wrote that Era 1 of medicine goes back to ancient times, to Hippocrates and beyond. In Era 1 the profession and practice of medicine was noble. Medicine had special knowledge, inaccessible to those who are not doctors. Medicine was beneficent, and there seemed every reason to allow it to self-regulate. After all, given that medicine had special knowledge, how could an outsider judge the quality of care provided. Society conceded to the medical profession a privilege most other work groups do not get - the authority to judge the quality of its own work.

However, the basis of Era 1 was shaken when researchers found enormous unexplained variation in practice, rates of injury from errors in care high enough to make health care a public health menace, indignities and injustice related to race and social class, and that some of the soaring costs of care were wasteful and not producing better outcomes.

These findings meant a pure reliance on trusted professionalism seem naive. If medical professionals were so intelligent, so hard working and so scientific, why was there so much variation? If they were beneficent, how could they permit so much harm? If they are to self-regulate, how could they waste so much and sometimes - even if only a tiny number of exceptional cases - do tremendous harm?

The harms and inconsistency helped birth Era 2, which still dominates the present. Exponents of Era 1 believed in professional trust and prerogative; those who believe in Era 2 believe in accountability, scrutiny, measurement, incentives, and markets. The machinery of Era 2 is the manipulation of contingencies: rewards, punishments, and pay for performance. Don Berwick writes that "Numbers have become our tyrant, not our servant".

The collision of norms from these two eras - between professional autonomy on the one hand, and the various tools of external accountability on the other, has led to discomfort and self-protective reactions. Doctors, other health care professionals, and many health care managers feel angry, misunderstood, and overcontrolled, and the effort involved reduces the clinical capacity of people working in health systems. Patients, governments, and consumer groups feel suspicious, resisted, and often helpless.

Berwick wrote that it is time for Era 3 - guided by updated beliefs that reject both the protectionism of Era 1 and the reductionism of Era 2. He provides a framework which is most useful in summarising what medicine might do to move on from Era 2 to a rebalanced Era 3.

The first action should be to reduce mandatory measurements. This is not a new idea. Measurements are part of what economists call transaction costs. This thinking was introduced by the John Commons in 1931, and Oliver Williamson's Transaction Cost Economics article, published in 2008 popularised the concept. It probably helped that Williamson won the Nobel prize for economics the next year. In short institutions that have high transaction costs, perform worse. This is very important, but the reality is there can be no going back to Era 1 where there is no measurement. A reduction is needed in measurement, not a cessation. There have been far too many instances of poor quality care in the NHS and in other health systems.

But we are out of balance. I read recently that a GP in England must submit 233 bits of data to receive all the elements of reimbursement which form their practice income. If we exclude public holidays, it is about one submission for every working day. Many of these are the outdated, non-evidence-based, and harmful Quality and Outcomes Framework, but that is far from the only culprit. Era 2 has brought with it excessive measurement, much of which is useless but nonetheless mandated.

This includes measurement linked to inspection. Just as Ofsted has become tainted as the inspector of schools, so has the Care Quality Commission in healthcare. It gives an illusion that the care provided achieves a pre-specified, evidence-based standard. It does nothing of the sort. It encourages rules-following, population-based, defensive decision making in which everybody with disease X should get treatment Y, and if an organisation has a piece of paper setting out a protocol then everybody is assumed to be following it. That is not the intention of those who produce clinical guidelines or introduced inspection or who advocated pay for performance to incentivise following

428

the evidence-based guidelines. But it is how many doctors have come to see "quality" care. They think if they do not do what NICE or the CQC says they should be doing, they are letting patients down. Plenty of people inside and outside health systems think the same.

If this book has done anything I hope it has comprehensively made the case for individualising decisions and described the many limitations of population-based decisions. These include people going for screening tests when they do not truly understand their probabilities of being helped or harmed, people having tests and follow up tests when they do not realise the imprecision of such measurements, and much treatment of risk factors for diseases and actual diseases when again their probabilities of being helped or harmed are not even considered, never mind fully explained and understood. It all costs a lot of time and money and involves a lot of work for patients. These are part of the transaction costs. We can do better, and there are many doctors already doing their best - despite the health system working against them – to do just that. The rest need a helping hand. Good quality care with good access at reasonable cost is the aim, and none is helped by intemperate measurement. It is as unwise and irresponsible as intemperate health care. The aim should be to measure only what matters, and mainly for learning.

The National Institute of Care Excellence (NICE) are part of all that. They rightly make population-level decisions when they are appraising a new technology and recommending whether it meets the cost effectiveness threshold for use across the NHS. But if we recognise the importance of individualising healthcare decisions, then why in national guidelines are there usually lots, and sometimes more than a hundred, recommendations in a guideline that is written or is usually interpreted as though those recommendations apply to everybody with the condition? Leaving aside that no health system has the capacity to implement the volume of recommendations, it is surely preferable for guidelines to just describe in absolute terms the baseline rate of events without treatment and with treatment, and then leave the decision about whether that recommendation is applicable and relevant to an individual patient and their clinician.

It should be possible to support individual decision making with decision aids in a form appropriate to the decision and the evidence. It might be appropriate in some circumstances to give an indication of what proportion of the total population with the condition it might be reasonable to see a treatment used. But the current way guidelines are written actually works against decisions being tailored to individual patients, especially when they are linked to NICE-generated QOF targets, which in turn are responsible for a large chunk of GP practice income.

Before I leave the topic of NICE, one of the great strengths of NICE has been its independence. Mike Rawlins and his successor David Haslam frequently talked about the importance of the payers leaving NICE to do its job without influence. They meant "There must be no government interference in the workings or the decisions of NICE".

In recent times there has been at least one instance where it seems that pressure has been put on NICE's decision making by the government.cccxii In the post-Brexit era there was a government-backed desire to see the UK as a "pharmaceutical powerhouse" where the results of the latest science could be readily deployed to improve the health of the population. Inclisiran, developed by Novartis, improved cholesterol but there were and still are no published randomised trials showing patients live longer or better with fewer heart attacks or strokes. Despite much pharmaceutical company-driven huffing and puffing to encourage uptake, the embedding of an evidence-based culture within UK prescribers seem to have won the day. Whilst big claims were made for 300,000 patients being treated, only around 4,000 prescriptions have been written. It works against everybody's interests to have NICE's independence threatened in the way it seems to have been.

Berwick suggests in Era 3 there should be a shift in the strategy towards quality. That will not happen without an upskilling of consultation skills, and that cannot happen without traditional approaches to teaching consultation skills being upgraded. Appreciating and communicating uncertainty and probability, risk communication, assessing how much patients truly want to be involved in decisions, ensuring ideas concerns, and expectations are routinely explicit, being able to have a realistic and accurate conversation about test results and decisions about screening – all these are not separate issues but an intrinsic part of consultation skills.

If we are to rebalance medicine, we need a spiral curriculum covering all these aspects that flows seamlessly from undergraduate courses to postgraduate training and onwards into lifelong learning. This will require a significant effort but forms part of an important new concordat between those who work in the NHS, patients, and the government. If the NHS is to get the resources it needs, then it must commit to doing things differently with those resources. Proper shared decision making is one of the few options that might just enable great care to be provided that is also affordable. If we are to make that change as part of Era 3 it needs a proper plan – and it should be based on another of Berwick's strength. We should use his life's work in constructing such a plan – we know lots about how to spread better practice now. We should use Improvement Science to construct the plan to get shared decision making everywhere, every time, for everyone.

If we want an important outcome measure for Era 3 then surveying patients and asking them how much they were involved in decisions made about their healthcare would be an important thing to measure. However, before doing that, we should show the patients an example of what a shared decision-making consultation really looks like before they answer the survey - because sadly many of them will not yet have experienced one.

Berwick then talks about civility. "Everything possible begins in civility" he writes. I heard recently about a GP registrar to had come to the UK as an international medical graduate. Her sister was in the UK too, with the rest of her family far away. Both of

431

them were barely thirty years old. The sister got cancer, but with modern, scientific treatment she had a good chance of a complete cure. She started a gruelling course of chemotherapy and she needed her sister to look after her. Of course her sister was more than willing to do that, and she requested to reduce her work from full time to part time, with the appropriate reduction in her salary. When her sister was well again she would return as soon as possible to full time work and training in the NHS. Her request was refused by the NHS.

Until we get serious about looking after the NHS workforce, nothing is possible. Morale is rock bottom. Everywhere. It clearly is not just pay, although that is of course a big factor. But improving terms and conditions helps with retention. The NHS needs to keep as many of the newly qualified doctors in the UK that it can, and it needs to keep as many of the older doctors it can from retiring early. The NHS cannot train new people fast enough to make a quick difference to the workforce crisis and the vacancy rates. Many NHS employees think the NHS is a very poor employer. There was a time when people were very proud to do their jobs in the NHS. It felt like one made a real difference. We can get back to that, but it needs a whole new strategy.

It is not just relationships with colleagues that need attention. Sarah Abrams, a junior doctor from South London told this to the British Medical Journal in 2023[cccxiii]:

"In 2021 I worked the Christmas weekend on call. Just three juniors were covering the wards of 500 patients. Two of us were expected to review 175 of those patients. The bleep was non-stop, and before you'd have the chance to finish one job, three more had been added to the list. Two patients fell and weren't seen for at least two or three hours, and one patient received blood an hour after they should have done because we just didn't have time to do everything. We didn't have time to sit down or eat lunch.

"In the last hour of my third 13-hour shift in a row I went to review one last patient, who was fine. But the patient in the neighbouring bed was very angry that he hadn't been seen and wasn't due to be seen because he had been well over the weekend. He told me I was a bad doctor, that I didn't care for

my patients, that I wouldn't care like this for my family, and that I should be ashamed of my work. I tried to reason with him and apologised, but I left crying and sat in a broom cupboard to think about what had happened. I think that represents what it's like to work every day, not just for a weekend on call at Christmas. You're really, really trying your hardest, but it is thankless. And this moral injury inevitably leads to burnout.

"The workforce retention crisis numbers are truly staggering, and, anecdotally, many of my friends are planning to leave. Of the eight juniors I started with, only two of us are planning to stay in the NHS."

I think it is appropriate to criticise the political decisions which have resulted in the NHS crisis that we are now in, but a better and wider understanding of the efforts made by the NHS staff who remain is only fair. Things may not currently be as everyone would like them to be, but for the moment everyone needs to cut some slack for people who are caring for patients whilst being frazzled, tired, and often without hope.

Berwick concludes that in Era 3 we are seeking a new moral ethos. Part of that has to be a recognition that endlessly looking for the ever more expensive science and technology to be the only way forward to improve health needs a serious rethink.

In the UK, according to the Office of National Statistics, health spend in 1997/6 was £76billion. In 2013/14 it was £163billion, a 63% increase. However, over the same time the increase in costs was not associated with equivalent improvements in health. Every year the Chief Medical Officer for England issues an annual report. Professor Sir Chris Whitty's, in 2020, comprised a wide range of graphs describing the health of the nation and how it had changed over time.

Improvements in life expectancy at birth were at a rate well below the increase in health spend, this continued until about 2012, but then they stalled and are now falling A similar pattern can be seen in most other developed countries. If we take the timeframe much further back then clean water, better nutrition, vaccinations against infections and eventually antibiotics provided big improvements in life expectancy in the first half of the 20th century.

Longevity of older generations largely reflects their experiences over their entire lives. While health care is particularly important in later life, it is a wider mix of factors – better incomes and living conditions, changes in behaviour (e.g. smoking, exercise, diet), as well as medical advances – that has led to many of the improvements in life expectancy. These are large, long-term, population-level effects. Reductions in smoking rates from the mid-1970s, advances in treatment of heart disease in the 1990s and, more recently, getting better at diagnosing and treating cancer have contributed to the gains in the second half of the 20th century.

But a consequence of having already achieved large gains in life expectancy is that it is becoming increasingly difficult to achieve further big improvements using scientific advances. We have a 21st Century problem and we will not be able to tackle it with 20th Century approaches.

Future life expectancy will be shaped by the lifetime experiences of the population today. The strongest influences on people's health are the social, economic, environmental, and commercial conditions of people's lives – the "wider determinants" of health that Professor Sir Michael Marmot has spent his life's work describing.cccxiv The complex and interrelated nature of these determinants of health makes measuring the impact of any single one on mortality challenging. The current trends that are likely to affect future life expectancy are the widening mortality rates associated with people's socioeconomic status. Life expectancy is much worse in deprived communities.

Current approaches to prevention often concentrate on technology-based screening programmes – for example breast, cervical and bowel screening programmes - in many developed countries. These have their drawbacks with many false positive tests when populations with low prevalence are screened, as discussed in earlier chapters. The National Screening Committee does a great job in assessing screening programmes and rejecting those who do more harm than good, but even for those programmes that are approved it is remarkably difficult as a patient to find clear descriptions of the benefits and risks of screening. Such descriptions are essential for individual consent. Without them many people simply accept the invitation (or not) without being aware of the true positive and true negative probabilities inherent in such testing. Both of those results could be regarded ethically as a "good" result, but people should also have easy access to the probabilities of having a false positive or false negative test when screened. Both of those would be regarded as a "bad" result by many.

Much national communication about such screening programmes simply exhorts people to attend screening, and much effort is extended to measure "success" by an increase in the proportion of the target population screened – without a proportionate and dispassionate measurement of the good and the harms done by screening. Perhaps if we are going to measure the success of screening programmes we should measure the proportion of those screened who had read an unbiased summary of the probability of true /false, positive/ negative results before being screened and who demonstrably understood those probabilities?

The second plank of prevention is the identification and modification of risk factors for the future development of disease. Being a smoker is the obvious one, but there are many, many others - alcohol consumption, blood pressure, cholesterol, obesity, type 2 diabetes, inactivity, loneliness, poverty and so on. Over the last forty years identifying these risk factors has become established as part of the normal routine of clinical practice, especially in primary care, and in England at least this work is incentivised through the pay for performance scheme that is the Quality and Outcomes framework. To the uninitiated this seems entirely right and proper. Prevention just must be better.

But there are significant unintended consequences. This risk factor identification work requires time and effort, and if NHS

435

staff are doing this work they are not available for diagnosing and treating those who are acutely ill or believe themselves to be ill. Given the current difficulties in accessing help for acute illness, that alone means there is a need to examine how and why we have created this monster of risk identification work, and whether it is doing the good that was intended.

When we ask that question we find some difficulties. Brief conversations with people who smoke and providing advice about smoking has about a 98% failure rate – that is, only about two people in 100 who are given that brief advice in an NHS consultation stop smoking. On the face of it, it seems crazy to spend time doing something that fails 98 times out of 100 and may be not welcomed at that time by the recipient of the advice. But if there are still 6 million adults who smoke and the advice is provided to all of them, that translates into 120,00 fewer smokers – and that must be a good thing. How do we do this smarter?

So many risk factors have now been identified and so ubiquitous are recommendations in NICE guidelines for health care professionals to identify them in their patients and try to change their patients lifestyle and behaviours that the work has actually become impossible. Prevention may be very attractive, and we would all support it, but in its current guise it is out of balance.

So there is a real dilemma. No one would wish to return to the days when people died from a stroke never having had their blood pressure taken which would have identified their hypertension which they might have had for many years. Early detection would have meant years of taking tablets and the risk of their side effects, but that treatment would have reduced the probability of them having a stroke or a heart attack but not abolished those risks. Many people taking the tablets to lower blood pressure would have been fine without the tablets, and other people taking the tablets would still have had the stroke or heart attack despite taking them. It's a difficult decision requiring great data and great consultation skills to explain the probabilities and uncertainties in terms the patient understands.

No one would wish to cancel an established, National Screening Committee recommended cancer screening programme because there are too many acutely ill people. But there is an urgent need now to re-examine the risk factor detection approaches currently in place, and the good and harms it does they have done. Can we do less, or do the same only much less frequently, or do we concentrate our efforts on those of the population who might be more motivated to change? Health promotion experts have known for decades that if people are already thinking about making a change, and they are offered support and encouragement to support that change, then the numbers of people who successfully make the change is much higher than in the population who are not thinking about the issue (yet).

But as part of that review, there is a new consideration that astonishingly has not be considered when these polices were created. The new consideration is "capacity". If we do not have the people to do the work, we cannot do the work.

Whilst we are thinking about prevention, much NHS work in people with long term conditions involves reviewing their progress. What if we asked patients when they thought it might be useful to have their next review? For many stable, long-term conditions, would it be harmful to review every year instead of every six months if that is the established routine, or every two years instead of annually, or in six months instead of every three, or........well, you get the picture? In the 20th Century the doctor would always make the determination about the optimum time to see the patient again based solely on habit or clinical expertise or using some other magical form of guess. The patient was simply the passive accepter of such decisions about what the review period should be – or not, because many patients do not attend for their review appointments. Well, that was the 20th Century way. We are now in the 21st Century, and in a capacity crisis. If the patient has a legitimate view on when their next appointment should happen, finding that out has inherent merit just from the ethical perspective of autonomy. And I'd hazard a decent wager that the overall effect would help free up capacity rather than create additional workload pressures.

Michael Marmot does not exclude there being a place for more technical aspects of ill-health detection but places it in the context of other social determinants of health. These are early years development, employment and especially having some control over one's work, living standards, communities, discrimination and environmental sustainability. These seven social determinants, alongside ill health prevention, results in the gradient of health outcomes across a population.

Thanks to Professor Marmot we have known this for decades, his work is now recognised internationally and at the highest levels of governments – he is both a Knight and a Companion of Honour.

It is not as if everyone with a reasonable set of circumstances pertaining to social determinants of health is guaranteed compression of morbidity, but when social inequalities are not addressed, compression of morbidity is more common. There can be no debate on this. Not only is there a strong social justice case for addressing health inequalities, there is also a pressing economic case. In 2010 Professor Marmot estimated that the annual cost of health inequalities was between £36 billion and £40 billion through lost taxes, welfare payments and NHS costs.

If the NHS is to survive and even thrive in the 21st Century there needs to be concerted action by national and local governments to reduce the steepness of the social gradient of health inequalities. Action is required on employment, income, communities, active transport, housing and sustainability – and perhaps a little bit of sensible early detection of disease based on technology. To rebalance medicine, whilst the science and the technology is brilliant, it needs to be accompanied by a better understanding of evidence and its limitations, better consultation skills, and a better understanding of human decision making and how it operates.

This is not just a nice thing to do. As Don Berwick writes, there is a moral case. And if we want the NHS to survive and then thrive we need a rebalanced approach to measurement, to prevention and towards individualised outcomes.

CHAPTER TWENTY
EIGHT

Goldilocks Medicine

Most people know the story of the English fairy tale Goldilocks. The story was first written down by English writer and poet Robert Southey, and first published anonymously as "The Story of the Three Bears" in 1837 in a volume of his writings called "The Doctor". Goldilocks found the bears' cottage in the woods where there were three beds, one of which was too big, one too small and a third which was "just right". Then she found three bowls of porridge, one of which was too hot, one was too cold and one was "just right".

The Goldilocks phenomenon is used in science. In astronomy if a celestial object orbits too close to its star (like Mercury), water on its surface boils away. If it is too far away (like Pluto), if there is any water it freezes. The 'Goldilocks Zone,' or habitable zone, is the "just right" range of distance with the right temperatures for water to remain liquid. Discoveries in the Goldilocks Zone, like the distant Earth-size planet Kepler-186f, are what scientists hope will lead us to water on distant planets, and one day life outside the solar system.

David Shulman is widely considered the first to have used the Goldlicks analogy in economics in a 1992 article called "The Goldilocks Economy: Keeping the Bears at Bay." A Goldilocks economy is characterized by growth, employment, and inflation being in balance. Ideal conditions are low unemployment; a steady increase in the prices of stocks, derivatives, bonds, and real estate (asset price inflation); low market interest rates; low inflation as measured by a consumer price index; and steady growth in the economy overall (gross domestic product). It can be challenging for central bankers and governments to engineer a Goldilocks economy since many factors need to come together for this economic state to exist. A Goldilocks economy is considered by some to only be achievable as a temporary state.

If, and I accept it is a big if, some short-term stability is achieved in the NHS and the working environment for health care professionals is improved so people see some hope for a worthwhile, manageable, and satisfying career in the NHS, then there is a requirement to address the 21st Century problems

441

health services face. Whilst organisation and funding are essential requirements of a well-functioning health system, only consistent use of softer, individualised, skills-based medicine can begin to truly address the big challenges medicine faces. Goldilocks Medicine has plenty of science, technology and evidence. But that is balanced by kindness, individualised care, person-centred consultations, shared understanding, and shared decision making. And to create the cognitive space for health care professionals to practice Goldilocks medicine the health system and those who have responsibility for funding it and for its quality need to be mature enough to move away data collection for the sake of it, and coercive, centralised inspection approaches.

Many aspects of medicine are not black or white, do or not do. But some are. There is one option for a 10 year old girl with an undisplaced fracture of her ankle. She needs a few weeks in a plaster cast and her body will heal well pretty much every time. The management of the fractured ankle does not involve a preference-sensitive decision, so whilst kindness and empathy for the patient and her parents is a given, exploring her ideas, concerns and expectations is less of a priority than stabilising the fracture with the cast, easing the pain, and sensitive conversations about how to manage the next few weeks of reduced mobility.

But in a 70 year old man with what seems to be a low-risk, probably very slow growing prostate cancer there are several treatment choices including no active treatment but with active monitoring, at least a couple of approaches to radiotherapy, and several approaches to surgery. This is where the patient needs help in understanding their condition, and what the treatment options are, together with their pros and cons. The patient, hopefully once the shock of the initial diagnosis subsides a little, is likely to have preferences for one approach or the other. That may result in a different approach than the health care professional might have chosen for themselves, and different patients will choose different options one from another. This is simply different people assessing the pros and cons of different options individually.

This can be difficult because both patient and clinician seek certainty when there is none. No one can predict which will be the best approach for this individual prostate cancer. Goldilocks Medicine makes explicit the uncertainty that is sometimes uncomfortable for humans, and therefore is so often currently glossed over. It is a world away from an approach which determines for everybody what the treatment should be because there is a randomised controlled trial which says one approach works best for groups of people.

In multimorbidity Goldilocks Medicine really helps to solve problems. Take the example of Mavis, who a year ago was a 90 year old woman who has been taking medicines to control her blood pressure for many years without difficulties. But then she spent six weeks in hospital with a chest infection, a urinary infection, a positive test for coronavirus, and severe anxiety and depression. She was also diagnosed with Parkinson's disease. Slowly she recovers and is discharged to a care home. She is less anxious and depressed but nowhere near her usual feisty and cheery demeanour. She has lost a lot of weight, is now unable to walk, and because of weight loss and poor nutrition is at risk of her skin breaking down and pressure sores developing. How do we best manage her problems?

We might, if we were focused on the science, wonder what her blood pressure control is like. After all, at 90 years old she is, merely just considering her age, at high risk of stroke or heart attack, both of which are associated with hypertension. National guidelines and pay for performance incentivise robust management of hypertension. But what if we asked Mavis what mattered to her?

When Mavis arrived at the Care Home she told the staff she could only manage to eat mashed potato, gravy and custard-because that was all she could manage of the food offered her in hospital. Cath the Cook said "If I just give you that I'll lose my job". After negotiation Mavis started eating a varied but pureed diet. Her antidepressant medication was adjusted to help with anxiety, and when it subsided she agreed it could be stopped.

Slowly her weight increased, her skin improved, her risk of developing pressure sores reduced, and she negotiated the removal of her technology-based ripple mattress which she disliked. The ripple mattress was the technical approach top pressure sores; the food was the better approach.

Her old, often cheeky personality began to re-emerge. She began instructing the nurses on how she liked her glaucoma eye drops to be inserted. "I'll make a sign for your back. It will say GB" she told a nurse after the eye drops one night. "Why GB?" said the puzzled nurse. "Because you're Getting Better at it" said Mavis with a grin.

Then Mavis got an appointment to go for her diabetic eye screening photograph. She had diligently attended every annual appointment for this unpleasant procedure for twenty years. Every single photograph had been normal, but the unthinking system was going to arrange ambulance and precious hospital time and resources to take another picture, and someone needed to go with her.

Mavis did not want to go. She had had her fill of hospitals and dreaded the probable wait for several hours for the ambulance to bring her home. There was a bit of negotiation involved and the staff settled for "not this year, we'll see how I am next year" rather than "forget it forever".

Emboldened by this new approach, Mavis then decided that the separate hospital appointments for her glaucoma and cataracts to be checked, for the thyroid cancer now many years ago, and for the diabetes clinic could also all be put into the "let's see how I am in a year" category. What mattered to Mavis was getting as much enjoyment out each day as she could, rather than sitting in a hospital outpatient clinic to yet again to be told by a complete stranger that from a technical perspective "It all looks fine" by whichever specialist doctor she was seeing that day. Seeing a doctor she did not know, who had never seen her before, and would never see her again because her or she would be working in a different hospital before Mavis's next appointment was due was simply not her priority. Mavis's priorities now were to be in her new home where she had a social life, where the magnificent Julie organised crafts, or music or bingo, and where the nurses and care assistants were around for a bit of banter.

Then she turned again to her medicines. She was starting to get back on her feet with help from the care staff, a bit of physiotherapy and a walking frame. Goodness knows if she could possibly get back to walking a little, but at least people were trying. But her lower legs were swollen with fluid. That did not help the efforts to get back walking, and Mavis did not like the feeling of swollen legs nor how they looked. A common side effects of one of her blood pressure tablets (amlodipine) is swollen legs.

There was a review by her new general practitioner. He was not keen on stopping the blood pressure medicine. He had apparently done this before with other patients and it had not gone well. The new hero was the Care of the Elderly consultant who came to see Mavis about how her Parkinson's was doing. She successfully stopped the Parkinson's medicines which were not doing much other than giving her nightmares. And then she reassured the Care Home staff that the probabilities were Mavis was much more likely to be harmed from the blood pressure tablets than get benefit from them.

Goldilocks medicine was what mattered was to Mavis. Some science and technology. But mixed with kindness, care and focussed her priorities. In time that made lots of aspects of her nursing care easier and quicker, and the health costs were a little lower. Some trips out in a wheelchair in a minibus were possible for ice cream on the seafront or a whizz round a garden centre followed by coffee and cake. It wasn't great being 91 in a care home, but it was as good as it could be.

All this was possible by doing less medicine. The concept is difficult and counterintuitive. It just does not seem logical to minds trained to think that more science and more technology is better, that less medicine can be better for people. But the evidence says it is. In a 2021 systematic review of "deprescribing" - reviewing medicines and stopping those of limited or no current value as judged by clinician and patient jointly - found Mavis-like medicine to be safe, feasible, well tolerated and led to important benefits.[cccxv] By the way, Mavis-like medicine does not use the term "frailty". The F-word has negative connotations for many people with multiple health challenges. They very much prefer to be asked about "what matters to them", and "what would a good day look like to you?". Call Mavis-like patients "frail" and they might just ask to have someone else looking after them.

Now I am not saying for one moment that we should abandon all of the scientifically - based framework on which medicine rests, or that it is desirable to stop all measurement of clinical activity. But what I am saying is that for some - perhaps for many - current aspects of medicine we have become imbalanced. We need to be neither too close to our medical sun nor too far away from it.

Making a diagnosis and constructing a patient-centred management plan is one of the most cognitively complex tasks a human being can undertake.[cccxvi] Only by finding out what the values and preferences of that individual patient are and aligning those with the treatment options do we end up with high quality clinical care. Shared decision making actually takes the pressure off making decisions.

The good news is that there are early but significant efforts being made so that the current variation in approaches deployed by health care professionals to individualising care is reduced. In England the Personalised Care Institute[cccxvii] and the NICE Shared Decision Making guideline[cccxviii] are of course to be welcomed. The Realistic Medicine approach in Scotland[cccxix] and the Welsh Value in Health[cccxx] seem to be making some headway. Internationally, Victor Montori from the Mayo Clinic in Rochester, in the United States writes "We must transform healthcare from an industrial activity into a deeply human one". His book "Why We Revolt" is a best seller. I co-authored a paper with the less catchy title "Making evidence-based medicine work for individual patients" in the British Medical Journal in 2016.[cccxxi] Eight years on, progress is indeed slow, but the chorus of voices is getting louder.

The British Medical Journal's "Too Much Medicine" initiative describes similar aims - to highlight the threat to human health posed by overdiagnosis and the waste of resources on unnecessary care. They say *"We are part of a movement of doctors, researchers, patients, and policymakers who want to describe, raise awareness of, and find solutions to the problem of too much medicine. Causes of too much medicine include expanded disease definitions, uncritical adoption of population screening, disease mongering and medicalisation, commercial vested interest, strongly held clinical beliefs, increased patient expectations, litigation, and fear of uncertainty and new technology. Winding back the harms of too much medicine invites clinicians to focus on those who are sick, and only intervene with those who are well when there is a strong case to do so."*

People are living much longer and healthier lives, while being repeatedly told to be anxious about many symptoms that "could be cancer" or heart disease or dementia or a host of other things to worry about. We do not talk about what makes for good health so much. Health would be much improved by a better lifestyle – diet, exercise, reducing alcohol, and so on, but of course the issue is that poverty impedes access to this for many.

Western medicine is in an existential crisis.........over interfering, protocol driven, increasingly expensive and verging on the unaffordable, and most importantly creating unfulfillable expectations of control over disease and death. Science and technology has created false idols of certainty and control. The inevitable uncertainty of life and disease has come to feel like a failing; the best science can do is improve the probability of cure and life, yet death at some point will definitely happen.

In other words, medicine is out of balance. The challenge is whether there is leadership prepared to take on the complex challenge of rebalancing medicine in all its aspects. No doubt it will take time – at least ten years.

But there is an enormous prize for making changes to medicine, and it might be the economic argument that makes rebalancing medicine a reality. In 2017 the Organisation for Economic Co-operation and Development calculated that 20% of health expenditure makes no or minimal contribution to good health outcomes.[cccxxii] Public funding for health services in England comes from the Department of Health and Social Care's budget. The Department's spending in 2022/23 was £181.7 billion. So potentially over £36billion is spent each year by the NHS in England which is of little or limited value.

How could that be? Evidence shows that if people are fully informed about the risks and benefits of treatment options they choose less treatment of more conservative treatment. And yet the medico-legal and financial incentives are aligned against shared decision making which in itself has medico-legal precedent and professional regulatory requirements. Work is required to remove the perverse incentives to shared decision making, and work is required to improve the understanding of uncertainty and risk, and to improve consultation skills.

A removal of large portions of unnecessary measurement whilst retaining those few measures that have value would move medicine more towards Don Berwick's third age of medicine and free up the time of clinicians and support staff within the NHS. Some measurement will still be required, because the identification and rectifying of unwarranted variations (both under-use and over-use) remain key to the provision of high quality care.

But much more than that is required to support the most valuable asses health and social care has – the people who work in health and social care. It is not just about pay, but an urgent, realistic review of pay and conditions is required. Undoubtedly some sectors of the workforce remain disadvantaged in terms of salary, but there is much more to be done in supporting existing staff and encouraging ongoing recruitment to the huge number of current vacancies.

Just as one example, the current administrative arrangements for allocation of doctors' postgraduate training posts operate with gross insensitivity to the reasonable needs of the workforce far too often. Such doctors feel unsupported, and it is no surprise that many leave medicine or leave the UK to practice medicine in another country. We simply cannot afford to lose our most valuable assets, and it is obvious that we should therefore treat them like valuable assets. The people who look after us when we need looking after, need to be looked after much better. And when that is the case there can be an agreed push to increase the all-too-important continuity of care which matters so much to how care feels, but also has major benefits in terms of reducing unnecessary tests and referrals to hospitals, but also reduces premature mortality.

We could also rebalance our approach to prevention and gain a great deal. Far too little attention is paid to addressing Michael Marmot's social determinants of health, and arguably we think of prevention as primarily being scans and blood tests. We could flip this on its head and do much more to support healthy, productive lives. And in addition, whilst no one would want to take away existing screening programmes, better information to support the making of truly informed decisions is required. I have personally been the recipient of invitations to participate in a number of national screening programmes. Those invitations consist of encouragement to attend. I have never received materials that adequately set out the benefits and risks of the screening programme, for example with the probabilities explained in natural frequencies and with details of the false positive and false negative rates.

Above all, rebalancing medicine is not about failing to offer treatments that have been demonstrated to be reasonably safe, reasonably effective, and reasonably cost-effective. Indeed the opposite is true; if in health and social care there is not a move towards rebalancing medicine then the costs of an increasingly wasteful service become unaffordable, care becomes ever more rationed and even more fragmented, quality of care decreases and those delivering care become even more disenchanted with their work. This downward spiral has to be halted and soon.

I hope that with political will a new concordat can be created between politicians fully committed to the founding principles of the NHS, those who deliver care, and the patients and public. It will take time to restore the faith of all parties in the NHS, but for those of us who believe that the creation of the NHS is one of the greatest achievements of any civilisation, rebalancing medicine is a prospect truly worth pursuing.

ACKNOWLEDGENTS

I recently read "Walking Home" by the Poet Laureate, Simon Armitage. For some unfathomable reason - his wife suspects a mid-life crisis - he decided to walk the Pennine Way from north to south, and to finance his trip entirely from donations made at poetry recitals he gives on the way. The book is an account of his journey, all 250 miles of it from Kirk Yetholm just over the Scottish border in the Cheviot Hills to Edale in Derbyshire, along the spine of the Pennines and through some of the wildest country in England.

I particularly was struck by his retelling of a story about his mother who years previously was on walking holiday in Ireland. Her party set off for the days walk and as they left the village a black Labrador trotted up and accompanied them. To start with they enjoyed the playful dog's presence, but as the morning continued they became concerned that the dog was increasingly far from home. They began to shout at it to go back, and waved their arms ineffectually. The dog kept trotting along, all be it now at a distance because the party - in addition to continuing verbal and non-verbal discouragement - were now resorting to throwing sticks in its general direction, and even stones. And before anyone contacts the Royal Society for the Prevention of Cruelty to Animals, they were making sure to miss the dog because it was, after all, a Church walking holiday. Eventually, as the village at the end of the twenty mile walk hove into view, the dog scampered past them and nudged its way in through the back door of one of the first village houses. Despite the daunting journey, and all the obstacles placing in its way by well-meaning humans, the dog had found its way back home, and joy was unconfined at his safe return.

As a metaphor it works for me. I am very glad have finally nudged my own back door open and finished this book. I would like to thank many colleagues who have helped me down the years; there are too many of you to mention and it would be invidious to pick out any individuals. Thank you one and all. And thank you to the learners I have had, and still have, the privilege of attempting to teach. You have actually taught me far more than I have taught you. And of course, the patients who I tried to help, and who also taught me so much. I would be a better doctor for them now, because I understand more about human decision making, and because I am no longer so sleep-deprived. But I did the best that I could at the time, and did not make too many mistakes, thankfully.

It has taken me ten years to write this book, and there have been at least four previous versions. My aim was to keep the book as easy a read as possible, as "reference-light" as possible, and a long way from an academic tome. I hope with this version I have done some justice to the importance of both science and technology and the need for individualising care – alongside the complexity of health decision making, both at population, for localities, and for individuals. I have, of course, relied much on the work of others and that work should be properly acknowledged. With regret that means over 300 references. I hope I have not missed anyone out. If I have, *mea culpa*.

Dr Simon Tobin helped me with early clinical material for an earlier version of this book, and I am sorry that those efforts came to nought. I hope the eventual format is useful to you and yours. James McCormack in Vancouver generously gave of his time in reviewing the last but one edition of this book. It took me some time to realise that as usual he was right, and I hope this version meets with his approval. Julian Treadwell gave me permission to reproduce from "GP Evidence". My Yorkshire colleague Ramesh Mehay gave permission to reproduce some figures of consultation models chapter from his magnificent book "The Essential Handbook for GP Training and Education".

The Nicholas Timmins, Mike Rawlins and John Appleby book "A Terrible Beauty; A Short History of NICE" was an enormous help with Chapter 13. I hope combining my brief precis of that enlightening work with my own experiences of working with and then for NICE in those days has done it justice.

Richard Lehman, former Banbury GP, former Professor of Shared Understanding of Medicine at Birmingham University, and hero to many for his years of summarising the week's new research in the BMJ has been a constant supporter of this book. Without his nudges and gentle chidings I doubt I would ever have got to the end. Thank you, Richard.

There are many people who contribute to the "Overdiagnosis" e-mail discussion group of the Royal College of General Practitioners who in recent years have stimulated and encouraged me, even if many did not realise it. Thank you one and all. It's a great group.

And of course, thanks go to Joan, to Herbert, to Mavis, and to the dearly beloved Helen. There are indeed two cats in our yard, and everything is certainly easier because of you.

References

i

https://www.ons.gov.uk/peoplepopulationandcommunity/birthsdeat
hsandmarriages/lifeexpectancies/articles/howhaslifeexpectancychan
gedovertime/2015-09-09 (accessed 26th February 2024)

ii https://www.nice.org.uk/guidance/cg124/evidence/full-guideline-
pdf-183081997 (accessed 26th February 2024)

iii https://www.ncbi.nlm.nih.gov/pmc/articles/PMC4064952/
(accessed 26th February 2024)

iv https://academic.oup.com/eurheartj/article/25/19/1734/528714
(accessed 26th February 2024)

v https://pubmed.ncbi.nlm.nih.gov/12698012/ (accessed 26th
February 2024)

vi

https://www.ahajournals.org/doi/full/10.1161/strokeaha.115.01113
9 (accessed 26th February 2024)

vii Sommers L, Launer J. In: Sommers L, Launer J, eds. Clinical
uncertainty in primary care: the challenge of collaborative
engagement.Springer, 2013: 293-304. doi:10.1007/978-1-4614-6812-
7_13

viii Kissick WL. Medicine's Dilemmas: Infinite Needs versus Finite
Resources. Yale University Press; 1994.

ix Byock Ira. The Best Care Possible: A Physician's Quest to Transform
Care Through the End of Life. Avery, 2012.

x https://www.youtube.com/watch?v=dXGnvbsfuFM (accessed 26th
February 2024)

xi https://en.wikipedia.org/wiki/History_of_medicine (accessed 26th
February 2024)

xii https://bcmj.org/premise/history-bloodletting (accessed 26th
February 2024)

xiii Jessney B. Joseph Lister (1827-1912): a pioneer of antiseptic
surgery remembered a century after his death. J Med Biogr. 2012
Aug;20(3):107-10. doi: 10.1258/jmb.2011.011074. PMID: 22892302.

xiv Kadar N. Rediscovering Ignaz Philipp Semmelweis (1818-1865). Am J Obstet Gynecol. 2019 Jan;220(1):26-39. doi: 10.1016/j.ajog.2018.11.1084. Epub 2018 Nov 13. PMID: 30444981.

xv Cameron D, Jones IG. John Snow, the broad street pump and modern epidemiology. Int J Epidemiol. 1983 Dec;12(4):393-6. doi: 10.1093/ije/12.4.393. PMID: 6360920.

xvi Ellis H. Florence Nightingale: creator of modern nursing and public health pioneer. J Perioper Pract. 2020 May;30(5):145-146. doi: 10.1177/1750458919851942. Epub 2019 May 28. PMID: 31135282.

xvii Goodman NW. John Shaw Billings: creator of Index Medicus and medical visionary. J R Soc Med. 2018 Mar;111(3):98-102. doi: 10.1177/0141076818758615. PMID: 29521560; PMCID: PMC5846945.

xviii Duffy TP. The Flexner Report--100 years later. Yale J Biol Med. 2011 Sep;84(3):269-76. PMID: 21966046; PMCID: PMC3178858.

xix Misa, T. Computer science: Digital dawn. Nature 483, 32–33 (2012). https://doi.org/10.1038/483032a

xx Sharp D. Thomas Wakley (1795-1862): a biographical sketch. Lancet. 2012 May 19;379(9829):1914-21. doi: 10.1016/S0140-6736(12)60526-1. Epub 2012 May 16. PMID: 22595800.

xxi Tbakhi A, Amr SS. Ibn Al-Haytham: father of modern optics. Ann Saudi Med. 2007 Nov-Dec;27(6):464-7. doi: 10.5144/0256-4947.2007.464. PMID: 18059131; PMCID: PMC6074172.

xxii Sallam HN. Aristotle, godfather of evidence-based medicine. Facts Views Vis Obgyn. 2010;2(1):11-9. PMID: 25206962; PMCID: PMC4154333.

xxiii Harris JC. Galileo Galilei: scientist and artist. Arch Gen Psychiatry. 2010 Aug;67(8):770-1. doi: 10.1001/archgenpsychiatry.2010.95. PMID: 20679584.

xxiv Tröhler U (2003). James Lind and scurvy: 1747 to 1795. JLL Bulletin: Commentaries on the history of treatment evaluation. https://www.jameslindlibrary.org/articles/james-lind-and-scurvy-1747-to-1795/

xxv Hróbjartsson A, Gøtzsche, PC, Gluud, C. The controlled clinical trial turns 100 years: Fibiger's trial of serum treatment of diphtheria. BMJ 1998; 317: 1243 doi: https://doi.org/10.1136/bmj.317.7167.1243.

xxvi Tan SY, Tatsumura Y. Alexander Fleming (1881-1955): Discoverer of penicillin. Singapore Med J. 2015 Jul;56(7):366-7. doi: 10.11622/smedj.2015105. PMID: 26243971; PMCID: PMC4520913.

xxvii Bennett JW, Chung KT. Alexander Fleming and the discovery of penicillin. Adv Appl Microbiol. 2001;49:163-84. doi: 10.1016/s0065-2164(01)49013-7. PMID: 11757350.

xxviii Ligon BL. Penicillin: its discovery and early development. Semin Pediatr Infect Dis. 2004 Jan;15(1):52-7. doi: 10.1053/j.spid.2004.02.001. PMID: 15175995.

xxix Ligon BL. Sir Alexander Fleming: Scottish researcher who discovered penicillin. Semin Pediatr Infect Dis. 2004 Jan;15(1):58-64. doi: 10.1053/j.spid.2004.02.002. PMID: 15175996.

xxx Gaynes R. The Discovery of Penicillin—New Insights After More Than 75 Years of Clinical Use. Emerg Infect Dis. 2017 May;23(5):849–53. doi: 10.3201/eid2305.161556. PMCID: PMC5403050.

xxxi Michael Holroyd, The Guardian 13 July 2012, "Bernard Shaw and his lethally absurd doctor's dilemma". (Accessed 27th February 2024)

xxxii Walker NM. Edward Almroth Wright. J R Army Med Corps. 2007 Mar;153(1):16-7. doi: 10.1136/jramc-153-01-05. PMID: 17575871.

xxxiii Gelpi A, Gilbertson A, Tucker JD. Magic bullet: Paul Ehrlich, Salvarsan and the birth of venereology. Sex Transm Infect. 2015 Feb;91(1):68-9. doi: 10.1136/sextrans-2014-051779. PMID: 25609467; PMCID: PMC4318855.

xxxiv Wainright M, Swan HT. Medical History, 1986, 30: 42-56. https://www.ncbi.nlm.nih.gov/pmc/articles/PMC1139580/pdf/medhist00072-0046.pdf. (Accessed 27th February 2024)

xxxv Ligon BL. Sir Howard Walter Florey--the force behind the development of penicillin. Semin Pediatr Infect Dis. 2004 Apr;15(2):109-14. doi: 10.1053/j.spid.2004.04.001. PMID: 15185195.

xxxvi Fletcher C. The First Clinical Use of Penicillin. BMJ 1984; 289: 1721-4. https://www.bmj.com/content/bmj/289/6460/1721.full.pdf. (Accessed 27th February 2024).

xxxvii Florey ME, Florey H. General and local administration of penicillin. Lancet 1943; 389-397. https://www.jameslindlibrary.org/wp-data/uploads/2014/07/Floery_ME_1943.pdf. (Accessed 27th February 2024).

xxxviii
https://archive.ph/20120630175532/http://archive.sciencewatch.co
m/interviews/norman_heatly.htm (Accessed 27th February 2024).

xxxix Karamitsos DT. The story of insulin discovery. Diabetes Res Clin
Pract. 2011 Aug;93 Suppl 1:S2-8. doi: 10.1016/S0168-8227(11)70007-
9. PMID: 21864746.

xl Rosenfeld L. Insulin: discovery and controversy. Clin Chem. 2002
Dec;48(12):2270-88. PMID: 12446492.

xli Crystal P. A History of the World in 100 Pandemics, Plagues and
Epidemics. Pen & Sword Books,Yorkshire. 2021.

xlii Sakula A. Robert Koch: centenary of the discovery of the tubercle
bacillus, 1882. Thorax. 1982 Apr;37(4):246-51. doi:
10.1136/thx.37.4.246. PMID: 6180494; PMCID: PMC459292.

xliii Riesz PB. The life of Wilhelm Conrad Roentgen. AJR Am J
Roentgenol. 1995 Dec;165(6):1533-7. doi:
10.2214/ajr.165.6.7484601. PMID: 7484601.

xliv Glaziou P, Floyd K, Raviglione M.Trends in tuberculosis in the UK.
Thorax 2018;73:702-703.

xlv Wainwright M. Streptomycin: discovery and resultant
controversy. Hist Philos Life Sci. 1991;13(1):97-124. PMID: 1882032.

xlvi http://www.nytimes.com/2012/06/12/science/notebooks-shed-
light-on-an-antibiotic-discovery-and-a-mentors-
betrayal.html?ref=scienc

xlvii Schatz, A.: The True Story of the Discovery of Streptomycin:
Actinomycetes: Vol. IV, No. 2: 27-39: August 1993

xlviii Cramer RB (1992). What it takes : the way to the White
House (1st ed.). New York: Random House. pp. 110–111. ISBN 978-0-
394-56260-5.

xlix Crofton J. The MRC randomized trial of streptomycin and its
legacy: a view from the clinical front line. J R Soc Med. 2006
Oct;99(10):531-4. doi: 10.1177/014107680609901017. PMID:
17021304; PMCID: PMC1592068.

l Hill AB. Suspended judgment. Memories of the British Streptomycin
Trial in Tuberculosis. The first randomized clinical trial. Control Clin
Trials. 1990 Apr;11(2):77-9. doi: 10.1016/0197-2456(90)90001-i.
PMID: 2161313.

li https://www.gwern.net/docs/statistics/causality/1990-hill.pdf (accessed 29th May 2024)

lii http://select.nytimes.com/gst/abstract.html?res=F70D1EFF3E5D117 B93C2AA1789D95F448585F9 (accessed 29th May 2024)

liii https://www.theguardian.com/education/2002/nov/02/research.hig hereducation. (Accessed 27th February 2024).

liv Bothwell LE, Greene JA, Podolsky SH, Jones DS. Assessing the Gold Standard--Lessons from the History of RCTs. N Engl J Med. 2016 Jun 2;374(22):2175-81. doi: 10.1056/NEJMms1604593. PMID: 27248626.

lv Sepkowitz KA. One hundred years of Salvarsan. N Engl J Med. 2011 Jul 28;365(4):291-3. doi: 10.1056/NEJMp1105345. PMID: 21793743.

lvi Ross JE, Tomkins SM. The British reception of Salvarsan. J Hist Med Allied Sci. 1997 Oct;52(4):398-423. doi: 10.1093/jhmas/52.4.398. PMID: 9444923.

lvii Ferner RE, Aronson JK. Medicines legislation and regulation in the United Kingdom 1500-2020. Br J Clin Pharmacol. 2023 Jan;89(1):80-92. doi: 10.1111/bcp.15497. Epub 2022 Sep 23. PMID: 35976677.

lviii Barkan ID. Industry invites regulation: the passage of the Pure Food and Drug Act of 1906. Am J Public Health. 1985 Jan;75(1):18-26. doi: 10.2105/ajph.75.1.18. PMID: 3881052; PMCID: PMC1646146.

lix Wax PM. Elixirs, diluents, and the passage of the 1938 Federal Food, Drug and Cosmetic Act. Ann Intern Med. 1995 Mar 15;122(6):456-61. doi: 10.7326/0003-4819-122-6-199503150-00009. PMID: 7856995.

lx Greene JA, Podolsky SH. Reform, regulation, and pharmaceuticals--the Kefauver-Harris Amendments at 50. N Engl J Med. 2012 Oct 18;367(16):1481-3. doi: 10.1056/NEJMp1210007. PMID: 23075174; PMCID: PMC4101807.

lxi Watts G. Frances Oldham Kelsey. Lancet. 2015 Oct 3;386(10001):1334. doi: 10.1016/S0140-6736(15)00339-6. PMID: 26460767.

lxii https://www.bmj.com/content/bmj/2/5256/855.full.pdf (Accessed 27th February 2024).

lxiii Stavrou A, Challoumas D, Dimitrakakis G. Archibald Cochrane (1909-1988): the father of evidence-based medicine. Interact Cardiovasc Thorac Surg. 2014 Jan;18(1):121-4. doi: 10.1093/icvts/ivt451. Epub 2013 Oct 18. PMID: 24140816; PMCID: PMC3867052.

lxiv Hill GB. Archie Cochrane and his legacy. An internal challenge to physicians' autonomy? J Clin Epidemiol. 2000 Dec;53(12):1189-92. doi: 10.1016/s0895-4356(00)00253-5. PMID: 11146263.

lxv https://community.cochrane.org/archie-cochrane-name-behind-cochrane (Accessed 27th February 2024).

lxvi Cochrane AL. Sickness in Salonica: my first, worst, and most successful clinical trial. BMJ 289:1726-1727.

lxvii Cochrane AL (1950). Methods of investigating the connections between dust and disease. In: The application of scientific methods to industrial and service medicine. London: Medical Research Council, p 97-100.

lxviii
https://www.bmj.com/content/bmj/suppl/2015/05/18/bmj.h2639.DC1/David_L_Sackett_Interview_in_2014-15.pdf (Accessed 29th May 2024)

lxix Chalmers TC, Eckhardt RD, Reynolds WE, Cigarroa JG, Jr, Deane N, Reifenstein RW, Smith CW, Davidson CS (1955). The treatment of acute infectious hepatitis. Controlled studies of the effects of diet, rest, and physical reconditioning on the acute course of the disease and on the incidence of relapses and residual abnormalities. Journal of Clinical Investigation 34:1163-1235.

lxx https://www.ncbi.nlm.nih.gov/pmc/articles/PMC1705173/ (Accessed 27th February 2024)

lxxihttps://www.linkedin.com/pulse/worlds-most-cited-scientists-dr-john-morley/ (Accessed 27th February 2024)

lxxii https://jamanetwork.com/journals/jama/article-abstract/400956?redirect=true (Accessed 27th February 2024)

lxxiii Macher D, Papousek I, Ruggeri K, Paechter M. Statistics anxiety and performance: blessings in disguise. Front Psychol. 2015 Aug 4;6:1116. doi: 10.3389/fpsyg.2015.01116. PMID: 26300813; PMCID: PMC4523713.

lxxiv Connor H. John Graunt F.R.S. (1620-74): The founding father of human demography, epidemiology and vital statistics. J Med Biogr. 2022 Feb 15:9677720221079826. doi: 10.1177/09677720221079826. Epub ahead of print. PMID: 35167377.

lxxv Stone MJ. The wisdom of Sir William Osler. Am J Cardiol. 1995 Feb 1;75(4):269-76. doi: 10.1016/0002-9149(95)80034-p. PMID: 7832137.

lxxvi Winkelstein W Jr. Vignettes of the history of epidemiology: Three firsts by Janet Elizabeth Lane-Claypon. Am J Epidemiol. 2004 Jul 15;160(2):97-101. doi: 10.1093/aje/kwh185. PMID: 15234929.

lxxvii Winkelstein W Jr. Janet Elizabeth Lane-Claypon: a forgotten epidemiologic pioneer. Epidemiology. 2006 Nov;17(6):705. doi: 10.1097/01.ede.0000239729.38570.10. PMID: 17068415.

lxxviii Paneth N, Susser E, Susser M. Origins and early development of the case-control study: Part 1, Early evolution. Soz Praventivmed. 2002;47(5):282-8. doi: 10.1007/pl00012638. PMID: 12512221.

lxxix https://api.pageplace.de/preview/DT0400.9781498768597_A374064 86/preview-9781498768597_A37406486.pdf (Accessed 29th May 2024)

lxxx Press DJ, Pharoah P. Risk factors for breast cancer: a reanalysis of two case-control studies from 1926 and 1931. Epidemiology. 2010 Jul;21(4):566-72. doi: 10.1097/EDE.0b013e3181e08eb3. PMID: 20498604.

lxxxi Frost WH. Risk of persons in familial contact with pulmonary tuberculosis. Am J Public Health 1933; 23: 426–32.

lxxxii https://www.bmj.com/content/suppl/2005/07/28/331.7511.295.DC1 (Accessed 27th February 2024)

lxxxiii Doll, R. 1936. Medical Statistics. St.Thomas's Hosp. Gaz., 294–97.

lxxxiv https://www.bmj.com/content/300/6733/1183 (Accessed 27th February 2024).

lxxxv https://www.bmj.com/content/300/6734/1256 (Accessed 27th February 2024).

lxxxvi https://www.bmj.com/content/300/6735/1324 (Accessed 27th February 2024).

lxxxvii https://www.bmj.com/content/300/6736/1385 (Accessed 27th February 2024).

lxxxviii https://www.bmj.com/content/300/6737/1449 (Accessed 27th February 2024).

lxxxix https://www.stats.ox.ac.uk/~snijders/Doll2002.pdf (Accessed 27th February 2024).

xc Wynder EL, Graham EA. Tobacco smoking as a possible etiologic factor in bronchiogenic carcinoma; a study of 684 proved cases. J Am Med Assoc. 1950 May 27;143(4):329-36. doi: 10.1001/jama.1950.02910390001001. PMID: 15415260.

xci Doll R, Hill AB. Smoking and carcinoma of the lung; preliminary report. Br Med J. 1950 Sep 30;2(4682):739-48. doi: 10.1136/bmj.2.4682.739. PMID: 14772469; PMCID: PMC2038856.

xcii van Hecke O, Smith BH, Sullivan FM. Lessons from Mackenzie that still resonate. Br J Gen Pract. 2013 Mar;63(608):158-9. doi: 10.3399/bjgp13X664423. PMID: 23561780; PMCID: PMC3582972.

xciii Kodama K, Mabuchi K, Shigematsu I. A long-term cohort study of the atomic-bomb survivors. J Epidemiol. 1996 Aug;6(3 Suppl):S95-105. doi: 10.2188/jea.6.3sup_95. PMID: 8800280.

xciv Mahmood SS, Levy D, Vasan RS, Wang TJ. The Framingham Heart Study and the epidemiology of cardiovascular disease: a historical perspective. Lancet. 2014 Mar 15;383(9921):999-1008. doi: 10.1016/S0140-6736(13)61752-3. Epub 2013 Sep 29. PMID: 24084292; PMCID: PMC4159698.

xcv Dawber TR, Moore FE, Mann GY. Coronary heart disease in the Framingham study. Am J Public Health Nations Health. 1957 Apr;47(4 Pt 2):4-24. doi: 10.2105/ajph.47.4_pt_2.4. PMID: 13411327; PMCID: PMC1550985.

xcvi Bergman NA. Michael Faraday and his contribution to anesthesia. Anesthesiology. 1992 Oct;77(4):812-6. doi: 10.1097/00000542-199210000-00027. PMID: 1416178.

xcvii López-Valverde A, Montero J, Albaladejo A, Gómez de Diego R. The discovery of surgical anesthesia: discrepancies regarding its authorship. J Dent Res. 2011 Jan;90(1):31-4. doi: 10.1177/0022034510385239. Epub 2010 Oct 12. PMID: 20940364.

xcviii Edwards ML, Jackson AD. The Historical Development of Obstetric Anesthesia and Its Contributions to Perinatology. Am J Perinatol. 2017 Feb;34(3):211-216. doi: 10.1055/s-0036-1585409. Epub 2016 Jul 19. PMID: 27434694.

xcix World Medical Association. World Medical Association Declaration of Helsinki: ethical principles for medical research involving human subjects. JAMA. 2013 Nov 27;310(20):2191-4. doi: 10.1001/jama.2013.281053. PMID: 24141714.

c https://pharmaphorum.com/r-d/a_history_of_the_pharmaceutical_industry (Accessed 29th May 2024).

ci Druss BG, Marcus SC. Growth and decentralization of the medical literature: implications for evidence-based medicine. J Med Libr Assoc. 2005 Oct;93(4):499-501. PMID: 16239948; PMCID: PMC1250328.

cii Covell DG, Uman GC, Manning PR (1985). Information needs in office practice: are they being met? Annals of Internal Medicine 103:596-599.

ciii Osheroff JA, Forsythe DE, Buchanan BG, Bankowitz RA, Blumenfeld BH, Miller RA (1991). Physicians' information needs: analysis of questions posed during clinical teaching. Annals of Internal Medicine 114:576-581.

civ Antman EM, Lau J, Kupelnick B, Mosteller F, Chalmers TC (1992). A comparison of results of meta-analyses of randomised control trials and recommendations of clinical experts. Treatments for myocardial infarction. JAMA 268:240-248.

cv Oxman AD, Guyatt GH (1993). The science of reviewing research. Annals of the New York Academy of Sciences 703:125-134.

cvi Davis D, O'Brien MA, Freemantle N, Wolf FM, Mazmanian P, Taylor-Vaisey A (1999). Impact of formal continuing medical education: do conferences, workshops, rounds, and other traditional continuing education activities change physician behaviour or health care outcomes? JAMA 282:867-874.

cvii Haynes RB (1993). Where's the meat in clinical journals? ACP Journal Club 119:A-22-23.

cviii Alison Glover J. The incidence of tonsillectomy in school children. 1938. Vol. 31. Proceedings of the Royal Society of Medicin (pg. 1219-36). (Reprinted Int J Epidemiol) 2008;37:09–19

cix John E. Wennberg Tracking Medicine: A Researcher's Quest to Understand Health Care 1st Edition. 2010.Oxford University Press.

cx https://www.kingsfund.org.uk/publications/whats-happening-life-expectancy-england (Accessed 29th February 2024)

cxi https://data.worldbank.org/indicator/SP.DYN.CBRT.IN?locations=GB (Accessed 29th February 2024)

cxii https://www.nuffieldtrust.org.uk/chapter/inheritance (Accessed 29th February 2024)

cxiii Weisz G, Cambrosio A, Keating P, Knaapen L, Schlich T, Tournay VJ. The emergence of clinical practice guidelines. Milbank Q. 2007 Dec;85(4):691-727. doi: 10.1111/j.1468-0009.2007.00505.x. PMID: 18070334; PMCID: PMC2690350.

cxiv Samanta A, Samanta J. Legal standard of care: a shift from the traditional Bolam test. Clin Med (Lond). 2003 Sep-Oct;3(5):443-6. doi: 10.7861/clinmedicine.3-5-443. PMID: 14601944; PMCID: PMC4953641.

cxv https://en.wikipedia.org/wiki/MEDLINE

cxvi O'Rourke K. An historical perspective on meta-analysis: dealing quantitatively with varying study results. J R Soc Med. 2007 Dec;100(12):579-82. doi: 10.1177/0141076807100012020. PMID: 18065712; PMCID: PMC2121629.

cxvii Antman EM, Lau J, Kupelnick B, Mosteller F, Chalmers TC. A comparison of results of meta-analyses of randomized control trials and recommendations of clinical experts. Treatments for myocardial infarction. JAMA. 1992 Jul 8;268(2):240-8. PMID: 1535110.

cxviii Sackett DL, Rosenberg WM, Gray JA, Haynes RB, Richardson WS. Evidence based medicine: what it is and what it isn't. BMJ. 1996 Jan 13;312(7023):71-2. doi: 10.1136/bmj.312.7023.71. PMID: 8555924; PMCID: PMC2349778.

cxix 9 Ways To Reduce Unwarranted Variation Managed Care Magazine, November 2003. (Accessed 29th February 2024) cxx Donabedian A. Evaluating the quality of medical care. 1966. Milbank Q. 2005;83(4):691-729. doi: 10.1111/j.1468-0009.2005.00397.x. PMID: 16279964; PMCID: PMC2690293.

cxxi Lunny C, Ramasubbu C, Puil L, Liu T, Gerrish S, Salzwedel DM, et al. (2021) Over half of clinical practice guidelines use non-systematic methods to inform recommendations: A methods study. PLoS ONE 16(4): e0250356. https://doi.org/10.1371/journal.pone.0250356

cxxii Robbins, Lionel. An Essay on the Nature and Significance of Economic Science. Ludwig von Mises Institute. p. 15. ISBN 978-1-61016-039-1.

cxxiii https://en.wikipedia.org/wiki/The_Wealth_of_Nations (Accessed 29th February 2024).

cxxiv Savedoff WD. Kenneth Arrow and the birth of health economics. Bull World Health Organ. 2004 Feb;82(2):139-40. Epub 2004 Mar 16. PMID: 15042237; PMCID: PMC2585899.

cxxv Greenhalgh, T., Snow, R., Ryan, S. et al. Six 'biases' against patients and carers in evidence-based medicine. BMC Med 13, 200 (2015). https://doi.org/10.1186/s12916-015-0437-x

cxxvi Foundations of Cost-Effectiveness Analysis for Health and Medical Practices. Milton C. Weinstein and William B. Stason, New England Journal of Medicine, March 31 1977 pp 716 -721

cxxvii Maynard A. Alan Williams. BMJ. 2005 Jul 2;331(7507):51. PMCID: PMC558550.

cxxviii Richmond C, Teasdale G. William Bryan Jennett. BMJ. 2008 Mar 1;336(7642):512. doi: 10.1136/bmj.39500.632384.BE. PMCID: PMC2258384.

cxxx Timmins N, Rawlins M, Appleby J. A Terrible Beauty; A Short History of NICE. https://f1000research.com/documents/6-915 (Accessed 29th February 2024)

cxxxi https://assets.publishing.service.gov.uk/government/uploads/system/uploads/attachment_data/file/259812/ambition.pdf (Accessed 30th May 2024).

cxxxii Shaw Q. On aphorisms. Br J Gen Pract. 2009 Dec 1;59(569):954–5. doi: 10.3399/bjgp09X473312. PMCID: PMC2784544.

cxxxiii Goldacre Ben. Bad Pharma: How Drug Companies Mislead Doctors and Harm Patients. Harper Collins. London. 2012.

cxxxiv McGettigan P, Golden J, Fryer J, Chan R, Feely J. Prescribers prefer people: The sources of information used by doctors for prescribing suggest that the medium is more important than the message. Br J Clin Pharmacol. 2001 Feb;51(2):184-9. doi: 10.1111/j.1365-2125.2001.01332.x. PMID: 11259994; PMCID: PMC2014444.

cxxxv Verhoeven AA, Boerma EJ, Meyboom-de Jong B. Use of information sources by family physicians: a literature survey. Bull Med Libr Assoc. 1995 Jan;83(1):85-90. PMID: 7703946; PMCID: PMC226003.

cxxxvi Straus SE, Sackett DL. Using research findings in clinical practice. BMJ. 1998 Aug 1;317(7154):339-42. doi: 10.1136/bmj.317.7154.339. PMID: 9685286; PMCID: PMC1113635.

cxxxvii Covell DG, Uman GC, Manning PR. Information needs in office practice: are they being met? Ann Intern Med. 1985 Oct;103(4):596-9. doi: 10.7326/0003-4819-103-4-596. PMID: 4037559.

cxxxviii Slawson DC, Shaughnessy AF, Bennett JH. Becoming a medical information master: feeling good about not knowing everything. J Fam Pract. 1994 May;38(5):505-13. PMID: 8176350.

cxxxix Slawson DC, Shaughnessy AF. Teaching information mastery: creating informed consumers of medical information. J Am Board Fam Pract. 1999 Nov-Dec;12(6):444-9. doi: 10.3122/jabfm.12.6.444. PMID: 10612362.

cxl Shaughnessy AF, Slawson DC, Bennett JH. Teaching information mastery: evaluating information provided by pharmaceutical representatives. Fam Med. 1995 Oct;27(9):581-5. PMID: 8829983.

cxli Shaughnessy AF, Slawson DC. POEMs: patient-oriented evidence that matters. Ann Intern Med. 1997 Apr 15;126(8):667. doi: 10.7326/0003-4819-126-8-199704150-00032. PMID: 9103150.

cxlii https://www.unboundmedicine.com/medline/citation/17152761/[History_of_opium_poppy_and_morphine] (accessed 25th March 2024) cxliii Khan MA, Raza F, Khan IA. Pain: history, culture and philosophy. Acta Med Hist Adriat. 2015;13(1):113-30. PMID: 26203543.

cxliv DeLeo JA. Basic science of pain. J Bone Joint Surg Am. 2006 Apr;88 Suppl 2:58-62. doi: 10.2106/JBJS.E.01286. PMID: 16595445.

cxlv Juvin P, Desmonts JM. The ancestors of inhalational anesthesia: the Soporific Sponges (XIth-XVIIth centuries): how a universally recommended medical technique was abruptly discarded. Anesthesiology. 2000 Jul;93(1):265-9. doi: 10.1097/00000542-200007000-00037. PMID: 10861170.

cxlvi Schmitz R. Friedrich Wilhelm Sertürner and the discovery of morphine. Pharm Hist. 1985;27(2):61-74. PMID: 11611724.

cxlvii https://en.wikipedia.org/wiki/Alkaloid (accessed 25th May 2024)

cxlviii Mahdi JG, Mahdi AJ, Mahdi AJ, Bowen ID. The historical analysis of aspirin discovery, its relation to the willow tree and antiproliferative and anticancer potential. Cell Prolif. 2006 Apr;39(2):147-55. doi: 10.1111/j.1365-2184.2006.00377.x. PMID: 16542349; PMCID: PMC6496865.

cxlix Prescott LF. Paracetamol: past, present, and future. Am J Ther. 2000 Mar;7(2):143-7. PMID: 11319582.

cl https://en.wikipedia.org/wiki/Nonsteroidal_anti-inflammatory_drug (accessed 25th March 2024)

cli Vane JR. Inhibition of prostaglandin synthesis as a mechanism of action for aspirin-like drugs. Nat New Biol. 1971 Jun 23;231(25):232-5. doi: 10.1038/newbio231232a0. PMID: 5284360.

clii Painful lessons. *Nat Struct Mol Biol* **12**, 205 (2005). https://doi.org/10.1038/nsmb0305-205

cliii Simmons DL, Botting RM, Hla T. Cyclooxygenase isozymes: the biology of prostaglandin synthesis and inhibition. Pharmacol Rev. 2004 Sep;56(3):387-437. doi: 10.1124/pr.56.3.3. PMID: 15317910.

cliv Krumholz HM, Ross JS, Presler AH, Egilman DS. What have we learnt from Vioxx? BMJ. 2007 Jan 20;334(7585):120-3. doi: 10.1136/bmj.39024.487720.68. PMID: 17235089; PMCID: PMC1779871.

clv Mukherjee D, Nissen SE, Topol EJ. Risk of cardiovascular events associated with selective COX-2 inhibitors. JAMA. 2001 Aug 22-29;286(8):954-9. doi: 10.1001/jama.286.8.954. PMID: 11509060.

clvi Dieppe PA, Ebrahim S, Martin RM, Jüni P. Lessons from the withdrawal of rofecoxib. BMJ. 2004 Oct 16;329(7471):867-8. doi: 10.1136/bmj.329.7471.867. PMID: 15485938; PMCID: PMC523096.

clvii Fries JF. Letter to Raymond Gilmartin re: physician intimidation. 9 Jan, 2001. Merck. www.vioxxdocuments.com/Documents/Krumholz_Vioxx/Fries2001.pdf

clviii Breslaier et al. Cardiovascular Events Associated with Rofecoxib in a Colorectal Adenoma Chemoprevention Trial N Engl J Med 2005; 352:1092-1102 DOI: 10.1056/NEJMoa050493

clix Topol EJ, Falk GW. A coxib a day won't keep the doctor away. Lancet. 2004 Aug 21-27;364(9435):639-40. doi: 10.1016/S0140-6736(04)16906-7. PMID: 15325809.

clx https://onlinelibrary.wiley.com/doi/full/10.1046/j.1365-2036.2003.01454.x October 2002. Subsequently published in Alimentary Pharmacology and Therapeutics Vol 17 Issue 3 on 04 Feb 2003. (accessed 25th March 2024)

clxi https://pharmaceutical-journal.com/article/feature/still-feeling-the-vioxx-pain (accessed 25th March 2024)

clxii Jüni P, Nartey L, Reichenbach S, Sterchi R, Dieppe PA, Egger M. Risk of cardiovascular events and rofecoxib: cumulative meta-analysis. Lancet. 2004 Dec 4-10;364(9450):2021-9. doi: 10.1016/S0140-6736(04)17514-4. PMID: 15582059.

clxiii Horton R. Vioxx, the implosion of Merck, and aftershocks at the FDA. Lancet. 2004 Dec 4-10;364(9450):1995-6. doi: 10.1016/S0140-6736(04)17523-5. PMID: 15582041.

clxiv Dieppe PA, Ebrahim S, Martin RM, Jüni P. Lessons from the withdrawal of rofecoxib. BMJ. 2004 Oct 16;329(7471):867-8. doi: 10.1136/bmj.329.7471.867. PMID: 15485938; PMCID: PMC523096.

clxv Jüni P, Reichenbach S, Egger M. COX 2 inhibitors, traditional NSAIDs, and the heart. BMJ. 2005 Jun 11;330(7504):1342-3. doi: 10.1136/bmj.330.7504.1342. PMID: 15947376; PMCID: PMC558270.

clxvi Krumholz HM, Ross JS, Presler AH, Egilman DS. What have we learnt from Vioxx? BMJ. 2007 Jan 20;334(7585):120-3. doi: 10.1136/bmj.39024.487720.68. PMID: 17235089; PMCID: PMC1779871.

clxvii https://www.ahajournals.org/history/aae48e4b-936b-46ba-ac33-79cdfaa15e9d/10.1161_hc4401.100078_5e9d.pdf (accessed 25th March 2024)

clxviii https://www.acpjournals.org/doi/10.7326/0003-4819-139-7-200310070-00005 (accessed 25th March 2024)

clxix Silverstein FE, Faich G, Goldstein JL, Simon LS, Pincus T, Whelton A, Makuch R, Eisen G, Agrawal NM, Stenson WF, Burr AM, Zhao WW, Kent JD, Lefkowith JB, Verburg KM, Geis GS. Gastrointestinal toxicity with celecoxib vs nonsteroidal anti-inflammatory drugs for osteoarthritis and rheumatoid arthritis: the CLASS study: A randomized controlled trial. Celecoxib Long-term Arthritis Safety Study. JAMA. 2000 Sep 13;284(10):1247-55. doi: 10.1001/jama.284.10.1247. PMID: 10979111.

clxx Jüni P, Rutjes AW, Dieppe PA. Are selective COX 2 inhibitors superior to traditional non steroidal anti-inflammatory drugs? BMJ. 2002 Jun 1;324(7349):1287-8. doi: 10.1136/bmj.324.7349.1287. Erratum in: BMJ 2002 Jun 29;324(7353):1538. PMID: 12039807; PMCID: PMC1123260.

clxxi Solomon SD, McMurray JJ, Pfeffer MA, Wittes J, Fowler R, Finn P, Anderson WF, Zauber A, Hawk E, Bertagnolli M; Adenoma Prevention with Celecoxib (APC) Study Investigators. Cardiovascular risk associated with celecoxib in a clinical trial for colorectal adenoma prevention. N Engl J Med. 2005 Mar 17;352(11):1071-80. doi: 10.1056/NEJMoa050405. Epub 2005 Feb 15. PMID: 15713944.

clxxii Kearney PM, Baigent C, Godwin J, Halls H, Emberson JR, Patrono C. Do selective cyclo-oxygenase-2 inhibitors and traditional non-steroidal anti-inflammatory drugs increase the risk of atherothrombosis? Meta-analysis of randomised trials. BMJ. 2006 Jun 3;332(7553):1302-8. doi: 10.1136/bmj.332.7553.1302. PMID: 16740558; PMCID: PMC1473048.

clxxiii https://webarchive.nationalarchives.gov.uk/ukgwa/20141205150130/http://www.mhra.gov.uk/home/groups/plp/documents/websiteresources/con2025036.pdf. (accessed 25th March 2024)

clxxiv National Prescribing Centre Cardiovascular and gastrointestinal safety of NSAIDs. MeReC Extra 30 (2007) https://www.centreformedicinesoptimisation.co.uk/a-reminder-about-cardiovascular-risks-with-some-traditional-nsaids-as-well-as-with-coxibs/ (accessed 25th March 2024)

clxxv https://wchh.onlinelibrary.wiley.com/doi/epdf/10.1002/psb.795 (Accessed 30th May 2024).

clxxvi Greenhalgh T, Robert G, Macfarlane F, Bate P, Kyriakidou O. Diffusion of innovations in service organizations: systematic review and recommendations. Milbank Q. 2004;82(4):581-629. doi: 10.1111/j.0887-378X.2004.00325.x. PMID: 15595944; PMCID: PMC2690184.

clxxvii Gabbay J, le May A. Evidence based guidelines or collectively constructed "mindlines?" Ethnographic study of knowledge management in primary care. BMJ. 2004 Oct 30;329(7473):1013. doi: 10.1136/bmj.329.7473.1013. PMID: 15514347; PMCID: PMC524553.

clxxviii Allen D, Harkins KJ. Lancet 2005; 365: 1768

clxxix Smith R. All changed, changed utterly. BMJ 1998: 316: 1917. http://www.bmj.com/content/316/7149/1917.long (accessed 25th March 224)

clxxx Di Pietrantonj, C; Rivetti, A; Marchione, P; Debalini, MG; Demicheli, V (April 2020). "Vaccines for measles, mumps, rubella, and varicella in children". Cochrane Database of Systematic Reviews. 4: CD004407. doi:10.1002/14651858.CD004407.pub4. PMC 7169657. P MID 32309885.

clxxxi Godlee F, Smith J, Marcovitch H. Wakefield's article linking MMR vaccine and autism was fraudulent. BMJ. 2011 Jan 5;342:c7452. doi: 10.1136/bmj.c7452. PMID: 21209060.

clxxxii Peckham S. The new general practice contract and reform of primary care in the United Kingdom. Health Policy. 2007 May;2(4):34-48. PMID: 19305731; PMCID: PMC2585462.

clxxxiii https://www.pulsetoday.co.uk/news/contract/government-auditors-call-for-revamp-to-qof-exception-reporting/ (accessed 25th March 2024) clxxxiv Doran T, Kontopantelis E, Valderas JM et al.. Effect of financial incentives on incentivised and non-incentivised clinical activities: longitudinal analysis of data from the UK quality and outcomes framework. *BMJ* 2011; 342. doi: 10.1136/bmj.d3590

clxxxv Campbell SM, Reeves D, Kontopantelis E, Sibbald B, Roland M. Effects of pay for performance on the quality of primary care in England. *N Engl J Med* 2009; 361: 368–78.

clxxxvi Roland M, Campbell S. Successes and failures of pay for performance in the United Kingdom. *N Engl J Med* 2014; 370: 1944–9.

clxxxvii Ryan AM, Krinsky S, Kontopantelis K, Doran T. Long-term evidence for the effect of pay-for-performance in primary care on mortality in the UK: a population study. *Lancet* 2016. doi: 10.1016/S0140-6736(16)00276-2

clxxxviii Petersen LA, Woodard LD, Urech T, Daw C, Sookanan S. Does pay-for-performance improve the quality of health care?*Ann Intern Med* 2006; 145: 265–72.

clxxxix http://www.sspc.ac.uk/media/media_486342_en.pdf (accessed 25th March 2024)

cxc Chan, KS., Wan, E.YF., Chin, WY. *et al.* Effects of continuity of care on health outcomes among patients with diabetes mellitus and/or hypertension: a systematic review. *BMC Fam Pract* **22**, 145 (2021). https://doi.org/10.1186/s12875-021-01493-x

cxci Pereira Gray DJ, Sidaway-Lee K, White E, Thorne A, Evans PH. Continuity of care with doctors-a matter of life and death? A systematic review of continuity of care and mortality. BMJ Open. 2018 Jun 28;8(6):e021161. doi: 10.1136/bmjopen-2017-021161. PMID: 29959146; PMCID: PMC6042583.

cxcii O'Mahony S. Medicine and the McNamara fallacy. J R Coll Physicians Edinb 2017; 47: 281–7 | doi: 10.4997

cxciii Kneebone Roger. Expert: Understanding the Path to Mastery. Viking. ISBN-13: 978-0241392034.

cxciv Kahneman Daniel. Thinking Fast and Slow. Penguin. ASIN: B005MJFA2W

cxcv https://en.wikipedia.org/wiki/Jeanne_Calment (accessed 25th March 2024) cxcvi Christiaens TC, De Meyere M, Verschraegen G, Peersman W, Heytens S, De Maeseneer JM. Randomised controlled trial of nitrofurantoin versus placebo in the treatment of uncomplicated urinary tract infection in adult women. Br J Gen Pract. 2002 Sep;52(482):729-34. PMID: 12236276; PMCID: PMC1314413.

cxcvii Endo A. A historical perspective on the discovery of statins. Proc Jpn Acad Ser B Phys Biol Sci. 2010;86(5):484-93. doi: 10.2183/pjab.86.484. PMID: 20467214; PMCID: PMC3108295.

cxcviii Randomised trial of cholesterol lowering in 4444 patients with coronary heart disease: the Scandinavian Simvastatin Survival Study (4S) Lancet. 1994 Nov 19;344(8934):1383–9.

cxcix Long-Term Intervention with Pravastatin in Ischaemic Disease (LIPID) Study Group Prevention of cardiovascular events and death with pravastatin in patients with coronary heart disease and a broad range of initial cholesterol levels. N Engl J Med. 1998 Nov 5;339(19):1349–57.

cc Sacks FM, Pfeffer MA, Moye LA et al. The effect of pravastatin on coronary events after myocardial infarction in patients with average cholesterol levels. Cholesterol and Recurrent Events Trial investigators. N Engl J Med. 1996 Oct 3;335(14):1001–9.

cci Shepherd J, Cobbe SM, Ford I et al. Prevention of coronary heart disease with pravastatin in men with hypercholesterolemia. West of Scotland Coronary Prevention Study Group. N Engl J Med. 1995 Nov 16;333(20):1301–7.

ccii Shepherd J, Blauw GJ, Murphy MB et al. PROspective Study of Pravastatin in the Elderly at Risk. Pravastatin in elderly individuals at risk of vascular disease (PROSPER): a randomised controlled trial. Lancet. 2002 Nov 23;360(9346):1623–30; PROSPER study group.

cciii Downs JR, Clearfield M, Weis S et al. Primary prevention of acute coronary events with lovastatin in men and women with average cholesterol levels: results of AFCAPS/TexCAPS. Air Force/Texas Coronary Atherosclerosis Prevention Study. JAMA. 1998 May 27;279(20):1615–22.

cciv Colhoun HM, Betteridge DJ, Durrington PN et al. Primary prevention of cardiovascular disease with atorvastatin in type 2 diabetes in the Collaborative Atorvastatin Diabetes Study (CARDS): multicentre randomised placebo-controlled trial. Lancet. 2004 Aug;364(9435):21–27. 685–96.

ccv Sever PS, Dahlöf B, Poulter NR et al. Prevention of coronary and stroke events with atorvastatin in hypertensive patients who have average or lower-than-average cholesterol concentrations, in the Anglo-Scandinavian Cardiac Outcomes Trial–Lipid Lowering Arm (ASCOT-LLA): a multicentre randomised controlled trial. Lancet. 2003 Apr 5;361(9364):1149–58; ASCOT Investigators.

ccvi Heart Protection Study Collaborative Group. MRC/BHF Heart Protection Study of cholesterol lowering with simvastatin in 20, 536 high-risk individuals: a randomised placebo-controlled trial. Lancet. 2002 Jul 6;360(9326):7–22.

ccvii Cannon CP, Braunwald E, McCabe CH et al. Intensive versus moderate lipid lowering with statins after acute coronary syndromes. N Engl J Med. 2004 Apr 8;350(15):1495–504; Pravastatin or Atorvastatin Evaluation and Infection Therapy-Thrombolysis in Myocardial Infarction.

ccviii LaRosa JC, Grundy SM, Waters DD et al. Intensive lipid lowering with atorvastatin in patients with stable coronary disease. N Engl J Med. 2005 Apr 7;352(14):1425–35.

ccix https://qrisk.org (accessed 25th March 2024)

ccx https://gpevidence.org (accessed 25th March 2024)

ccxi Kessels RP. Patients' memory for medical information. J R Soc Med. 2003 May;96(5):219-22. doi: 10.1177/014107680309600504. PMID: 12724430; PMCID: PMC539473.

ccxii Leahey TH. Herbert A. Simon: Nobel Prize in Economic Sciences, 1978. Am Psychol. 2003 Sep;58(9):753-5. doi: 10.1037/0003-066X.58.9.753. PMID: 14584993.

ccxiii Bate L, Hutchinson A, Underhill J, Maskrey N. How clinical decisions are made. Br J Clin Pharmacol. 2012 Oct;74(4):614-20. doi: 10.1111/j.1365-2125.2012.04366.x. PMID: 22738381; PMCID: PMC3477329.

ccxiv Croskerry P, Petrie DA, Reilly JB, Tait G. Deciding about fast and slow decisions. Acad Med. 2014 Feb;89(2):197-200. doi: 10.1097/ACM.0000000000000121. PMID: 24362398.

ccxv Croskerry P. A universal model of diagnostic reasoning. Acad Med. 2009 Aug;84(8):1022-8. doi: 10.1097/ACM.0b013e3181ace703. PMID: 19638766.

ccxvi Croskerry P. From mindless to mindful practice--cognitive bias and clinical decision making. N Engl J Med. 2013 Jun 27;368(26):2445-8. doi: 10.1056/NEJMp1303712. PMID: 23802513.

ccxvii Featherston R, Downie LE, Vogel AP, Galvin KL. Decision making biases in the allied health professions: A systematic scoping review. PLoS One. 2020 Oct 20;15(10):e0240716. doi: 10.1371/journal.pone.0240716. PMID: 33079949; PMCID: PMC7575084.

ccxviii Ludolph R, Schulz PJ. Debiasing Health-Related Judgments and Decision Making: A Systematic Review. Med Decis Making. 2018 Jan;38(1):3-13. doi: 10.1177/0272989X17716672. Epub 2017 Jun 25. PMID: 28649904.

ccxix https://www.nobelprize.org/prizes/economic-sciences/2002/kahneman/biographical/

ccxx Raffle, Angela E., Anne Mackie, and J. A. Muir Gray, *Screening: Evidence and Practice*, 2 edn
Oxford, 2019; https://doi.org/10.1093/med/9780198805984.001.0001,

ccxxi O'Sullivan JW, Muntinga T, Grigg S, Ioannidis JPA. Prevalence and outcomes of incidental imaging findings: umbrella review. BMJ 2018;361:k2387.

ccxxii https://apps.who.int/iris/bitstream/handle/10665/37650/WHO_PHP_34.pdf?sequence=17&isAllowed=y (accessed 25th March 2024)

ccxxiii https://www.hardingcenter.de/en (accessed 25th March 2024)

ccxxiv Ackerson K, Preston SD. A decision theory perspective on why women do or do not decide to have cancer screening: systematic review. J Adv Nurs. 2009 Jun;65(6):1130-40. doi: 10.1111/j.1365-2648.2009.04981.x. Epub 2009 Apr 3. PMID: 19374678.

ccxxv https://www.nice.org.uk/guidance/ng131/chapter/Recommendations#information-and-decision-support-for-people-with-prostate-cancer-their-partners-and-carers (accessed 25th March 2024)

ccxxvi https://www.nice.org.uk/guidance/ng158 (accessed 25th March 2024)

ccxxvii https://www.nice.org.uk/guidance/ng91/resources/visual-summary-pdf-4787282702 (accessed 25th March 2024) ccxxviii Gill CJ, Sabin L, Schmid CH. Why clinicians are natural bayesians. BMJ. 2005 May 7;330(7499):1080-3. doi: 10.1136/bmj.330.7499.1080. Erratum in: BMJ. 2005 Jun 11;330(7504):1369. PMID: 15879401; PMCID: PMC557240.

ccxxix McCormack J P, Holmes D T. Your results may vary: the imprecision of medical
measurements *BMJ* 2020; 368 :m149 doi:10.1136/bmj.m149

ccxxx Johansson M, GuyattG, Montori V. Guidelines should consider clinicians' time needed to
treat *BMJ* 2023; 380 :e072953 doi:10.1136/bmj-2022-072953

ccxxxi Safi, R.; Browne, G. J.; Jalali Naini, A. (2021). "Mis-spending on information security measures: Theory and experimental evidence". *International Journal of Information Management*. **57** (102291): 102291. doi:10.1016/j.ijinfomgt.2020.102291

ccxxxii Whitty C J M, SmithG, McBride M, Atherton F, Powis S H, Stokes-LampardH et al. Restoring and extending secondary prevention BMJ 2023; 380 :p201 doi:10.1136/bmj.p201

ccxxxiii https://blogs.bmj.com/bmj/2014/08/21/neal-maskrey-tipping-the-balance-towards-individualised-care/

ccxxxiv Ha JF, Longnecker N. Doctor-patient communication: a review. Ochsner J. 2010 Spring;10(1):38-43. PMID: 21603354; PMCID: PMC3096184.

ccxxxv Tongue JR, Epps HR, Forese LL. Communication skills for patient-centered care. J Bone Joint Surg Am 2005; 87: 652–58.

ccxxxvi Kyle S, Shaw D. Doctor–patient communication, patient knowledge and health literacy: how difficult can it all be? The Bulletin of the Royal College of Surgeons of England, Volume 96, Number 6 https://doi.org/10.1308/rcsbull.2014.96.6.e9

ccxxxvii Granger K. Healthcare staff must properly introduce themselves to patients. BMJ 2013; 347 : f5833 doi:10.1136/bmj.f5833

ccxxxviii https://www.england.nhs.uk/wp-content/uploads/2020/11/2018-Never-Events-List-updated-February-2021.pdf (accessed 26th March 2024)

ccxxxix https://www.gmc-uk.org/professional-standards/professional-standards-for-doctors/good-medical-practice/domain-2-patients-partnership-and-communication#treating-patients-fairly-and-respecting-their-rights-F5736F7E095D4E71A443F3C7AAB6C30C (accessed 26th March 2024)

ccxl Heritage J, Robinson JD, Elliott MN, Beckett M, Wilkes M. Reducing patients' unmet concerns in primary care: the difference one word can make. J Gen Intern Med. 2007 Oct;22(10):1429-33. doi: 10.1007/s11606-007-0279-0. Epub 2007 Aug 3. PMID: 17674111; PMCID: PMC2305862.

ccxli Bass LW,Cohen RL. Ostensible Versus Actual Reasons for Seeking Pediatric Attention: Another Look at the Parental Ticket of Admission Pediatrics 1982; 70: 870–874.https://doi.org/10.1542/peds.70.6.870

ccxlii Raftery A, Scowen P. A survey of communication skills teaching at medical school[suppl]. Ann R Coll Surg Engl2006;88:84-6doi:10.1308/147363506X97649.

ccxliii Maskrey N. Shared decision making: why the slow progress? An essay by Neal Maskrey.
BMJ 2019; 367 :l6762 doi:10.1136/bmj.l6762

ccxliv
https://www.ncbi.nlm.nih.gov/pmc/articles/PMC2158724/?page=1 (accessed 27th March 2024)

ccxlv Byrne PS, Long BEL. Doctors Talking to Patients. HMSO. 1976

ccxlvi Becker MH, Maiman LA. Sociobehavioral determinants of compliance with health and medical care recommendations. Med Care. 1975 Jan;13(1):10-24. doi: 10.1097/00005650-197501000-00002. PMID: 1089182.

ccxlvii Stewart M et al. Patient-centred medicine: transforming the clinical method. 2003. Radcliffe Medical Press Abingdon Oxford

ccxlviii Neighbour R. The Inner Consultation. 1987. CRC Press. London.

ccxlix Silverman J, Kurtz S, Draper J. Skills for Communicating with Patients. CRC Press London. 2013.

ccl Kurtz S, Silverman J, Draper J. Teaching and Learning Communication skills in Medicine. Radcliffe Publishing. Oxford. 1998.

ccli Cooper V, Hassell A. Teaching consultation skills in higher specialist training: experience of a workshop for specialist registrars in rheumatology, Rheumatology, Volume 41, Issue 10, October 2002, Pages 1168–1171, https://doi.org/10.1093/rheumatology/41.10.1168

cclii Jacklin S, Chapman S, Maskrey N. Virtual patient educational intervention for the development of shared decision-making skills: a pilot study. BMJ Simul Technol Enhanc Learn. 2019 Sep 19;5(4):215-217. doi: 10.1136/bmjstel-2018-000375. PMID: 35521483; PMCID: PMC8936636.

ccliii Jacklin S, Maskrey N, Chapman S. Improving Shared Decision Making Between Patients and Clinicians: Design and Development of a Virtual Patient Simulation Tool. JMIR Med Educ. 2018 Nov 6;4(2):e10088. doi: 10.2196/10088. PMID: 30401667; PMCID: PMC6246962.

ccliv Thompson J, White S, Chapman S. Interactive Clinical Avatar Use in Pharmacist Preregistration Training: Design and Review. J Med Internet Res. 2020 Nov 6;22(11):e17146. doi: 10.2196/17146. PMID: 33155983; PMCID: PMC7679212.

cclv Haslam DA. Who cares? The James Mackenzie Lecture 2006. Br J Gen Pract. 2007 Dec;57(545):987-93. doi: 10.3399/096016407782604884. PMID: 18252075; PMCID: PMC2084139.

cclvi Singh Ospina, N., Phillips, K.A., Rodriguez-Gutierrez, R. et al. Eliciting the Patient's Agenda- Secondary Analysis of Recorded Clinical Encounters. J GEN INTERN MED 34, 36–40 (2019). https://doi.org/10.1007/s11606-018-4540-5

cclvii https://www.hee.nhs.uk/our-work/person-centred-care (Accessed 27th March 2024)

cclviii https://www.nice.org.uk/guidance/ng197

cclix https://www.gmc-uk.org/professional-standards/professional-standards-for-doctors/good-medical-practice/about-good-medical-practice (accessed 28th March 2024)

cclx https://www.gmc-uk.org/ethical-guidance/learning-materials/blog---montgomery--judgement (accessed 28th March 2024)

cclxi https://www.bmj.com/content/357/bmj.j2224 (accessed 28th March 2024) cclxii Kneebone R. Expert: Understanding the Path to Mastery. Penguin. Dublin. 2021

cclxiii Schmidt HG, Norman GR, Boshuizen HP. A cognitive perspective on medical expertise: theory and implication. Acad Med. 1990 Oct;65(10):611-21. doi: 10.1097/00001888-199010000-00001. Erratum in: Acad Med 1992 Apr;67(4):287. PMID: 2261032.

cclxiv Dreyfus HL, Dreyfus SE. Mind over Machine. Macmillan. New York. 1988.

cclxv Dobson J, Linderholm T, Perez J. 2018. Retrieval practice enhances the ability to evaluate complex psychology information. Med Educ. 52(5):513–525.

cclxvi https://aktprep.co.uk/making-decisions-better/#studyskills (accessed 28th March 2024)

cclxvii Ericsson, K. A., Krampe, R. T., & Tesch-Römer, C. (1993). The role of deliberate practice in the acquisition of expert performance. *Psychological Review, 100*(3), 363–406. https://doi.org/10.1037/0033-295X.100.3.363

cclxviii Graber ML, Franklin N, Gordon R. 2005. Diagnostic error in internal medicine. Arch Intern Med. 165(13):1493–1499.

cclxix Graber ML, Rencic J, Rusz D, Papa F, Croskerry P, Zierler B, Harkless G, Giuliano M, Schoenbaum S, Colford C, et al. 2018. Improving diagnosis by improving education: a policy brief on education in healthcare professions. Diagnosis (Berl). 5(3):107–118.

cclxx
Whiting PF, Davenport C, Jameson C, Burke M, Sterne JAC, Hyde C, Ben-Shlomo Y. 2015. How well do health professionals interpret diagnostic information? A systematic review. BMJ Open. 5(7):e008155.

cclxxi https://nap.nationalacademies.org/catalog/21794/improving-diagnosis-in-health-care (accessed 27th March 2024)

cclxxii Nicola Cooper, Maggie Bartlett, Simon Gay, Anna Hammond, Mark Lillicrap, Joanna Matthan, Mini Singh & On behalf of the UK Clinical Reasoning in Medical Education (CReME) consensus statement group (2021) Consensus statement on the content of clinical reasoning curricula in undergraduate medical education, Medical Teacher, 43:2, 152-159, DOI: 10.1080/0142159X.2020.1842343 cclxxiii Kissick WL. Medicine's Dilemmas: Infinite Needs versus Finite Resources. Yale University Press; 1994.

cclxxiv https://www.health.org.uk/publications/long-reads/health-care-funding (accessed 27th March 2024)

cclxxv https://www.kingsfund.org.uk/blog/2022/03/public-satisfaction-nhs-falls-25-year-low (accessed 27th March 2024)

cclxxvi https://ifs.org.uk/collections/nhs-waiting-lists (accessed 27th March 2024)

cclxxvii Watt T, Charlesworth A, Gershlick B. Health and care spending and its value, past, present and future. Future Healthc J. 2019 Jun;6(2):99-105. doi: 10.7861/futurehosp.6-2-99.

cclxxviii Getzen TE. Healthcare is an individual necessity and a national luxury: Applying multilevel decision models to the analysis of healthcare expenditures. J Health Econ2000;19:259–70.

cclxxix de la Maisonneuve C, Martins JO. Public spending on health and long-term care: a new set of projections. OECD Economic Policy Papers2013;6.

cclxxx Charlesworth A, Johnson P. (eds). Securing the future: funding health and social care to the 2030s. London: The Institute for Fiscal Studies, 2018.

cclxxxi https://lordslibrary.parliament.uk/staff-shortages-in-the-nhs-and-social-care-sectors/ (accessed 28th March 2024)

cclxxxii https://www.bbc.co.uk/news/health-62594141 (accessed 28th March 2024)

cclxxxiii https://www.ft.com/content/fac8062a-bd83-486b-ac6f-582f1931750b (accessed 28th March 2024)

cclxxxiv https://www.gmc-uk.org/news/news-archive/action-needed-to-stop-senseless-waste-of-nhs-talent---gmc-chief-warns

cclxxxv https://www.gmc-uk.org/professional-standards/professional-standards-for-doctors/good-medical-practice

cclxxxvi https://www.nuffieldtrust.org.uk/chart/number-of-gps

cclxxxvii Appleby J. What's happened to NHS spending and staffing in the past 25years? BMJ 2023; 380 :p564 doi:10.1136/bmj.p564 cclxxxviii https://www.bma.org.uk/advice-and-support/nhs-delivery-and-workforce/pressures/pressures-in-general-practice-data-analysis (accessed 15th April 2024)

cclxxxix https://www.manchester.ac.uk/discover/news/a-third-of-gps-plan-to-quit-within-five-years-finds-survey/ (accessed 15th April 2024)

ccxc Starfield B, Shi L, Macinko J. Contribution of primary care to health systems and health. Milbank Q. 2005;83(3):457-502. doi: 10.1111/j.1468-0009.2005.00409.x.

ccxci Pereira Gray DJ, Sidaway-Lee K, White E, Thorne A, Evans PH. Continuity of care with doctors - a matter of life and death? A systematic review of continuity of care and mortality. BMJ Open. 2018 Jun 28;8(6):e021161. doi: 10.1136/bmjopen-2017-021161. PMID: 29959146; PMCID: PMC6042583.

ccxcii https://www.ama-assn.org/practice-management/scope-practice/amid-doctor-shortage-nps-and-pas-seemed-fix-data-s-nope (accessed 28th March 2024)

ccxciii Whitaker P. What is a Doctor? A GP's Prescription for the Future. Cannongate. 2023. ASIN : B0BRQLZ69G

ccxciv https://www.rcplondon.ac.uk/projects/outputs/focus-physicians-2017-18-census-uk-consultants-and-higher-specialty-trainees (accessed 15th April 2024)

ccxcv https://www.bmj.com/bmj/section-pdf/954278?path=/bmj/359/8128/Careers.full.pdf (accessed 15th April 2024)

ccxcvi https://ifs.org.uk/publications/nhs-funding-resources-and-treatment-volumes (accessed 15th April 2024)

ccxcvii Watt TLS. The 'do nothing' option: How public spending on social care in England fell by 13% in 5 years. *London: The Health Foundation*, 2018.

ccxcviii LSE–Lancet Commission on the future of the NHS: re-laying the foundations for an equitable and efficient health and care service after COVID-19. Lancet, 221. ISSN: 0140-6736, Vol: 397, Issue: 10288, Page: 1915-1978.

ccxcix https://www.digitalhealth.net/2023/07/epr-frontline-digitisation-target-declared-unachievable/ (accessed 15th April 2024) ccc https://www.manchestereveningnews.co.uk/news/greater-manchester-news/ambulance-10-hour-wait-hip-21515895 (accessed 17th April 2024)

ccci https://www.independent.co.uk/news/health/nhs-delays-waiting-times-a-e-b2236788.html (accessed 17th April 2024)

cccii https://www.theguardian.com/society/2022/dec/20/93-year-old-left-screaming-in-pain-on-floor-during-25-hour-ambulance-wait (accessed 17th April 2024)

ccciii https://www.itv.com/news/westcountry/2022-08-18/woman-aged-90-waited-almost-two-days-for-an-ambulance-after-falling-at-her-home (accessed 17th April 2024)

ccciv https://www.nhfd.co.uk/20/NHFDcharts.nsf/vwCharts/BestPractice (accessed 17th April 2024)

cccv https://bjgplife.com/chatgpt-prepares-for-the-akt-and-does-rather-well/ (accessed 17th April 2024)

cccvi Ayers JW, Poliak A, Dredze M, Leas EC, Zhu Z, Kelley JB, Faix DJ, Goodman AM, Longhurst CA, Hogarth M, Smith DM. Comparing Physician and Artificial Intelligence Chatbot Responses to Patient Questions Posted to a Public Social Media Forum. JAMA Intern Med. 2023 Jun 1;183(6):589-596. doi: 10.1001/jamainternmed.2023.1838. PMID: 37115527; PMCID: PMC10148230.

cccvii https://www.thelancet.com/journals/lanonc/article/PIIS1470-2045(23)00298-X/abstract (accessed 28th May 2024)

cccviii https://www.thelancet.com/journals/eclinm/article/PIIS2589-5370(23)00518-7/fulltext#:~:text=The%20use%20of%20artificial%20intelligence,have%20been%20observed%20across%20studies. (accessed 28th May 2024)

cccix https://www.today.com/health/mom-chatgpt-diagnosis-pain-rcna101843 (accessed 28th May 2024)

cccx https://www.thelancet.com/journals/landig/article/PIIS2589-7500(23)00225-X/fulltext (accessed 28th May 2024)

cccxi Berwick DM. Era 3 for medicine and health care. JAMA 2016; 315: 1329–30.

cccxii https://www.bmj.com/content/384/bmj.q90 (accessed 28th May 2024)

cccxiii https://www.bmj.com/content/380/bmj.p708 (accessed 28th May 2024)

cccxiv https://www.health.org.uk/sites/default/files/2020-03/Health%20Equity%20in%20England_The%20Marmot%20Review%2010%20Years%20On_executive%20summary_web.pdf (Accessed 5th June 2024)

cccxv Ibrahim, K., Cox, N.J., Stevenson, J.M. et al. A systematic review of the evidence for deprescribing interventions among older people living with frailty. BMC Geriatr21, 258 (2021). https://doi.org/10.1186/s12877-021-02208-8.

cccxvi Graber ML, Franklin N, Gordon R. Diagnostic Error in Internal Medicine. Arch Intern Med.2005;165(13):1493–1499. doi:10.1001/archinte.165.13.1493

cccxvii https://www.personalisedcareinstitute.org.uk (accessed 28th May 2024)

cccxviii https://www.nice.org.uk/guidance/ng197 (accessed 28th May 2024)

cccxix https://www.realisticmedicine.sco (accessed 28th May 2024)

cccxx https://vbhc.nhs.wales (accessed 28th May 2024)

cccxxi McCartney M, Treadwell J, Maskrey N, Lehman R. Making evidence based medicine work for individual patients. BMJ 2016; 353 :i2452 doi:10.1136/bmj.i2452

cccxxii https://read.oecd-ilibrary.org/social-issues-migration-health/tackling-wasteful-spending-on-health_9789264266414-en#page1 (accessed 10th May 2024)

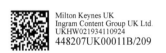
Milton Keynes UK
Ingram Content Group UK Ltd.
UKHW021934110924
448207UK00011B/209